Monographs on Endocrinology

Volume 20

Robert Volpe

Auto-immunity in the Endocrine System

With 32 Figures and 15 Tables

Springer-Verlag
Berlin Heidelberg NewYork 1981

Robert Volpé, M. D., F.R.C.P. (C), F.A.C.P.

Professor, Department of Medicine,
University of Toronto;
Physician-in-Chief,
The Wellesley Hospital,
Toronto, Ontario M4Y 1J3,
Canada

ISBN-13:978-3-642-81626-0 e-ISBN-13:978-3-642-81624-6
DOI: 10.1007/978-3-642-81624-6

Library of Congress Cataloging in Publication Data.
Volpé, Robert, 1926– . Auto-immunity in the endocrine system.
(Monographs on endocrinology; v. 20) Includes bibliographies and index.
1. Endocrine glands – Diseases – Immunological aspects. 2. Autoimmune diseases. I. Title. II. Series.
[DNLM: 1. Autoimmune diseases. 2. Endocrine diseases – Etiology. 3. Endocrine diseases – Immunology.
WL MO57 v. 20 / WK 100 A9396]
RC649.V64 616.4'079 81-9090
ISBN-13:978-3-642-81626-0 (U.S.) AACR2

Softcover reprint of the hardcover 1st edition 1981

2125/3020 – 543210

Preface

The present monograph will concern itself with those disorders of the endocrine system, either associated with destruction, interference with function or hyperfunction, which are considered to be due to auto-immune processes.

Endocrinopathies	Non-endocrine auto-immune disorders associated with the endocrinopathies
Graves' (Basedow's, Parry's) disease	Pernicious anaemia
Hashimoto's thyroiditis	Vitiligo
Idiopathic Addison's disease	Myaesthenia gravis
Insulinopenic diabetes mellitus	Sjögren's syndrome
Auto-immune oophoritis and orchitis	Rheumatoid arthritis
Auto-immune hypoparathyroidism	Idiopathic thrombocytopenic purpura
Auto-immune hypophysitis	Chronic active hepatitis
Possibly some cases of infertility due to anti-sperm antibodies	Primary biliary cirrhosis

Reproduced with permission from Volpé (1977)

The above table indicates those organ-specific endocrinopathies considered to be due to auto-immune factors, as well as those non-endocrine, organ-specific auto-immune disorders which may be associated with them (Volpé 1977). It is evident that such disorders, occurring without any obvious external cause, raise the very elementary question of how immune processes directed against self-constituents could be initiated. Generally, of course, the immune system acts as a regulatory and defence mechanism, and disorders of auto-immunity represent breakdowns in this regulatory system. The following chapters will be concerned with the individual components of the endocrine system so affected by auto-immune processes; it will first be necessary to provide an initial chapter for the purpose of summarizing some general principles of immunology, in order to place the immune disorders of the endocrine system in context.

It is commonplace to observe that the field of immunology is of very great magnitude and is evolving very rapidly. The chapter on general principles therefore will not be all-embracing, but will select those elements which will be necessary for a comprehension of the disorders to be discussed later. Moreover, the chapters which follow will not offer comprehensive citations of the literature, but rather references will be made to studies considered most appropriate, most important or representative or to many of the extensive and excellent reviews which have recently appeared on topics appropriate to this text.

While the reviews of the endocrinopathies which follow the introductory chapter will cite the views of many workers, the perspectives will not be neutral. The author will infuse his own interpretations on the various observations collated herein, in an effort to derive a unitary hypothesis which will then encompass most, if not all, of the auto-immune organ-specific endocrinopathies (and those non-endocrine, organ-specific auto-immune disorders associated with them). These views have evolved from consideration of studies in the author's laboratory and of many others, as distilled through innumerable discussions between the present writer and many colleagues. Particular gratitude is expressed to Vas V. Row, my research associate, and many previous research fellows: Drs. Jean Dussault, Eric Laryea, Joseph McConnon, Lamk Lamki, Peter Clarke, Robert Munro, John O'Donnell, Andrew Knox, Merrill Edmonds, Christian von Westarp, Jay Silverberg, Akira Sugenoya, Krinos Trokoudes, Arthur Kidd, Nobumitsu Okita, Mark Lewis, Jacques How, and Duncan Topliss. These young men have been a source of constant stimulation over the years, for which the author is greatly indebted.

It is important also to express gratitude to the unsung heroes of this monograph; to my secretaries, Mrs. Sarah McLaughlin and Mrs. Ursula Besteman, for their efforts in typing, arranging and organizing this work; to Mrs. V. Empey, Medical Librarian, Wellesley Hospital, and her staff for their assistance with the background references; to the Medical Art Department, Wellesley Hospital, for the diagrams; and finally, to my wife and family, and my skiing and tennis partners for their forbearance during the long months of preparation of this manuscript.

Toronto, July 1981 Robert Volpé

Contents

1 General Principles of Immunology (as Related to Auto-immune Disease)

1.1 Immunity and the Immune Response

The term "immunity" may be defined as those physiological mechanisms which endow the organism with the capacity to recognize substances as foreign, and to neutralize, eliminate or metabolize them without injury to its own tissues. Responses to such foreign substances may be divided into two types, i.e. those which are non-specific, and those which are specific immunological responses. Non-specific responses may occur following the initial and even subsequent exposure to foreign antigen, and are not dependent on specific recognition. A non-specific response involves the participation of cellular and chemical mediators, such as macrophages, lysozymes, properdin, interferon, prostaglandins and complement (Playfair 1975).

Although the term "complement" was originally designated to imply an auxiliary factor in serum that, acting upon an antibody-coated cell, would lead to lysis of the cell, the complement system is now known to be a complex cascade of interacting proteins. It is evident that the complement sequence consists of nine functional entities or eleven discrete proteins. These have a variety of different molecular weights and properties. The terms applied to these components include Clq, Clr, Cls, C2, C3, C4, C5, C6, C7, C8 and C9. The components of complement cause the accumulation of neutrophils from the circulation (chemotaxis). Complement products are capable of neutralizing viruses, producing kinin-like substances which contract smooth muscle and cause increased vascular permeability, producing immune adherence, intensifying an inflammatory reaction, and perhaps affecting cell surfaces, thus resulting in cell damage or death. The phenomenon of rapid red cell destruction may be closely related to that of immune adherence.

Specific immunological response (also called adaptive immunity) is restricted primarily to chordates (Hildemann and Reddy 1973). In this form of immune response, the organism demonstrates its ability to select from the entire spectrum of possible foreign substances those to which it is actually exposed, and to react against them in a specific manner. Moreover, this specific response can then be expanded, either to combat a continuing invasion, or for subsequent use, by means of immunological memory (Bellanti 1978). The specific response is mediated by lymphocytes; the crucial role of lymphocytes in the immune response will be discussed below.

Terminology to be employed in this chapter and monograph is of importance. A substance giving rise to antibody is called an antigen. A determinant not antigenic on its own, but against which antibody can be formed, is called a hapten. The additional determinant required to convert a hapten into an antigen (usually by stimulating a T-lymphocyte) is called a carrier. The term "immunogen" refers to substances capable of giving rise to actual immunity or protection. A substance capable of non-specifically stimulating the formation of antibody to unrelated antigens is termed an adjuvant (Playfair 1975).

1.1.1 The Role of Lymphocytes in the Immune Response

Immunological responses serve three functions – defence, homeostasis and surveillance (Fudenberg et al. 1976). The first function, defence against invasion by micro-organisms, was a matter of scientific inquiry over many generations, and was the route by which the explosion in knowledge regarding immunological processes has occurred. The second function, homeostasis, allows the organism to preserve uniformity of a given cell type. Removal of damaged cellular elements, such as circulating erythrocytes or leucocytes, may be performed by ordinary degradative or catabolic functions, which are immune in nature.

Finally, immune surveillance is a function which monitors the recognition of abnormal cell types which constantly arise within the body. This immunoregulatory system is complex and will be discussed in the latter portion of this chapter.

1.1.2 Types of Lymphocytes

There appear to be two major categories of lymphocytes. While all lymphocytes are initially produced in the bone marrow, some are processed by the micro-environment of the thymus [possibly by a thymic hormone, thymopoietin (Goldstein 1975), thymosin (Goldstein et al. 1972), thymic serum factor (Bach et al. 1977, 1978)], and are thus termed thymus-dependent or T-lymphocytes. Most of the remainder of bone marrow-derived lymphocytes are not processed by the thymus, but rather in another specific inducing micro-environment, probably within the bone marrow itself, and are considered analogous to those lymphocytes which come from the avian bursa of Fabricius (bursa-equivalent or B-lymphocytes) (Bellanti 1978) (Fig. 1.1). There is evidence that some cells which appear to be lymphocytes morphologically may be neither T- nor B-lymphocytes, e.g. null cells. Moreover, it is now evident that there are many subclasses of T-lymphocytes which have different function.

T-lymphocytes have specific surface components which permit identification with specific antisera (Elliott et al. 1980). The first demonstration of this means of identification was with the theta-isoantigen system in mice, but identification of the T-lymphocytes in other species (including humans) by similar techniques has been accomplished (Miescher and Muller-Eberhard 1976). T-lymphocytes are responsible for "cell-mediated immunity", and have a variety of functions in the immune response. While the T-lymphocyte cannot produce antibodies itself (except as surface receptors), it can cooperate with appropriate B-lymphocytes which in consequence then do produce such antibodies (Katz and Benacerraf 1972). The production of IgG in particular always requires the participation by T-lymphocytes in addition to B-lymphocytes. When T-lymphocytes co-operate with and direct groups of B-lymphocytes in this manner to produce antibodies, they are termed helper T-lymphocytes. T-lymphocytes may also be involved in the direct killing of target cells, the activation of some functions of macrophages, and the production of a variety of soluble products (lymphokines); the variety of functions of these lymphokines may be mediated by structural specificity for each function or for a few related functions (Dumonde and Maini 1971). Lymphokines include macrophage

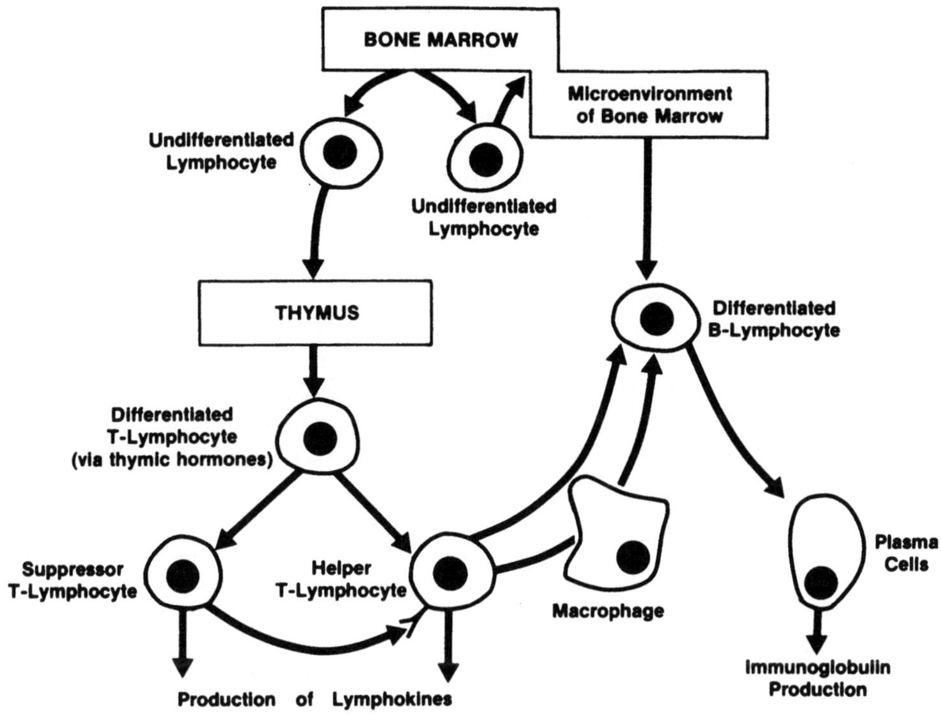

Fig. 1.1. Simplified version of lymphocyte differentiation. (See text for discussion.) (Okita et al. 1981)

migration inhibition factor, macrophage aggregation factor, macrophage-spreading inhibitory factor, migration inhibition factor for other cells (T-lymphocytes, polymorphonuclear leucocytes), chemotactic factor, mitogenic factor, lymphotoxic factor, skin reactive factor, interferon, inhibitors of proliferation and DNA synthesis and lymph node permeability factor. Secondly, T-lymphocytes belonging to a subset act as suppressor T-lymphocytes, i.e. they suppress other T-lymphocytes (such as helper T-lymphocytes), as well as B-lymphocytes. Finally, T-lymphocytes exert a regulatory function, which is considered to be by the action of a third subset of T-lymphocytes, and affect feedback regulation of helper and suppressor T-lymphocytes. These cells, which are also involved in self-recognition, will be the subject of a fuller discussion below. In any event, deficiency of T-lymphocytes can result in severe infections, and possibly malignancy (Bellanti 1978; Miescher and Muller-Eberhard 1976). New techniques are gradually becoming available to identify the three subsets of T-lymphocytes by means of conventional hetero-antibodies, monoclonal antibodies produced by hybridomas, auto-antibodies from patients with systemic lupus erythematosus, allo-antibodies, and receptors for isotype specific Fc receptors (Evans et al. 1977; Moretta et al. 1977; Reinherz and Schlossman 1979; Reinherz et al. 1979).

B-lymphocytes are the precursors of the cells which secrete antibody. A deficiency in B-lymphocytes generally results in bacterial infections. It appears that antibody production can come directly from B-lymphocytes, or via transformation of B-lymphocytes to plasma cells. B-lymphocytes may be identified by their surface immunoglobulin molecules, which are being produced by these cells, although primitive B-lymphocytes may not have such markings (Fudenberg et al. 1976). The latter, however, have the ability to transform into cells capable of producing immunoglobulins. Immunoglobulins are of several types, namely, IgA, IgE, IgG, IgM and IgD (Bernier 1978). IgG, the most abundant of the immunoglobulins, is thought to contribute to immunity against many infecting agents, including bacteria, viruses, parasites and some fungi. In addition, most auto-antibodies are of this type, and thus the IgG class of immunoglobulins is of particular interest in relation to auto-immune disorders, and will receive most attention in this volume. IgA, the second most abundant serum immunoglobulin, contributes to the immunity of the individual in the external secretory system (gastro-intestinal, respiratory and genito-urinary tracts). IgM, the largest of the immunoglobulin molecules, is restricted almost entirely to the intravascular space. These macromolecules are capable of agglutinating particulate antigen, such as bacteria and red blood cells, and of fixing complement efficiently. IgD has not yet been assigned a clear biological role, but may act as a specific B-lymphocyte surface receptor in the initiation of the immune response (Elliott et al. 1980). Finally, IgE, the reaginic antibody, is present in only trace amounts in the serum; it appears to initiate aspects of the "acute allergic reaction".

All antibodies are immunoglobulins (Ig), and the terms are virtually interchangeable. A singlc organism can produce millions of slightly different antibodies of different specificities, producing a wide repertoire of antibodies capable of responding to an equally wide range of antigens that may possibly be encountered (Bernier 1978).

IgG antibody molecules consist of two heavy polypeptide (H) chains and two light (L) chains, which are linked by disulphide bonds. The molecular weight of IgG is approximately 160 000. Differences between antibodies which permit response to different antigens are attributable to differences, which may be very extensive, in the N-terminal parts of the H and L chains. Thus, this part of the molecule is termed the variable (V) region, and each region is called a domain. Indeed, less marked differences in other domains of the H chain permit the mediation of other biological functions, such as fixation to macrophages. The "antigen-binding site" or "antibody-active site" of the immunoglobulin molecule is the region that combines with a specific antigen. An antigen can only select from the already available molecules those which happen to fit it best, and thus the production of antibody is selective. After such an antigen-antibody union, there is preferential amplification of the response though selective stimulation and multiplication of the specific clone of B-lymphocytes. The B-lymphocytes producing the highest affinity antibody bind the greatest amount of antigen, leading to their being most highly stimulated. This results in multiplication of clones with high affinity antibodies, leading to a progressive increase in the avidity of the specific antibody for the antigen in question (Katz and Benacerraf 1972). Since this also involves specific helper T-lymphocytes, it is presumed that these too are sensitized, and also take part in the amplification process (Waldman and Munro 1973). Such "high avidity" antibody is generally found late in the primary immune response to an invading antigen, but more quickly in a secondary response, i.e. when the same antigen is encountered again.

Auto-antibodies are those antibodies which react against self-constituents, and are at the core of the discussion in the latter part of this chapter and in later chapters. A special form of auto-antibody is the anti-idiotypic antibody, which is an antibody reacting against an antibody produced by self or against an immunocompetent cell in the same organism (Wigzell et al 1978). It is now felt that auto-anti-idiotypic immunity is a normal part of the conventional immune process, and may have as a consequence potentiation or elimination of a select immune function if this is dependent on the presence of a given clone of idiotype-positive cells. Such antibodies may thus be important as one of the means of normal regulation of the immune processes, but also, under some circumstances, may mimic auto-antigens. Thus there may be a complex network of anti-idiotypic antibodies, not only participating in immuno regulation (along with other mechanisms), but possibly activating or potentiating an immune process (Jerne 1975). Thus these specialized antibodies carry the potential to selectively change the immune course in already immune individuals. For example, anti-idiotypic antibodies formed against auto-antibodies could theoretically prevent certain biological effects of the original auto-antibody, while perhaps producing another biological effect resulting from the immune complex so formed.

In the circulation T-lymphocytes constitute about 55%–60% of the total. In the thymus, over 90% of the cells are T-lymphocytes, whereas in the bone marrow the majority of the cells are B-lymphocytes. In lymph nodes and spleen, the ratio is approximately equal. Cells of both types appear to be capable of recognizing individual foreign substances, so that only one clone of cells from each type ultimately responds to a given foreign antigen. (Actually, as mentioned above, several clones initially respond, but the clone with the highest affinity for the antigen is selected on the basis of that affinity.) Each B-lymphocyte carries only one type of surface antibody molecule, and thus is apparently capable of responding to only one specific antigen (or perhaps a few very closely related antigens). T-lymphocytes, on the other hand, may have the capacity of recognizing a slightly broader range of closely related antigens, although this point is controversial. Once they have come into contact with their complementary antigen, the reacting cells amplify the response quickly, replicating in both the T- and B-lymphocyte series. Even after the antigenic challenge has disappeared, this amplification of response may be recalled, presumably either by an expanded population of cells or by a clone of memory cells (Fudenberg et al 1976; Bellanti 1978).

1.1.3 Processing of Antigen

Antigen itself may be considered the part of the cellular environment that induces the development of immune responsiveness. Following the introduction of an antigen, a variety of sequential steps occurs. The antigen is first met by a macrophage, which appears to be important, even essential, for the processing of antigen, so that the antigen can interact with the cells of the lymphoid series (Möller 1978). Macrophages, which are activated by means of surface receptors, have many functions, which are beyond the scope of this brief review; for further discussion of the various roles of the macrophage, the reader is referred elsewhere (Möller 1978; Elliott et al. 1980). Following this processing by the macrophages, the antigen stimulates specific lymphocytes to proliferate and differentiate into immunocompetent cells; both T-lymphocytes capable of producing lymphokines and B-lymphocytes capable of forming antibody. Some of the T-lymphocytes so induced assist or help the B-lymphocyte response. Thus, not only is the response specific, but it is soon amplified so as to produce a completely appropriate response to the introduction of the antigen. When the antigen subsequently disappears, the population of immunocompetent cells undergoes involution. Some of these cells persist as "memory" cells, which are capable of carrying out certain functions if the same antigen is encountered at a later time. These functions consist of calling forth a much more rapid response (secondary response) of the same clones of T- and B-lymphocytes required once again to elicit a specific response to a specific antigen (Herscowitz 1978; Williams 1975).

Specific antigen receptors exist on the surface of both T- and B-lymphocytes (Davie and Paul 1972; Elliott et al. 1980). While certain antigens can directly stimulate B-lymphocytes so that they can consequently transform into plasma cells and produce antibody, most antigens require the interaction of helper T-lymphocytes, which co-operate with and direct groups of appropriate B-lymphocytes to then produce antibody, as previously briefly discussed. Another subpopulation of T-lymphocytes (suppressor T-lymphocytes) is capable of suppressing the immune response. This subpopulation will be discussed further below.

1.1.4 Genetic Control of the Immune Response

Many aspects of the immune response have now been shown to have a genetic basis. The immune system consists of a highly complex network of components, both cellular and soluble, most of which are specifically encoded for by genes. It is evident that a large number of specific immune response genes exist that control the specific responses to a variety of antigens. It is equally clear that genes may control the cellular interactions within the immune system, as well as the transmission of antigenic specificities from generation to generation.

The major histocompatibility complex (MHC) which is found in mammals is a single genetic region having a major influence on graft rejection. This region has been found to control not only the rejection of heterologous grafts, but also such immunological processes as the immune responsiveness to certain antigens and (more germane to the present discussion) susceptibility to the development of auto-immune diseases. The two MHC systems most extensively studied include the histocompatibility (H-2) system in the mouse and the human leucocyte antigen (HLA) system in man (Bach and van Rood 1976; Dausset 1978; Dausset and Contu 1980; Mc Devitt 1980; McDevitt and Landy 1972; Ritzmann 1976; Rose et al 1978; Svejgaard et al. 1980). The HLA system in man is located on the short arm of chromosome 6 (see Fig. 1.2). A recent excellent review deals with the relationship of HLA to endocrine disease specifically (Farid and Bear 1981).

In addition to the function listed above, this system is also involved in the killing of virus-infected cells and the synthesis of several complement components. However, the various complicated effects of these genes are not directly assessed when testing for disease associations in man. For such purposes, the HLA cell-suface "antigens" are used, because they are relatively easy to identify and because many frequent alternative genes (i. e. many common alleles) are know for each locus. At least four loci determine the classic transplantation antigens identified by

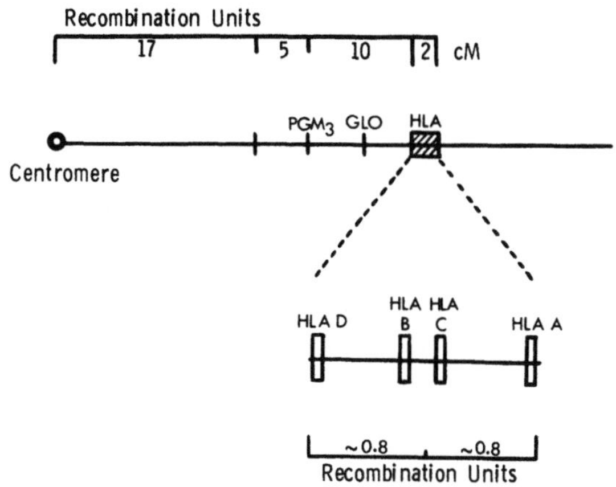

Fig. 1.2. The HLA complex on chromosome 6. This HLA complex is shown relative to other markers (PGM_3, phosphoglucomutase-3; *GLO*, glycoxylase). These markers are all on the short arm of chromosome 6 and distance are indicated in centimorgans (*cM*). The *lower part* of the figure depicts an expanded version of the HLA complex; again, distances between the HLA loci are indicated in centimorgans

serological methods. Eight well-defined and 11 provisional antigens are recognized as A-locus products, and 8 well-defined and 12 provisional antigens as B-locus products (WHO-IUIS Terminology Committee, 1975). The C-locus determines another series of serologically detected antigens, but their functions are not yet clarified, and only a few of the alternative alleles at this locus have been provisionalle defined. D-locus antigens (formerly called mixed-leucocyte culture or MLC antigens) cannot be detected by conventional serological typing. However, lymphocytes from two individuals with different D-locus antigens become activated and form large "blast" cells when cultured together in vitro, while lymphocytes from two D-locus compatible individuals generally will not activate each other in mixed cultures. By using "typing cells" of known specificity in mixed cultures set up so that only the unknown lymphocytes can proliferate, D-locus antigens of the unknown cells can be determined (Svejgaard et al. 1975). Recently, methods have been developed which allow the serological definition of a set of antigens which are closely related to, if not identical with, the HLA-Dw antigens as defined by mixed lymphocyte culture; these are termed HLA-D related (HLA-DR) (van Rood et al. 1975).

Genetic loci are linked if they occur together on the same chromosome in such approximation that they are not separated from each other during meiosis as often as genes on different chromosomes. Linkage can be demonstrated by analysing experimental crosses or the segregation of genes in family studies. HLA complexes are generally inherited intact. Each person receives one HLA complex from his father (his paternal haplotype) and the other from his mother (his maternal haplotype).

Linked alleles which occur together in the same haplotype more frequently than expected are said to be in linkage disequilibrium. Linkage disequilibrium is frequently observed amongst HLA genes, and its occurrence may be necessary to demonstrate certain disease associations. Currently, since it is not yet possible to state that a particular HLA gene is *responsible* for a disease, the HLA antigens should only be considered as convenient inherited markers of disease susceptibility. Incidentally, linkage disequilibrium may be detected in population studies, but not in family studies.

There are two general approaches to investigating associations between HLA antigens and disease (Friedman and Fialkow 1978). In population studies, frequencies of HLA antigens are compared in patients and matched control persons. In assessing apparent population associations between HLA antigens and a disease, it is necessary to determine the strength of the associations and their statistical significance. The strength of the association is generally expressed as relative risk, i. e. the chance of the disease appearing in a person with a given antigen compared to the chance in a person lacking that antigen. On the other hand, family studies are valuable in evaluating HLA disease associations since they illuminate the inheritance of disease susceptibility.

Family studies require kinships in which two or more siblings or other relatives (but not a parent and a single child, who always share one haplotype) are affected with the same disorder. Since complete HLA haplotypes are almost always inherited as units, family studies can be used to demonstrate HLA-linked disease-predisposing genes, even if they are not associated with any detectable antigen in the population (i. e. there is no linkage disequilibrium). In contrast, detection of an HLA disease association in population studies may sometimes depend on the occurrence of linkage disequilibrium.

It is striking that so many of the organ-specific endocrinopathies are associated with the same HLA-D antigen, at least in Caucasians (Table 1.1). It is not yet known whether these disorders all have different Dw3-associated susceptibility genes or whether the susceptibility for these conditions depends on a common Dw3-associated factor, which could conceivably encode a defect in immune regulation. The fact that in none of the Dw3-associated diseases is there an excess of HLA homozygotes indicates that the mode of inheritance of the susceptibility gene is rather a dominant one (with relatively low penetrance) (Albert and Scholz 1979). From this it may be concluded that the mechanism of pathogenesis is not the lack of reactivity, but rather some abnormality in immune activity. Since it is known that

Table 1.1. Some HLA-associated diseases[a]

Disorder	HLA-A	HLA-B	HLA-D/DR
Acute lymphocytic leukaemia	A2		
Haemochromatosis	A3	B14	
Ankylosing spondylitis		B27	
Behcet's syndrome		B5	
Subacute thyroiditis		Bw35	
Multiple sclerosis			Dw2/DRw2
Type I (insulinopenic diabetes)			
Irl (Ib)		B8	Dw3/DRw3 (Caucasian)
Ir2 (Ia)		B15	Dw4/DRw4 (Caucasian)
		BJ22	DYT (Japanese)
Addison's disease		B8	Dw3/DRw3
Chronic active hepatitis		B8	Dw3/DRw3
Myaesthenia gravis		B8	Dw3/DRw3
Graves' (Basedow's) disease		B8	Dw3/DRw3 (Caucasian)
		Bw35	Dw12 (Japanese)
		B46	– (Chinese)
Hashimoto's thyroiditis			DR5
Rheumatoid arthritis			Dw4/DRw4
Coeliac disease			Dw3/DRw3

[a] In Caucasians unless otherwise stated.

controlled self-reactivity is a physiological feature of the immune system, one could view the auto-immune phenomena in Graves' disease and in the other organ-specific auto-immune endocrinopathies as a reflection of a defect in immunological regulation. Thus it is possible that the disease susceptibility gene is coding for a defect in the regulation of certain immune responses, which leads to auto-immune processes (Albert and Scholz 1979).

1.1.5 Significance of HLA Disease Associations

It is evident that the disease predisposition could be due either to the HLA antigen itself or to the presence of another gene or genes carried in the same haplotype as the associated HLA allele. HLA antigens might produce disease susceptibility by serving as virus receptors or if they produce or precipitate an immunopathic response. However, it is more probable that linkage of defined HLA loci to disease-predisposing genes is responsible for the HLA associations observed with the organ-specific auto-immune diseases. Susceptibility to auto-immune disease might be due to human homologues of the murine Ir (immune response) or, even more likely, Is (immune suppression) genes, which modulate the strength and characteristics of the immune response to certain specific antigens (Katz and Benacerraf 1972; Rose et al. 1978). Ir genes appear to be important in experimental auto-immune thyroiditis in mice, but as yet neither Ir nor Is genes have been unequivocally demonstrated in man.

In animals, particularly in mice, there is now a large body of evidence linking the MHC with immune responsiveness, both with respect to experimentally induced and spontaneous auto-immune disease in animals. In some instances, there is evidence that at least some of the spontaneous models of auto-immune disease, such as the thyroiditis in Obese strain (OS) chickens, do not depend solely on the B haplotype (analogous to HLA genes in man), but appear to be polygenic (Rose et al. 1978).

1.1.6 Cell Interactions and Immunoregulation

The clonal selection theory of antibody formation proposed by Burnet (1959) stated that a given immunologically responsive cell (small lymphocyte) contains within its genome the genetic information needed to respond specifically to a single immunogen (or a few closely related immunogens), even before the cell encounters the foreign configuration. Thus, the lymphocyte population of an individual is differentiated so as to contain a diverse repertoire of clones of lymphocytes, each one capable of responding to a given antigen. The encounter between the immunogen and the precommitted clone of lymphocytes results in the proliferation of the latter and the amplification of that clone of differentiated antibody-forming cells. This hypothesis implies that an antiserum prepared against a complex immunogen (such as a bacterial immunogen) consists of a population of different antibodies, each produced by separate clones programmed to respond to a particular antigenic determinant on the complex micro-organism.

It is now clear that this hypothesis is essentially correct (Jerne 1971). Single plasma cells make only one class and allotype of H chain, and one type (lambda or kappa) and allotype of L chain, which display unique variable regions (idiotypes): one cell produces one antibody. As pointed out by Bellanti (1978), the uniformity in primary structure of the antibody produced by a single cell is similar to that of the myeloma protein produced in multiple myeloma, and suggests that the immunoglobulin molecule is subject to allelic exclusion; that is, the cell expresses only one of its several alleles for the different polypeptide chains of the immunoglobulin molecule. One possible exception to the one-cell–one-antibody rule is the finding of a small number of single cells in a population that produces both IgM and IgG or that have IgM on their surface and IgG internally. Since the early immune reponse is characterized by the predominance of IgM followed later by IgG, it has been suggested that cells may undergo an IgM→IgG switch in the course of an immune response.

An important and central feature of the immune system is that it usually manages to distinguish precisely between normal tissues of the body and foreign antigens. For example, immunological cells will react violently to host cells that harbour viruses during the course of a viral infection, and ignore surrounding uninfected cells. To reconcile the clonal selection theory with this observation, Burnet suggested that severe reactions which occur occasionally against one's own tissues could be blamed on the appearance of "forbidden" clones of self-reactive lymphocytes ("renegade" cells) which carry forbidden receptors that escaped elimination during the development of the immune system. The corollary of this proposal was that "forbidden" clones of self-reactive lymphocytes were normally deleted as the immune system developed (the clonal deletion theory) (Burnet 1959; Lederberg 1959). Tolerance was ascribed to a deletion of clones through contact between immature lymphocytes with their corresponding antigen. However, Dresser in 1961 discovered that small amounts of de-aggregated protein could induce tolerance in adult mice. Moreover, in some tolerance models, tolerance was confined to the T-lymphocyte compartment (Weigle et al. 1972). Burnet (1979) has recently reviewed the history of this theory in an interesting discussion. In consequence, Nossal (1979) has found it necessary to expand Burnet's model into the clonal abortion theory. He has proposed that during the maturation of lymphocytes into immunocompetent cells there is a sensitive differentiation stage at which contact with antigen capable of interacting with the lymphocyte receptors results in specific inactivation of the cell. This concept of clonal selection of specific antibody-forming cells by antigen has certainly become generally accepted, and auto-immune diseases are thought to result from a defect in the deletion process. However, as noted by Teale and Mackay (1979) and Gershon (1979), it has become evident recently that the immune system with its amplifying and controlling processes is far more complex than was previously suspected. There are now several known regulatory mechanisms, such as T-lymphocyte dependent suppression, receptor blockade, and idiotype anti-idiotype networks. Moreover, antiself antibodies may be found to be present in normal populations, along with B-lymphocytes which are capable of binding self-antigens. The question of whether clonal abortion really exists has recently been taken up by Teale and Mackay (1979) in an interesting hypothesis article. They point out that immature B-lymphocytes are either stimulated or inhibited by antigen, depending on the availability of T-lymphocyte help. That is, in the absence of helper T-lymphocytes B-lymphocytes are eliminated by exposure to even very low concentrations of multivalent antigen, whereas in the presence of helper T-lymphocytes, the B-lymphocytes are capable of mounting a response. Thus it seems possible that autoreactivity antibodies arise through stimulation of immature B-lymphocytes by means of helper T-lymphocytes or polyclonal B-cell activators (PBAs) and thus, immunization rather than tolerance develops.

The appearance of new clones of B-lymphocytes may occur as a result of the germ line theory or the theory of somatic mutations, or a combination of the two.

The germ line theory postulates that the structure of every variable (V) region that an animal can produce is encoded in its DNA. In this context, every vertebrate genome contains many thousands of different V genes, with divergence owing to natural selection of favourable point mutations, duplications and recombinations (Adams 1978). While this theory might be acceptable for the appearance of self-reactive *B-lymphocytes*, it could not account for the emergence of "forbidden" clones of helper T-lymphocytes, which would be necessary to activate the appropriate self-reactive B-lymphocytes. The lack of concordance (about 50%) in identical twins with Graves' disease and type I diabetes mellitus (see Chaps. 2, 3), as well as the variable timing of concordance (a random event), clearly adds a non-genetic random event. This event occurs in addition to the genetic basis for these conditions, suggesting strongly that the "forbidden" clones of T-lymphocytes are arising due to random somatic mutations.

The B-lymphocytes may also arise as a result of somatic mutation, rather than by the germ line. This question has yet to be resolved. In this model, a small number of germ line genes are hypothesized. These genes mutate during mitotic cell division and increase rapidly during ontogeny, either by antigenic-driven selection or by random drift of selective neutral mutations. Both the germ line theory and the somatic mutation theory agree that separate genes encode for the variable (V) and constant (C) regions of the immunoglobulin molecule. The somatic mutation model for B-lymphocyte diversity assumes that, in order to be transcribed, a V gene must be brought adjacent to a C gene, to form a single functioning cistron (V-C gene). The joining mechanism is not known, although it may be equivalent to a genetic translocation. The sequences of DNA coding for the V region and the sequences of DNA coding for the C region of an immunoglobulin L chain have been shown to be separate from one another (Parker 1980). The two nucleotide segments move closer together during differentiation of lymphocyte precursors to form a single transcription unit that will produce the final immunoglobulin chain.

It has been shown that normal individuals possess selfreactive B-lymphocytes, but not self-reactive T-lymphocytes (Wick 1975). It is also evident that there is a pivotal role for helper T-lymphocytes in regulating the B-lymphocytic production of antibody. How helper T-lymphocytes which stimulate B-lymphocytes to produce auto-antibodies arise is unresolved. When auto-immune manifestations follow drug administration, the drug may well have coupled to self-antigen, thus providing the necessary foreign carrier determinant for helper T-lymphocytes. The helper T-lymphocytes so stimulated by the drug determinant are then able to co-operate with developing self-reactive B-lymphocytes, thus overriding the tolerance signal, i. e. immunization rather than tolerance results. In addition, it has been suggested that infection with viruses may sometimes stimulate auto-immune processes, although the nature of this stimulation remains unclear. It has been proposed that viral antigens may become associated with self-constituents, thereby changing them to "non-self", thus stimulating helper T-lymphocytes. Indeed, there has been widespread speculation that viruses may be implicated in the pathogenesis of several immunologically mediated human diseases, although proof is still lacking.

Moreover, it is possible that viral infection may actually affect lymphocytes, and thus through this alternative pathway, viruses may also be implicated in human auto-immune disorders.

Finally, as mentioned above, the possibility must be entertained that a self-directed "forbidden" clone of helper T-lymphocytes may arise by normal random mutation of spontaneously generated new lymphocytes in a person who lacks the particular immune mechanisms capable of suppressing this particular "forbidden" clone of helper T-lymphocytes. The corollary is that clonal abortion is almost certainly a relevant physiological mechanism of self-tolerance (Nossal and Pike 1975). Teale and Mackay (1979) have suggested that it may be most important during the ontogeny of the immune system, i. e. at the embryological or neonatal stage when newly developing lymphocytes mature, probably in the absence of specific helper T-lymphocytes. At this stage there may be an abundance of non-specific suppressor T-lymphocytes, but whatever the reason, the lymphoid micro-environment at that time cannot be stimulated by antigen, foreign or otherwise.

Presumably, protection against infection is provided by placental transfer of immunoglobulins or by immunoglobulins obtained during suckling. Consequently, the large number of developing B-lymphocytes will differentiate through the tolerance-sensitive stage, without any interference from helper T-lymphocytes, thus permitting the elimination of developing self-reactive lymphocytes which come in contact with self-antigens by the clonal abortion pathway. Teale and Mackay (1979) point out that auto-immune diseases have not been described in infants, but occur in early adult life or later. Moreover, auto-immune diseases can be induced experimentally only in mature animals, and the spontaneous auto-immune diseases described in various inbred strains of mice occur at least some weeks after birth.

While the functions of non-specific suppressor T-lymphocytes found in the neonate are unknown, Kolsch and Heuer (1979) have discussed the possible functions of those antigen-specific suppressor T-lymphocytes which arise a few weeks later in the neonatally tolerant animal or within days after tolerogenic treatment in the adult (Fig. 1.3). Their late appearance after neonatal tolerance induction could mean that they have bypassed the tolerance-sensitive phase around birth. Kolsch and Heuer (1979) thus suggest that it could be an intrinsic property of T-lymphocytes not to be tolerizable by clonal deletion. Specific suppressor T-lymphocytes would then function predominantly by suppressing the development of other T-lymphocytes (cytotoxic and helper T cells) directed against self-antigens or foreign antigens introduced in low doses. Suppression thus would be a lifelong safeguard against expression of newly arising B cell clones reacting with thymus dependent antigens (see Fig. 1.3).

Once the immune system has developed, there is evidence that there is a constant turnover of lymphocytes, with constant appearance of immature developing B-lymphocytes. Teale and Mackay (1979) estimate that approximately 10^{11} new lymphocytes are generated in the adult human daily. They suggest that many of the potentially self-reactive lymphocytes, particulary those of high affinity, are eliminated by a clonal abortion mechanism. However, at this stage in life (childhood or early adulthood), there is much greater risk of intervention by helper T-lymphocytes or polyclonal activators, such as bacterial endotoxins, which may circumvent the tolerance signal, allowing self-reactive clones of lymphocytes to appear. It is well-

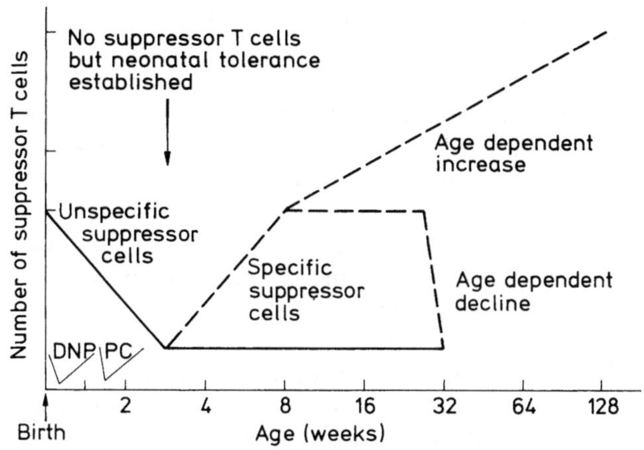

Fig. 1.3. Schema of the ontogeny of suppressor T-lymphocytes in the mouse. *DNP*, dinitrophenol; *PC*, phosphorylcholine. It is known that B cells from young animals can be rendered tolerant more easily than B cells from adult mice and that indeed tolerance susceptibility is a characteristic of developing clones. DNP- and PC-specific B cell clones appear in Balb/c mice in an ordered sequence. DNP-specific clones which arise during intra-uterine development are tolerable only in the first few days after birth and become resistant after 7 days of age, at a time when later developing PC-specific clones can still be rendered tolerant. (Kolsch and Heuer 1979)

known that the incidence of auto-antibodies in normal persons increases with age. However, with age, the immune system also acquires further ability to regulate itself, and it appears that specific suppressor T-lymphocytes arise as time goes on, as well as, perhaps, an idiotype network. As Gershon (1979) states, there is a cascade of cellular events which controls the intensity and type of immunological response. The immune system is not a collection of resting cells awaiting activation by foreign material. Instead, the immune response is controlled in a highly precise manner by messages continuously passed among at least three types of T-lymphocytes – inducer lymphocytes, regulatory lymphocytes and effector lymphocytes. Experiments in animal models have demonstrated that selective activation of regulatory T-lymphocytes is required to avoid immunological reactions against one's own tissues thoughout adult life. Immunity is therefore a regulatory web, with a delicately balanced system of stimulation and suppression capable of controlling (under normal circumstances) any self-reactive clones which may arise spontaneously or be stimulated to arise.

Thus, clonal abortion appears to be an important protection against auto-immunity (Nossal and Pike 1975; Nossal 1979). Auto-immune reactions and disease will occur only when there is a defect in some element of the immune regulatory mechanisms. A loss of suppressor T-lymphocytes has been implicated in certain of the spontaneous auto-immune diseases in animals and man.

Teale and Mackay (1979) deal with the problem that there is a general failure of lymphocytes to react to autologous albumin, transferrin, and other circulating proteins, i. e. monovalent self-antigens. They suggest that immature B-lymphocytes are simply not affected by monovalent antigens, being neither stimulated in the absence of helper T-lymphocytes nor eliminated by clonal abortion. They suggest the possibility that antigens must cross-link receptors in order to deliver an effective signal, either positive or negative, to the B-lymphocytes. If so, there would be little risk that monovalent antigens would evoke auto-immunity.

It is also likely that receptor blockade might contribute to the control of anti-self reactivity, in particular with self-antigens such as albumin which are present in high concentration. In any event, monovalent antigens aside, Teale and Mackay (1979) conclude that clonal abortion does play a physiological role in regulating the immune response, but suggest that it is most important in eliminating self-reactive lymphocytes during the early stages of development, before the appearance of ancillary regulatory systems. Clonal abortion would therefore limit the number of self-reactive lymphocytes in the system, until the more elaborate regulatory networks are developed.

Finally, it is evident that the development of auto-immune disorders is a complex matter. Firstly, the organism must have a genetic capability to be able to mount an immunological attack on its own tissues. This capability appears to be closely involved with the histocompatibility complex genes. The genetic abnormality inherited in many of the organ-specific auto-immune diseases may well be a specific defect in immunoregulation, possibly in many instances a single defect in a clone of suppressor T-lymphocytes. Secondly, T-lymphocyte help must occur, so as to circumvent the tolerogenic signal, and thus prevent the elimination of self-reactive clones. How such T-lymphocyte help is obtained is a matter of some controversy. The random appearance of some of the organ-specific auto-immune diseases in genetically predisposed populations may well indicate that the appearance of the specific "forbidden" organ-directed, self-reactive clone of T-lymphocytes may well be a random event, and unrelated to any specific antigenic stimulatory mechanism. Once randomly appearing in such a normal fashion, the inability to suppress such a "forbidden" clone of helper T-lymphocytes would be all that was necessary to initiate the disease. The self-reactive "forbidden" clone of helper T-lymphocytes (having thus escaped suppression and therefore surviving) would then react with its complementary auto-antigen (without any need for antigenic alteration); it would be amplified and stimulated to interact with and direct already present and appropriate clones of B-lymphocytes, consequently producing antibodies, and establishing the auto-immune process. Alternatively, the appearance of helper T-lymphocytes may not be truly spontaneous, but may occur as a result of viral interaction with lymphocytes. Another alternative is that the determinant recognized by the T-lymphocyte may be in the form of (a) viral antigens (incorporated into host-cell membranes), (b) drugs coupled to cell surfaces or other host determinants or (c) antigens which crossreact with self-constituents, such as some bacterial or viral antigens.

The nature of the defect in immunoregulation may not only be one of suppressor T-lymphocytes, since the role of the complementary anti-idiotype-bearing regulatory cells in the idiotype network remains to be clarified. (Moreover, the very idea that auto-immune disorders are due to defects in tolerance has been challenged by Adams and Knight (1980) in a provocative hypothesis paper on the H gene theory of auto-immune disease.)

Nevertheless, it is tempting to believe that in those organ-specific auto-immune disorders which occur more frequently than by chance in the same individuals or in their families and which may have a common or very closely related genetic basis, the mechanism(s) involved in their pathogenesis must be very closely related. Since later in this volume I will show evidence that there is indeed a defect in suppressor T-lymphocytes in Graves' and Hashimoto's diseases, the following hypothesis will be proposed to account for most, if not all, of the organ-specific auto-immune diseases which are listed on page V.

It is proposed that each of the diseases listed on page V (with possible exceptions) is due to a specific abnormality in a clone of suppressor T-lymphocytes. Each of these defects allows a specific organ-directed "forbidden" clone of helper T-lymphocytes, normally arising at random throughout life, to survive. (In a normal organism these self-same "forbidden" clones of helper T-lymphocytes are also arising, but are being immediately suppressed by normal immunoregulatory mechanisms). The random appearance of some such spontaneously generated "forbidden" clones of helper T-lymphocytes in the persons genetically incapable of regulating them would account for the random appearance of these diseases in the genetically predisposed persons (see Chap. 2). In any event, once the specific "forbidden" clone has arisen in this spontaneous and random manner, it not only survives, but interacts with its complementary antigen (on the target cell membrane) and possibly sets up a localized cell-mediated immune reaction. This would require no abnormality in the target cell membrane, merely the presence and availability of that antigen. The clone of "forbidden" helper T-lymphocytes which has then survived in this manner would be amplified and stimulated by interaction with the specific antigen, and in turn would help groups of already present appropriate B-lymphocytes, which would then in consequence produce the appropriate antibody. This last phase, along with the formation of immune complexes, as well as other

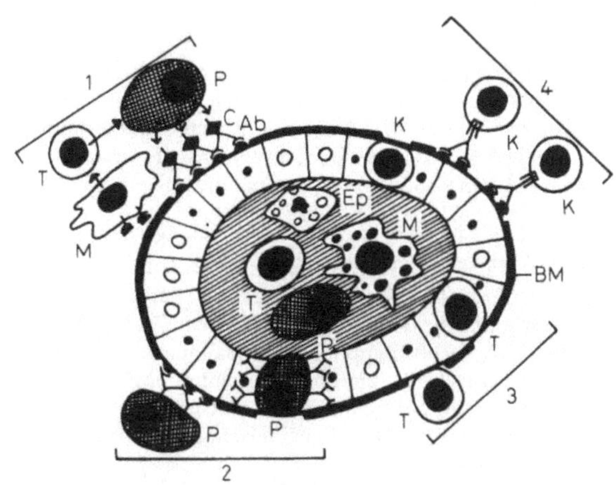

Fig. 1.4. Schematic representation of some possible pathogenetic immunological effector mechanisms in auto-immune thyroiditis. *Mechanism 1:* Cytotoxic antibody needs T-lymphocyte help for its formation and complement for induction of damage. *Mechanism 2:* Periopolesis by plasma cells. These cells produce antibody (with T-lymphocyte help) and act like "killer" (*K*) cells. *Mechanism 3:* Direct cytotoxicity by sensitized T-lymphocytes. *Mechanism 4:* Antibody-dependent cellular cytotoxicity. K cells either attached to thyroid auto-antibodies in situ or sensitized by immune complexes in antibody excess in circulation. Penetration of antibodies or effector cells through basement membrane and periopolesis entail damage of epithelial cells. All types of cells may be found in lumen of destroyed follicles. *P*, plasma cell; *T*, T-lymphocyte; *M*, macrophage; *Ep*, epithelial cell; *Ab*, auto-antibody to thyroglobulin or other thyroid antigen; *C*, complement; *BM*, basement membrane. (Wick et al. 1978)

ancillary, although secondary and often even non-specific, immunological and chemical events, would serve to complete the pathophysiological picture. Where cell damage is the paramount feature, possible mechanisms of cell damage are depicted on Fig. 1.4. In the course of this volume I will be applying this hypothesis to each of the organ-specific auto-immune endocrinopathies in turn.

It may well be that there are defects in immunoregulation which are "complete" in some patients, in which the appearance of the specific "forbidden" clone of helper T-lymphocytes will certainly initiate the particular disease. In others, the defect may be partial and even minimal. In such persons, one could postulate that, even after appearance of the particular "forbidden" clone of helper T-lymphocytes, there would be partial suppression, and the disease would remain occult, perhaps manifesting itself only by the presence of specific auto-antibodies. However, the disease might then become overt if some event occurred which further adversely affected the already partially defective immunoregulatory mechanism (see Sect. 2.2.11). Moreover, it is known that aging gradually reduces immunosuppression, and certainly appears to be a factor in increasing the expression of auto-immune disease with age (Inkeles et al 1977; Makinodan 1977; Roberts-Thomson et al. 1974; Weksler 1978; Kyewski and Wekerle 1978). This proposal could then account for those apparently healthy persons who manifest various auto-antibodies during life; these auto-antibodies are known to vary in titre and even disappear and reappear. Some, but not all, of these subjects may ultimately develop the particular overt disease. Others may develop auto-antibodies de novo in old age, and never develop any clinical evidence of the particular disorder.

1.2 References

Adams, DD (1978) The V gene theory of inherited autoimmune disease. J Clin Lab Immunol 1:17–24

Adams DD, Knight JG (1980) H gene theory of inherited autoimmune disease. Lancet 1:396–398

Albert ED, Scholz S (1979) Genetic aspects of autoimmunity in thyroid diseases. In: Klein E, Horster FA, Beysel D (eds) Autoimmunity in thyroid diseases. Schattauer, Stuttgart, pp 17–22

Bach FH, van Rood JJ (1976) The major histocompatibility complex, genetics and biology. N Engl J Med 295:806–813, 872–878, 927–936

Bach JF, Bach MA, Carnaud C, Dardenne M, Monier JC (1977) Thymic hormones and autoimmunity. In: Talal N (ed) Autoimmunity. Academic Press, New York, pp 207-230

Bach JF, Bach MA, Blanot D, Bricas E, Charreire J, Dardenne M, Fournier C, Pléau JM (1978) Thymic serum factor (FTS). Bull Inst Pasteur 76:325–398

Bellanti JA (1978) Immunology II. Saunders, Philadelphia

Bernier GM (1978) Antibody and immunoglobulins: structure and function. In: Bellanti JA (ed) Immunology II. Saunders Philadelphia, pp 115–137

Burnet FM (1959) The clonal selection theory of acquired immunity. Vanderbilt University Press, Nashville

Burnet FM (1979) Clonal selection and after. In: Bell GI, Perelson AS, Pimbley GH Jr (eds) Theoretical immunology. Dekker, New York, pp 63–85

Dausset J and Svejgaard A (1977) HLA and disease. Munksgaard, Copenhagen

Dausset J, Contu L (1980) The MHC and immune response in man. In: Fougereau M, Dausset J (eds) Immunology 80. Progress in immunology IV. Academic Press, London, pp 513–539

Davie JM, Paul WE (1972) Receptors on immunocompetent cells. V. Cellular correlates of the "maturation" of the immune response. J Exp Med 135:660–674

Dumonde DC, Maini RN (1971) The clinical significance of mediators of cellular immunity. Clin Allergy 1:123:139

Elliott BE, Kerbel RS Nagy ZA (1980) Surface receptors on the lymphoreticular cells; sensory devices for host recognition of foreign antigens and neoplasia. Can Med Assoc J 122:1361–1374

Evans RL, Breard JM, Lazarus H, Schlossman SF, Chess L (1977) Detection, isolation and functional characterization of two human T cell subclasses bearing unique differentiation antigens. J Exp Med 145:221–233

Friedmann JM, Fialkow PJ (1978) The genetics of Graves' disease. Clin Endocrinol Metab 7:47–65

Farid NR, Bear JC (1981) The human major histocompatibility complex and endocrine disease. Endocrine Rev 2:50–86

Fudenberg HH, Stites DP, Caldwell JL, Wells JV (1976) Basic and clinical immunology. Lange Medical Publications, Los Altos

Gershon RK (1979) "Clonal selection and after" and after. N Engl J Med 300:1105–1107

Goldstein AL, Guha A, Zatz MM, Hardy MA, White A (1972) Purification and biological activity of thymosin, a hormone of the thymus gland. Proc Natl Acad Sci USA 60:1800–1803

Goldstein G (1975) The isolation of thymopoietin (thymin). Ann NY Acad Sci 249:177–185

Herscowitz HB (1978) Immunophysiology: cell function and cellular interactions. In: Bellanti JA (ed) Immunology II. Saunders Philadelphia, pp 151–202

Hildemann WH, Reddy AL (1973) Phylogeny of immune responsiveness: marine invertebrates. Fed Proc 32:2188–2194

Inkeles B, Innes JB, Kurtz MM, Kadish AS, Weksler ME (1977) Immunological studies of aging. III. Cytokinetic basis for the impaired response from aged patients to plant lectins. J Exp Med 145:1176–1181

Jerne NK (1971) The somatic generation of immune recognition. Eur J Immunol 1:1–9

Jerne NK (1975) The immune system: a web on V-domains. Harvey Lect 70:93

Katz DH, Benacerraf B (1972) The regulatory influence of activated T cells on B cell responses to antigen. Adv Immunol 15:1–94

Kolsch E, and Heuer J (1979) Tolerance and autoimmunity – an introductory survey. In: Klein E, Horster FA, Beysel D (eds) Autoimmunity in thyroid diseases. Schattauer, Stuttgart, pp 3–16

Kyewski B, Wekerle H (1978) Increase of T lymphocyte self reactivity in aging inbred rats: in vitro studies with a model of experimental autoimmune orchitis. J Immunol 120:1249–1255

Lederberg J (1959) Genes and antibodies: do antibodies bear instructions for antibody specificity or do they select cell lines that arise by mutation? Science 129:1649–1653

Makinodan R (1977) Immunity and ageing. In: Finch CE, Hayflick L (eds) Handbook of the biology of ageing. Van Nostrand & Reinhold, New York, pp 379–408

McDevitt HO (1980) The role of H-2 I region genes in regulation of the immune response. In: Fougereau M, Dausset J (eds) Immunology 80. Progress in immunology IV. Academic Press, London, pp 503–512

McDevitt HO, Landy M (1972) Genetic control of immune responsiveness: relationship to disease susceptibility. Academic Press, New York

Miescher PA, Muller-Eberhard HJ (1976) Textbook of immunopathology, 2nd edn. Grune & Stratton, New York

Möller G (1978) Role of macrophages in the immune response. Immunol Rev 40:3–255

Moretta L, Webb SR, Gross CE, Lydyard PM, Cooper MD (1977) Functional analysis of two human T cell subpopulations: help and suppression of B cell responses by T cells bearing receptors for IgM or IgG. J Exp Med 146:184–200

Nossal GJV (1979) Differentiation of B cells and the clonal abortion theory. Adv Exp Med Biol 114:253–258

Nossal GJV Pike BL (1975) Evidence for the clonal abortion theory of B-lymphocyte tolerance. J Exp Med 141:904–917

Parker CW (1980) Clinical immunology. Saunders, Philadelphia

Playfair JHL (1975) Introduction (to autoimmunity in endocrine disease). Clin Endocrinol Metab 4:229–239

Reinherz EL, Schlossman SF (1979) Con A-inducible suppression of MLC: Evidence for mediation by the TH_2 T cell subset in man. J Immunol 122:1335–1341

Reinherz EL, Kung PC, Goldstein G, Schlossman SF (1979) Separation of functional subsets of human T cells by a monoclonal antibody. Proc Natl Acad Sci USA 76:4062–4065

Ritzmann SE (1976) HLA patterns and disease associations. JAMA 236:2305–2309

Roberts-Thomsen IC, Whittinham S, Youngchaiyud U, Mackay IR (1974) Ageing, immune response and mortality. Lancet 2:368–370

Rose NR, Bigazzi PE, Warner NL (1978) Genetic control of autoimmune disease. Elsevier/North Holland, New York

Svejgaard A, Hauge M, Jersild C, Platz R, Ryder LP, Staub Nielsen L, Thomsen M (1975) The HLA system: an introductory survey. Karger, New York (Monographs in human genetics, vol 7)

Svejgaard A, Morling N, Platz P, Ryder LP, Thomsen M (1980) HLA and disease. In: Fougereau M, Dausset J (eds) Immunology 80. Progress in immunology IV. Academic Press, London, pp 1065–1092

Teale JM, Mackay IR (1979) Autoimmune disease and the theory of clonal abortion. Is it still relevant? Lancet 2:284–287

van Rood JJ, van Leeuwen A, Parlevlist J, Termijtelen A, Keuning JJ (1975) In: Kissmeyer-Nielsen F (ed) Histocompatibility testing, report of the VI international histocompatibility workshop and conference. Munksgaard, Copenhagen, pp 629–636

Volpé R (1977) The role of autoimmunity in hypoendocrine and hyperendocrine function with special emphasis on autoimmune thyroid disease. Ann Intern Med 87:86–99

Waldman H, Munro A (1973) T-cell dependent mediator in the immune response. Nature 243:356–357

Weigle WO, Chiller JM, Habicht GS (1972) Effect of immunological unresponsiveness on different cell populations. Transplant Rev 8:3–25

Weksler ME (1978) The influence of immune function on life-span. Bull NY Acad Med 54:964–969

WHO-IUIS Terminology Committee (1975). Nomenclature for factors of the HLA system. Eur I Immunol 5:889–891

Wick G (1975) Experimental animal models in autoimmune endocrine disease. Clin Endocrinol Metab 4:241–266

Wick G, Kofler R, Gundolf R, Muller PU, Boyd R (1979) The nature of effector cells in experimental and spontaneous autoimmune thyroiditis. In: Milgrom F, Albini B (eds) Immunopathology. Karger, Basel, pp 101–106

Wigzell H, Binz H, Frischknecht H, Peterson P, Sege K (1978) Possible roles of auto-anti-idiotypic immunity in autoimmune disease. In: Rose NR, Bigazzi PE, Warner NL (eds) Genetic control of autoimmune disease. Elsevier/North Holland, New York, pp 327–342

Williams RC (1975) Lymphocytes and their interactions. Raven, New York

2 Auto-immunity in Thyroid Disease

2.1. Introduction

This chapter will discuss the immunological aspects of two clinically disparate disorders of the thyroid, namely, Graves' disease and Hashimoto's thyroiditis (and its variants) (see Table 2.1). While the clinical expression of these two disorders may be markedly different, there are many genetic and pathogenetic elements which are similar if not common to them both, and indeed some workers (although not this author) consider that these two conditions are merely opposite ends of a spectrum of the same condition (Bastenie and Ermans 1972; Fisher and Beall 1976).

Graves' disease (Parry 1825; Graves 1835; von Basedow 1840) is currently defined as a form of hyperthyroidism with a diffuse hyperplastic goitre associated frequently with other extrathyroidal manifestations, such as exophthalmos and occasionally pretibial myxoedema; the excess production of thyroid hormones in this disorder is generally considered to be due to the stimulation of the thyrotrophin (TSH) receptor by an immunoglobulin, termed thyroid-stimulating antibody (Volpé 1978 a).

The second auto-immune thyroid disorder, lymphocytic (Hashimoto's) thyroiditis, was first described by Hashimoto (1912); he reported four patients with goitre in whom the histology of the thyroid was characterized by diffuse lymphocytic infiltration, atrophy of the parenchymal cells, fibrosis and an eosinophilic change in some of the parenchymal cells. There is some variation in this histological picture in the variants as listed in Table 2.1. In the "chronic fibrous" thyroiditis variant, fibrosis predominates and lymphocytic infiltration is less marked (Hazard 1955). In the lymphocytic thyroiditis group in childhood and adolescence, fibrosis, Askanazy cells and even germinal centres are less obvious than in the adult form (Hazard 1955). Moreover, the titres of thyroid auto-antibodies are generally lower in this category, when compared with the adult forms (or may be negative) (Loeb et al. 1973). In "idiopathic myxoedema", the gland is characterized by atrophy, rather than hypertrophy of the thyroid gland. The atrophic asympto-

Table 2.1. Human auto-immune thyroid disease

A. Graves' disease (synonyms include: Parry's disease, Basedow's disease, exophthalmic goitre, auto-immune thyrotoxicosis)
B. Chronic auto-immune thyroiditis
   Variants:
   1. Hashimoto's (lymphocytic) thyroiditis
   2. Lymphocytic thyroiditis of childhood and adolescence
   3. Chronic fibrous variant
   4. Idiopathic myxoedema
   5. Atrophic, asymptomatic thyroiditis

matic form is clinically occult and often discovered at necropsy (Bastenie et al. 1967). Indeed, proof is not yet completely forthcoming to establish the various forms of chronic auto-immune thyroiditis as variants of an identical process. There may be subtle genetic factors inducing atrophy in some patients, as opposed to hypertrophy of the gland in others (Doniach et al. 1979; Volpé 1979 b), and such differences will be mentioned below. Nevertheless, there is also considerable genetic, functional and immunological evidence to indicate that all of the variants have a similar pathogenesis, and it is thus perhaps now time to utilize the term "chronic auto-immune thyroiditis" as the generic term for this group (Volpé 1979 b).

For many years this disorder was thought to be uncommon, and the diagnosis was often first made at thyroidectomy. Increased awareness, coupled with improved diagnostic procedures, has resulted in improved recognition. There is also some evidence that the disease may actually have increased in frequency, and this increase has been ascribed to increased iodine intake (Volpé 1979 b). It is now estimated that approximately 3%–4% of the population has chronic thyroiditis (Fisher and Beall 1976). Thyroid function in auto-immune thyroiditis may be normal, slightly reduced or severely deficient (Fisher and Beall 1976). About 3% of the population has some functional deficiency of the thyroid secondary to auto-immune thyroiditis (Tunbridge 1979), whereas up to 16% of elderly females have at least some degree of lymphocytic infiltration in their thyroid glands, although this cannot be recognized clinically (Yoshida et al 1978). About two-thirds of goitres in euthyroid children and adolescents prove to be due to lymphocytic infiltration (Hung et al. 1973). Graves' disease is also a common disorder and is estimated to occur in about 1% of the population (Tunbridge 1979).

In both Graves' and Hashimoto's diseases there are several aspects which suggest the participation of an auto-immune process (Solomon and Chopra 1972; Volpé et al. 1974) (see Table 2.2). Patients with Graves' disease occasionally have an enlarged spleen and lymphadenopathy and commonly have a relative lymphocytosis (Werner and Ingbar 1978). Patients with Hashimoto's thyroiditis commonly have hypergammaglobulinaemia (McConahey et al. 1961). In both conditions there is thymic enlargement (Michie and Gunn 1966) and lymphocytic infiltration within the thyroid stroma (Doniach et al. 1979; Werner and Ingbar 1978). Moreover, various immunoglobulins may be demonstrated within the thyroid in each of these conditions (Werner and Fierer 1972; Kalderon and Bogaars 1977). Thyroid auto-antibodies may be detected in nearly all cases of Hashimoto's thyroiditis, and (at least with sensitive radioassays) in virtually all cases of Graves' disease as well (Mori and Kriss 1971). Immune complexes have been detected in the plasma of both Graves' and Hashimoto's diseases (Brohee et al. 1979; Hopf et al. 1978; Calder et al. 1974 a; Cano et al. 1976; Mariotti et al 1979). Moreover, rheumatoid factors have been demonstrated in Graves' disease (Silverberg et al. 1978 b; Scherbaum et al. 1978). Thyroid auto-antibodies may be demonstrated in about 50% of asymptomatic relatives of patients with either disorder (Doniach et al. 1979; Chopra et al. 1977).

The overlap between Graves' and Hashimoto's diseases has been recognized for years (Hahn et al. 1965; Fisher and Beall 1976). Indeed, Graves' and Hashimoto's diseases frequently aggregate in the same families (Friedman and Fialkow 1978). There are several reports of identical twins, one with Graves' disease and the other with Hashimoto's thyroiditis (Jayson et al. 1967; Chertow et al. 1973). In fact, both

Table 2.2. Immune stigmata associated with Graves' and Hashimoto's diseases

Stigma	Graves' disease	Hashimoto's thyroiditis
Lymphocytic infiltration in thyroid	Frequently present	Almost invariable
Immunoglobulins in thyroid stroma	Yes	Yes
Type of infiltrating lymphocytes in thyroid	B- and T-lymphocytes, some unidentified lymphocytes	B- and T-lymphocytes, some unidentified lymphocytes
Immune complexes in circulation	Common	Common
Thymic enlargement	Common	Common
Lymphadenopathy and splenomegaly	Infrequent	–
Relative lymphocytosis	Common	–
Hypergammaglobulinaemia	–	Common
Benefit from corticosteroid therapy	Yes	Yes
Thyroid-stimulating immunoglobulin	Almost all	Infrequent
Exophthalmos	Common	Occasional
Evidence of cell-mediated immunity	Yes	Yes
Evidence for a defect in suppressor T-lymphocytes	Yes	Yes
Other auto-immune diseases in patients	Hashimoto's thyroiditis, exophthalmos, pernicious anaemia, diabetes mellitus, myaesthenia gravis, Addison's disease, vitiligo, chronic active hepatitis, idiopathic thromocytopenic purpura	Graves' disease, exophthalmos, pernicious anaemia, diabetes mellitus, myaesthenia gravis, rheumatoid arthritis, Addison's disease, Sjögren's syndrome, vitiligo, chronic active hepatitis
Thyroid antibodies in relatives	50%	50%
Thyroid and other auto-immune diseases in relatives	Common	Common
HLA genes (Caucasians)	HLA-B8-Dw3	Atrophic form: HLA-B8 and HLA-DRw3. Goitrous form: HLA-DR5
Animal models	–	Yes

Graves' and Hashimoto's diseases can cohabit the same thyroid gland (Fatourechi et al. 1971; Doniach et al. 1979). and the clinical expression will depend on which condition predominates.

In addition, other auto-immune diseases e. g. pernicious anaemia (Ungar et al. 1977), diabetes mellitus (Irvine 1975; Friedmann and Fialkow 1978), myaesthenia gravis (Simpson 1968; Aarli et al. 1978), rheumatoid arthritis (Monroe 1935), Addison's disease (Irvine 1975), Sjögren's syndrome (Martinez-Lavin et al. 1979; Shearn 1971; Whaley et al. 1973), vitiligo (Cunliffe et al. 1968; Ochi and DeGroot 1969), chronic active hepatitis (Elling at al. 1966) and idiopathic thrombocytopenic purpura (Dunlap et al. 1974) occur more frequently than expected in the same patients, or occur in the relatives of patients with either Graves' or Hashimoto's disease (Friedman and Fialkow 1978). Moreover, evidence of sensitization of T-lymphocytes is present in both disorders to the same thyroidal antigenic preparations, and evidence for a defect in supressor T-lymphocytes is likewise common to both (Okita et al. 1980 a, b and 1981 a, b).

Nevertheless, there are a few elements which are different in each condition, and it is thus the author's perspective that the two disorders should be considered separate entities (Kidd et al. 1980). These views will be amplified below, as will many of the comments made above.

2.2 Studies of the Immunological Aspects of Thyroid Disease

2.2.1 Initial Observations

The pioneer observations in the area of auto-immunity in the thyroid field were made in widely separated centres in one year, namely, 1956. In that year, Roitt et al (1956) in London, described the detection of thyroid auto-antibodies in the serum of patients with Hashimoto's thyroiditis. Almost simultaneously, Rose and Witebsky of Buffalo, New York, reported the induction of experimental thyroiditis in rabbits; they mixed one lobe of the rabbit's thyroid gland with Freund's adjuvant (a mixture of killed tubercle bacilli and oil) and reinjected this antigenic material into the footpad of the same rabbit. They were able to demonstrate thyroiditis in the contralateral (remaining) lobe of the animal's thyroid gland; since the lesion appeared to be organ-specific, it appeared that the Freund's adjuvant had conferred antigenic specificity to the thyroid auto-antigen (Rose and Witebsky 1956). In addition, during that same year, Adams and Purves (1956) in Dunedin, New Zealand, reported the presence of an abnormal thyroid stimulator in the serum of some patients with Graves' disease, which was capable of stimulating the guinea-pig thyroid. This was later termed long-acting thyroid stimulator (LATS) (McKenzie 1960) and proved to be an immunoglobulin G (IgG), i.e. an antibody (Kriss et al. 1964). [It is now termed thyroid-stimulating immunoglobulin or antibody (see below).]

These pioneer observations were monumental in catalysing studies of auto-immune endocrinopathies, and indeed investigations of thyroid immunology have continued to be models of auto-immunity in general. The innumerable reports which followed these original publications attest to the intense interest that this field has generated in the past two decades or more. In the following pages, an attempt will be made to collate this voluminous material, and perhaps more importantly, to interpret it in the light of the author's perspective.

2.2.2 Experimental and Spontaneous Animal Models in Auto-immune Thyroid Disease

In order to cast light on the human disorders which comprise the bulk of this chapter, there have been many studies of animal auto-immune thyroid disease, both in the form of experimentally induced thyroiditis and spontaneous thyroiditis in certain animals. One important reason for commencing such studies was in order to conform to the rigid criteria first postulated by Milgrom and Witebsky (1962), which have been utilized to define auto-immune disease in general. These are listed below:

1. A circulating antibody or a cellular immune reaction in patients with the disease.
2. A specific antigen in the human tissue or organ involved in the disease.

3. Production of antibody in experimental animals by immunization with the antigen.
4. Reproduction of the disease in an immunized experimental animal.
5. Passive transfer of the disease with immunologically competent cells or serum.

2.2.2.1 Experimental Auto-immune Thyroiditis

The first report on the experimental induction of auto-immune disease in an endocrine organ was that of experimental auto-immune thyroiditis by Witebsky and Rose (1956), as noted above. In these classic experiments, a pool of homologous thyroglobulin was prepared, emulsified with complete Freund's adjuvant, and injected intradermally into rabbits. These animals not only responded by the formation of thyroglobulin auto-antibodies, but also by the derangement of the thyroid architecture by infiltrating lymphocytes, neutrophils, plasma cells and histiocytes. The exact mode of action of adjuvants still remains to be clarified. In some manner, however, they confer antigenic capacity to the injected material.

The origin of the immunizing antigen was subsequently found to be of importance. Vladutiu and Rose (1972) have found that thyroid antigen prepared from syngeneic donors is less potent for the production of experimental auto-immune thyroiditis than allogeneic material. Auto-immune thyroiditis has been produced in many different species, including the rabbit, the guinea-pig, rat, mouse, dog, monkey and chicken (Rose and Witebsky 1971).

Wick (1975) has reviewed the pathological picture observed in this form of experimental thyroiditis. Histologically, focal (later confluent) infiltration first arises around small blood vessels between thyroid follicles. Early stages are characterized by the presence of eosinophils, neutrophils and small lymphoid cells. Later, mononuclear cells prevail, accompanied by histiocytes and macrophages. Small lymphoid cells penetrate the follicular basement membrane between epithelial cells, rupturing the epithelial lining and finally leading to complete destruction of the follicle. Epithelial cells, lymphocytes and macrophages merge into the follicular lumen. In later stages, strands of regenerating epithelium are found, but new follicles do not form and considerable interstitial fibrosis may be seen. Unlike the human disease [or spontaneous thyroiditis in Obese strain (OS) chickens], plasma cells are not predominant, and germinal centres usually fail to develop within the infiltrated thyroid gland. Moreover, self-perpetuation in the absence of a continuous antigenic stimulus does not occur and complete thyroid destruction is not found. In addition, electron-microscopic studies have failed to show the large Hurthle cells packed with mitochondria as seen in the human disease of Hashimoto's thyroiditis.

Antithyroglobulin antibodies are demonstrable by a variety of serological procedures (Wick 1975). Generally speaking, however, antimicrosomal antibodies are non-reactive.

There is considerable evidence to suggest that these lesions are mediated by T-lymphocytes, i.e. cell-mediated immunity. Paget et al. (1976) found that the predominant infiltrating lymphocytes within the thyroid of experimental auto-immune thyroiditis in guinea pigs were T-lymphocytes. Yet, despite the demonstrated excess of T-lymphocytes within this lesion, it appeared that the proportion of T-lymphocytes that were specifically sensitized to the thyroid antigen was small. These workers also showed considerable numbers of immunoglobulin-bearing B-lymphocytes, as well as cells capable of mediating antibody-dependent cell-mediated cytotoxicity (Van Boxel et al. 1973). These results were considered compatible with a role for cell-mediated immunity in the pathogenesis of experimental auto-immune thyroiditis. Moreover, delayed-type skin reactions to thyroglobulin are demonstrable in guinea-pigs with experimental auto-immune thyroiditis, and correlate well with the severity of the lesions (McMaster and Lerner 1967). Additionally, the transfer of lymph node cells from an animal with experimental auto-immune thyroiditis to a histocompatible recipient resulted in experimental auto-immune thyroiditis developing in the recipient (McMaster and Lerner 1967). In addition, Jepsen et al. (1979) have shown that neonatal thymectomy inhibits the production of the lesions of experimentally induced thyroiditis in guinea-pigs; this indicates that a T-lymphocyte subpopulation (which is sensitive to neonatal thymectomy) is required for the development of experimental auto-immune thyroiditis in the guinea pig.

However, delayed-type skin reactions found in guinea pigs with experimental auto-immune thyroiditis could not be produced in rabbits (Weigle and Romball 1975). Furthermore, experimental auto-immune thyroiditis cannot be produced in neonatally thymectomized chickens or rats or "nude" mice (Wick at al. 1979). Moreover, with considerable difficulty, Nakamura and Weigle (1967) and Vladutiu and Rose (1971) have succeeded in transferring experimental auto-immune thyroiditis by means of the transfer of serum in rabbits and mice respectively. Wick et al. (1979) argue that experimental auto-immune thyroiditis is likely to be a result of a termination of normal T-lymphocyte unresponsiveness to thyroglobulin in the presence of autoreactive B-lymphocytes. Bypassing specific regulatory T-lymphocytes can be achieved by injection of altered autologous or complexed homologous thyroglobulin. The T-lymphocytes activated via the bypass of specific regulatory T-lymphocytes may provide the second signal to thyroglobulin-reactive B-lymphocytes for further differentiation into effector cells. Recent studies indicate that antibody-dependent cellular cytotoxicity (i. e. K cell activity) may be the more likely effector mechanism in experimental auto-immune thyroiditis (Allison 1976; Clinton and Weigele 1972). There is no indication that complement is involved in the pathogenesis of these lesions (Fig. 2.1).

Moreover, the experimentally induced disease in animals is also greatly influenced by genetic factors. The severity of thyroiditis is dependent upon the genetic constitution of the animal and is H-2 linked. There appear to be immune response (Ir) genes which control antibody production and immune suppressive (Is) genes which control the level of immunosuppression. Such genes are clearly important in determining whether an animal is a "good responder" or a "poor responder" to the injection of auto-antigen (Braley-Mullen at al. 1978; Kong et al. 1978; Christadoss et al. 1978). Since this genetic control is likely to be exerted at the suppressor T-lymphocyte level (Vladutiu and Rose 1975), it would appear that self-recognizing T-lymphocytes also exist in the same way as do self-reactive precursors for K "killer" cells (Osband and Parkman 1978; Wekerle and Begemann 1978). Therefore, suppression of self-reactive T helper and B-lymphocytes must be considered as a mechanism by which auto-antibody formation is prevented. Indeed, for a variety of tolerance phenomena and other immunological reactions, involvement of suppressor T-lymphocytes has been demonstrated, which is distinct from and acts antagonistically to helper T-lymphocytes (Kolsch and Heuer 1979) (see Chap. 1). The antibodies produced in experimental auto-immune thyroiditis are

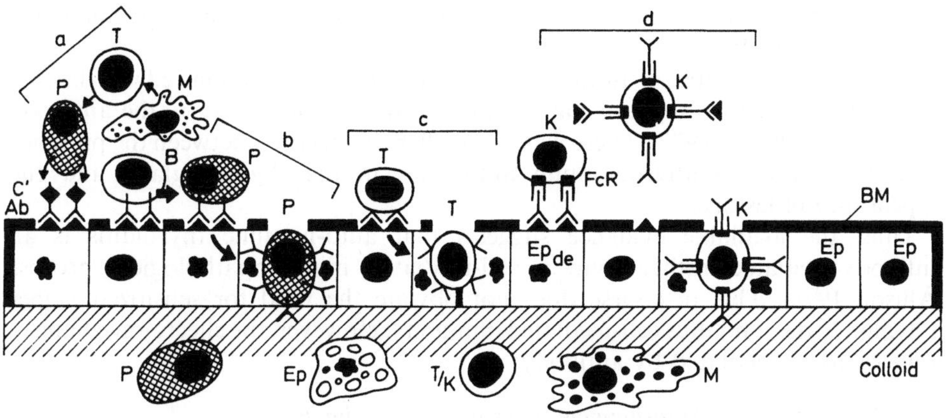

Fig. 2.1. Possible effector mechanism in spontaneous auto-immune thyroiditis of Obese strain chickens. *P*, plasma cells; *T*, T-lymphocytes; *M*, macrophage; *C'*, complement; *Ab*, antibody = auto-antibody to thyroid antigens, e. g. thyroglobulin; *B*, thyroglobulin binding B-lymphocytes; *EP*, epithelial cell; EP_{de}, degenerated epithelial cell; *K*, "killer" cell; *FcR*, Fc receptor; *BM*, basement membrane. *Mechanism a:* Cytotoxic antibody leading to damage by activation of complement. T-lymphocyte help is necessary for the production of this antibody in chickens. *Mechanism b:* Thyroglobulin binding B-lymphocytes attach to the homologous antigen and differentiate into plasma cells which may perform periopolesis and act in an antibody-dependent cellular cytotoxic-like fashion. *Mechanism c:* Direct cytotoxicity may be due to sensitized T-lymphocytes. *Mechanism d:* Antibody-dependent cellular cytotoxicity "killer" cells, triggered by attachment to either auto-antibodies in situ or immune complex in antibody excess in the circulation. The cytotoxic effect is symbolized by pyknotic nuclei of degenerated epithelial cells. After breakdown of the thyroid epithelial lining, all types of cells including desquamated epithelial cells can be found in the follicular lumen. (Wick and Boyd 1979)

predominatly, but not exclusively, IgG antibodies. The fact that IgG antibodies are produced suggests that the antigens in question are thymus-dependent antigens, for which collaboration between thymus-derived T-lymphocytes and B-lymphocytes is neccesary for mounting a response. Thus, functions of helper T-lymphocytes and B-lymphocytes are required for antibody formation (Kolsch and Heuer 1979).

Once IgG antibodies are formed, they may damage the cells through a variety of mechanisms. These may include immune complexes as well as "killer" (K) cells which have receptors for the allosterically-altered Fc part of IgG antibodies complexed with antigen. If the antigens are cells, then K cells are able to destroy them. Though K cells are primarily immunologically unspecific, they acquire "transient" specificity through binding of immune complexes (Kolsch and Heuer 1979). Nevertheless, since experimental auto-immune thyroiditis involves the use of an adjuvant and occurs in animals with normal suppressor T-lymphocyte function which has to be bypassed, it cannot be accepted as a truly analogous model for the situation in human Hashimoto's thyroiditis (Wick et al. 1979).

The traditional way to distinguish between cell-mediated and antibody-mediated immune reactions is adoptive transfer. If immune serum is capable of transferring the reaction, it is antibody-mediated, whereas if the reaction is transferred by immune lymphocytes to syngeneic recipients but not by serum it is assumed to be cell-mediated (Allison 1976). Experimental auto-immune thyroiditis has been transferred by immune serum in rabbits, guinea-pigs, mice and monkeys, although the cell infiltration observed has usually been less severe than in actively immunized animals (Allison 1976).

Moreover, the kinetics of antibody formation is in rabbits immunized with bovine thyroglobulin further suggest that the thyroiditis was produced by the antibody (Clinton and Weigle 1972). There was an excellent correlation between the presence of cells making antithyroglobulin antibodies in the thyroid gland and the appearance of lesions.

Thus, the available evidence suggests that auto-immune thyroiditis is an antibody-mediated rather than a cell-mediated immunopathological process (Allison 1976). This of course does not obviate the need for sensitized helper T-lymphocytes, and thus cell-mediated immunity. However, the effector mechanism appears to be mediated by antibody.

2.2.2.2 Spontaneous Auto-immune Thyroiditis in Animals

Since the experimentally induced animal model is not considered closely analogous to the human disorder, spontaneous models have been sought and found. Spontaneous development of auto-immune thyroiditis can be shown to occur in neonatally thymectomized mice (Kojima et al. 1976 a). It can be prevented, however, by the grafting of a neonatal thymus, or cell injection from adult thymus, spleen and lymph nodes, but not from bone marrow (depending on the timing of treatment) (Kojima et al. 1976 b). Spontaneous chronic thyroiditis with antibodies to thyroglobulin can readily be induced in rats by thymectomy combined with repeated sublethal irradiation, and this disorder can be suppressed by reconstruction with normal lymphoid cells (Penhale et al. 1976).

However, the depletion of T-lymphocytes in these various experiments was not absolute. Moreover, since suppressor T-lymphocytes are radiosensitive, whereas helper T-lymphocytes are relatively radioresistant, it would appear that the thymectomized, irradiated mice have an considerable depletion of suppressor T-lymphocytes in the presence of sufficient helper T-lymphocytes to co-operate in antibody formation. Thymectomy alone also produces thyroiditis by virtue of removal of more suppressor activity than helper activity.

However, perhaps more valuable spontaneous models which have not required such manipulation have been observed in closed colonies of Beagle dogs (Fritz et al. 1970; Beierwaltes and Nishiyama 1968), Buffalo strain rats (Glover and Reuber 1968) and finally, and most importantly, in the OS chicken (Cole et al. 1968; Wick et al. 1974).

The morphology of spontaneous auto-immune thyroiditis in the OS chickens includes a predominant infiltration with plasma cells, and a high number of germinal centres. The plasma cells are amongst the first lymphoid cells to be found in the early stage of thyroid infiltration at about one week of age. These plasma cells are surrounded by immunoglobulin and electron-dense deposits on immunofluorescence and electron-microscopic preparations respectively. Smaller lymphoid cells can also be found both in the interstitium and penetrating between epithelial cells. The nature of these latter cells (whether B- or T-lymphocytes) has not yet been determined (Wick et al. 1974).

Chickens are convenient laboratory animals, since it is possible selectively to deplete B-lymphocytes by bursectomy and T-lymphocytes by thymectomy (Allison 1976). Hormonal bursectomy by injection of antigen into OS chick embryos or surgical bursectomy will abolish or markedly reduce the auto-immune thyroiditis characteristic of this strain; very few of the bursectomized chickens showed circulating antibodies to thyroglobulin. If bursa cells were given to the bursectomized irradiated chickens, the thyroiditis recurred. Whole body irradiation after hatching or thymectomy of newly hatched OS chickens accelerated and aggravated the lymphoid infiltration of the thyroid and increased the incidence of antibodies against thyroglobulin (Wick et al. 1974).

Wick et al. (1979) have shown evidence that the damage to the thyroid gland that occurs in spontaneous thyroiditis in OS chickens may occur as a result of thyroglobulin auto-antibodies binding to the primarily altered thyroid cells, leading to damage by complement-mediated cytotoxicity. Consequently, thyroglobulin leaking from the damaged follicles will bind (directly or via macrophages) to thyroglobulin binding cells and trigger their differentiation into plasma cells. Free thyroglobulin or thyroglobulin-antithyroglobulin complexes may be bound by reticulo-endothelial cells, thereby trapping thyroglobulin binding B-lymphocytes, evoking further differentiation and proliferation within germinal centres.

These mechanisms are primarily B-lymphocyte induced, although thyroglobulin auto-antibody production, at least of the IgG type (some is also of IgM class), will require helper T-lymphocyte co-operation. Destruction of target cells occurs either by the antibody-producing cells themselves acting as effector cells, without the need of Fc receptors, or by Fc receptor positive K cells. These K cells may have receptors for either IgG or IgM. Possible mechanisms of cellular damage are depicted in Fig. 2.1.

The possible genetic basis for the development of spontaneous auto-immune thyroiditis in OS chickens has also been studied carefully. In the studies of Bacon et al. (1973), the presence of the Bl allele (the B locus in chickens is analogous to HLA in man) was found to be correlated with high responsiveness in respect to both spontaneous auto-immune thyroiditis and thyroglobulin auto-antibody production, while B4 was associated with low responsiveness. B1/B4 heterozygotes appeared as intermediate responders (Wick 1975).

Wick et al. (1979) have studied their own OS colony, where B1/B1 chickens and B4/B4 chickens display severe mean degrees of spontaneous auto-immune thyroiditis and high thyroglobulin auto-antibody titres, while a line developed in their laboratory with the genotype B3/B3 appears to be low responding. However, the correlation was not absolute, as there were always several B1, B4 birds with mild spontaneous auto-immune thyroiditis and low thyroglobulin antibody titres, and also some B3/B3 chickens with severe disease. Wick at al. (1979) have thus suggested that the development of spontaneous auto-immune thyroiditis is dependent on the action of genes at (at least) three loci. Ir1 genes, associated with the B locus, code for high (B1, B4) or low (B3) responsiveness, respectively. Ir2, localized at a non-B locus, is also responsible for high responsiveness; this may be operative perhaps via a decrease in number and/or function of suppressor T-lymphocytes. There is also some evidence for a defect in the thyroid cell itself in the OS chicken, but whether this is an important factor in the genesis of the lesion remains unclear.

In any event, it is clear that this spontaneous model is much closer to the human disorder, and thus affords a very valuable opportunity for studies of the pathogenesis of auto-immune thyroiditis, which may well be applicable to the human disease.

2.2.2.3 Attempts to Produce Experimental Models for Graves' Disease

Experimental Graves' disease has not yet been produced. Attempts have been made to immunize animals with thyroid antigens, so as to produce thyroid-stimulating immunoglobulin, but the demonstration of this immunoglobulin has not been convincing, and the animals have not been hyperthyroid (McKenzie 1968). Recently, Ong et al. (1976) have been able to raise an antibody in rabbits against bovine thyroid cell membrane preparations which exhibited thyroid-stimulating properties in vitro. It is thus possible that in the previous studies, concomitant thyroiditis in the immunized animals prevented the functional expression of hyperthyroidism. The "nude" (athymic) mouse has also been used in an attempt to develop an experimental model for Graves' Disease (Kidd et al. 1978). Because this furless animal is athymic and lacks normal T cell function, it may tolerate tissue grafts, even when those are xenogeneic. When Graves' lymphycytes were injected into cyclophosphamide-treated "nude" mice, the blood thyroxine levels, as measured by a filter paper spot test, were higher over the following 3 weeks than those determined in a control group of mice who received lymphocytes from normal persons (see Fig. 2.2). This transient rise in blood thyroxine levels, however, barely reached a point of statistical significance, and needs further confirmation. It is therefore evident that no acceptable animal model for Graves' disease has yet been devised or discovered.

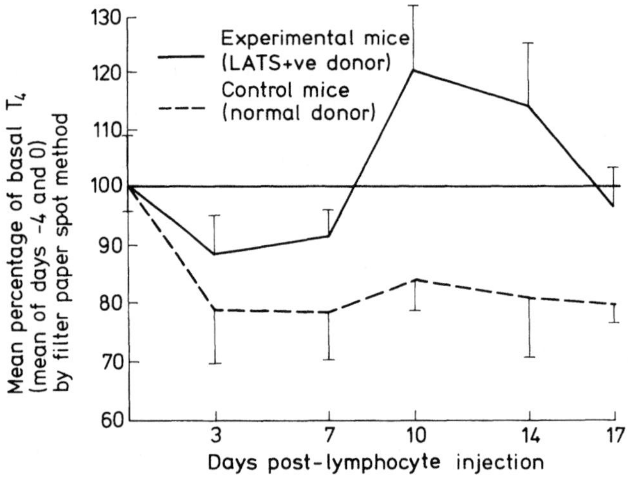

Fig. 2.2. Results of infusion of human lymphocytes from patients with Graves' disease or from normal controls into "nude" (athymic) mice. Results show the blood thyroxine values (from filter paper spot thyroxines) expressed as a percentage of the original baseline values. Each "nude" mouse received approximately twenty million human lymphocytes from either a patient with LATS-positive Graves' disease or from a normal control. Each animal was given cyclophosphamide (300 mg/kg) 4 days prior to the injection of the lymphocytes. After a drop in blood thyroxine values in both groups (possibly due to the cyclophosphamide), the animals receiving Graves' lymphocytes (experimental group) showed a rise in blood thyroxine levels reaching a peak at 10 days, falling to normal at 21 days. There were no significant changes in the blood thyroxine values in the animals receiving normal lymphocytes (control group). This suggests that the Graves' lymphocytes might have been capable of interacting with the normal thyroid of the mouse, and consequently producing thyroid-stimulating immunoglobulin in the "nude" mouse for at least several days. (Kidd et al. 1980)

2.2.3 Humoral Immunity in Human Thyroid Disease

As mentioned above, Roitt et al. first detected antibodies to thyroid antigens in the serum of some patients with Hashimoto's thyroiditis in 1956. They initially used the agar precipitin test which proved to be an excellent index of the chronic fibrous variant of Hashimoto's thyroiditis, where 96% of cases had positive precipitins, as opposed to 4% in the euthyroid lymphocytic variant (Doniach et al. 1979). The antigen then employed was thyroglobulin; however, five main antigen-antibody systems have now been identified, involving different constituents of the thyroid gland. These not only include thyroglobulin, but also include the "microsomal" antigen, the second antigen of the colloid, a cell surface antigen, the antigen related to the thyrotrophin (TSH) receptor, as well as antibodies reacting with thyroxine and triiodothyronine (Pinchera et al. 1979). The antigens involved, as well as the means of detection of the antibodies to these various antigens, are noted in Table 2.3.

To the various apparently normal constituents of the thyroid gland noted in Table 2.3, a variety of different antibodies may be produced by individual patients with auto-immune thyroid disease. The number of epitopes on autologous molecules is far smaller than for foreign antigens, but it nevertheless seems that antibodies with different properties may all play a part in determining the pathogenic mechanisms involved in the clinical variants of auto-immune thyroiditis and Graves' disease (Doniach 1975). Thyroid auto-antibodies have been found in all classes and subclasses of immunoglobulins (Hay and Torrigiani 1973). The complement-fixing "antimicrosomal" antibody has been shown to be cytotoxic (Pulvertaft et al. 1959), while there is no evidence that any other of the thyroid auto-antibodies has any deleterious effect on thyroid cells, at least acting alone. Thyroid auto-antibodies may also be non-complement fixing or may be precipitating antibodies, and IgE (reaginic) thyroid auto-antibodies are also detectable. Some antibodies may also be involved in the disposal of degraded antigens from normal turnover of thyroid cells (Grabar 1974). Others may be involved in immune complexes and may produce tissue damage in this manner (Kalderon and Bogaars 1977), or antibodies may co-operate with lymphocytes in producing an injury to thyroid tissue (lymphocyte-dependent cell-mediated cytotoxicity (Calder et al. 1974 b). "Killer" (K) cells may also have an adjunctive role in producing cell damage (Calder et al. 1976).

Each of the thyroid auto-antibodies has been shown to be polyclonal (Kriss 1968; Fahey and Goodman 1964; Adlkofer et al. 1973); while this was considered true for thyroid-stimulating antibody (TSAb, TSI) as well, more recent evidence adduced by Zakarija and McKenzie (1980) and Zakarija (1980) suggests that TSAb is oligoclonal at best, and may even be monoclonal.

2.2.3.1 Thyroglobulin Antibodies

It was once believed that thyroglobulin represented a "sequestered" antigen within the thyroid follicles, which was not recognizable to the organism as "self", and that destruction of the follicles with escape of the thyroglobulin might lead to auto-immune thyroiditis (Owen 1958). However, it is now known that thyroglobulin begins to leak into the circulation in utero in all persons, and in fact is a normal circulating constituent even before birth (Roitt and Torrigiani 1967). Thus, the

Table 2.3. Antigen-antibody systems involved in humoral responses of thyroid auto-immune disease. (Kidd et al. 1980)

Antigens	Antibody detection
Thyroglobulin	Precipitin technique Tanned red cell haemagglutination Immunofluorescence on fixed thyroid sections Competitive binding radioassay Coprecipitation with radio-iodinated thyroglobulin
Microsomal antigen	Complement fixation Immunofluorescence on unfixed thyroid sections Cytotoxicity test on culture thyroid cells Competitive binding radioassay Tanned red cell haemagglutination
Second colloid component	Immunofluorescence on fixed thyroid sections
Cell surface antigen(s)	Immunofluorescence on viable thyroid cells Mixed haemadsorption
Thyroxine and tri-iodothyronine	Antigen-binding capacity
Growth-stimulating and inhibiting antibodies	Effects on DNA content per thyroid cell nucleus, or G6PD activity per cell
TSH receptor-related antigen	a) Stimulatory assays: LATS bio-assay Colloid droplet formation in human thyroid slices Stimulation of human thyroid adenylate cyclase in vitro [Current terms employed for stimulatory assays include: human thyroid stimulator, human thyroid-stimulating immunoglobulin (TSI), thyroid-stimulating antibody (TSAb)] b) Binding assays: LATS protector assay Inhibition of 125I-thyrotrophin binding to human thyroid membranes (Thyrotrophin displacement activity (TDA), TSH-binding inhibitor immunoglobulin (TBII))

"secluded antigen" theory can be dismissed (Volpé et al. 1974). Moreover, thyroglobulin-binding B-lymphocytes can be shown to be present prior to birth (Roberts et al. 1973).

The concentration of thyroglobulin found normally in the plasma varies between 0 and 50 ng/ml; some normal persons have undetectable levels (Van Herle et al. 1973; Van Herle et al. 1979). Thyroglobulin is stored in the follicular colloid and physiologically re-enters the cell under the influence of thyroid-stimulating hormone, by a process of endocytosis. The colloid droplets merge with lysosomal droplets, and the thyroid hormones are split off by a protease, subsequently reaching the base of the thyroid cell and from there entering the capillaries. However, while proteolysis accounts for the metabolism of much of the thyroglobulin during its passage through the thyroid cells, some undegraded molecules frequently escape into the lymphatics (Van Herle et al. 1979).

Plasma thyroglobulin is increased in patients with a wide variety of thyroid disorders. These generally are those which are associated with increased thyroid cell activity (e.g. hyperthyroidism), thyroid cell damage (subacute thyroiditis or radioactive iodine) and thyroid tumours (adenomas and thyroid malignancy). Non-toxic nodular goitres are frequently associated with elevated levels as well (Van Herle et al. 1973; Van Herle et al. 1979). However increased concentrations of plasma thyroglobulin are not necessarily associated with the development of antibodies to thyroglobulin; these however are classically found in high titres in Hashimoto's and Graves' diseases, and occasionally in lower titres in other thyroid disorders (subacute thyroiditis, non-toxic goitre, thyroid malignancy), in asymptomatic relatives of patients with Graves' or Hashimoto's disease, in some non-thyroidal auto-immune conditions and in some otherwise apparently normal persons (Mori and Kriss 1971; Doniach 1975). These antibodies may be of any class, although precipitins belong mostly to class IgG. Thyroglobulin antibodies are non-complement fixing and for the most part are species specific but do show some cross-reactivity with monkey thyroglobulin (Doniach 1975). The tanned red cell agglutination test is the usual method for detecting these antibodies (Doniach 1975). Radioassay techniques (Mori and Kriss 1971; Peake et al. 1974; Salabé et al. 1974) will be discussed below.

Pinchera at al. (1979) have shown that on the basis of precipitin curves, thyroglobulin contains two pairs of antigenic sites, compared to the over 40 antigenic sites found in heterologous systems. Native thyroglobulin consists of a 19S protein, but thyroid extracts commonly contain variable amounts of a 12S dissociation product and 27S polymer. Pinchera at al. (1979) have shown that the antigenic determinants of thyroglobulin which will react with a potent antibody to thyroglobulin appearing in the serum of patients with Hashimoto's thyroiditis appear to be equally represented in these different molecular species.

By the common technique of tanned red cell haemagglutination significant titres of antithyroglobulin are found in about 70% of patients with Hashimoto's thyroiditis or newly diagnosed idiopathic myxoedema, about one-third of those with Graves' disease and in a smaller percentage of those with thyroid carcinoma and other thyroid disorders (Pinchera et al. 1979). However, by radioassay a large number of sera giving negative results by the haemagglutination technique was found to be positive by this same group. These workers could not explain this discrepancy by virtue of a greater sensitivity of the latter method. Discrepancies between the two methods were mostly found in sera from patients with metastatic thyroid carcinoma, Graves' disease or toxic adenoma. They suggested that these conditions may be associated with the presence in the serum of a substance which causes a positive radioassay response without producing haemagglutination. They further demonstrated that this substance could not be removed by immunoadsorption with thyroglobulin coupled to cepharose. They proposed that the interfering substance could be thyroglobulin itself, and indeed produced further data to indicate that increased serum thyroglobulin levels may produce false positive results in the measurement of antithyroglobulin antibodies by radioassays. This problem has also been encountered by Bayer and Kriss (1979 a, b), who have been able to identify falsely positive antithyroglobulin values by measuring the formation of thyroglobulin-antithyroglobulin complexes in the supernatant of the antithyroglobulin assay. Recently, a double antibody radio-immuno-assay technique has been developed for determination of these antibodies (Peake et al. 1974).

2.2.3.2 Antimicrosomal Antibodies

The thyroid microsomal antigen has been localized by immunofluorescence in the apical cytoplasm of follicular cells (Pinchera et al. 1979). Roitt et al. (1964) have provided evidence that this antigen is an inherent part of the smooth endoplasmic reticulum and is apparently composed of a lipoprotein of the membrane of exocytotic vesicles supporting newly synthesized thyroglobulin from the Golgi apparatus to the colloid.

The precise antigen or antigens have been a matter of considerable investigation. Roitt and his colleagues (1964) were unable to detect active antigen in solubilized preparations from human thyroid microsomes. However, Pinchera at al. (1979) have recently succeeded in solubilizing the appropriate antigen, using various detergents, high ionic strength solution and proteolytic enzymes as solubilizing agents. Despite continuing attempts to purify the solubilized microsomal antigen, the precise antigen has yet to be totally characterized. However, it is evident that an important component is cell membrane antigen(s) (Pinchera et al. 1979, 1980; Noguchi 1978).

In any event, antibodies to the microsomal antigen have been shown to be complement fixing (Doniach 1975) and have the ability to induce cytotoxic changes in monolayers of cultured thyroid cells (Pulvertaft et al. 1959). Correlation exists between the titres of this antibody and the histological lesions of Hashimoto's thyroiditis. The titres of thyroglobulin antibodies do not correlate as well. Antimicrosomal antibodies may be detected by immunofluorescence, complement fixation, haemagglutination (Fujita et al. 1970), or radioassay (Mori and Kriss 1971). Haemagglutination is rapidly becoming the favourite procedure. By these procedures antimicrosomal antibodies are detected in almost all patients with Hashimoto's thyroiditis, most of those with idiopathic myxoedema or Graves' disease, and much less frequently in other thyroid disorders. There are marked discrepancies between antimicrosomal and antithyroglobulin antibodies. Moreover, high levels of antithyroglobulin antibody may produce false positive results in measurements of antimicrosomal antibodies by haemagglutination (Pinchera et al. 1979), but these authors have shown that this interference may be easily overcome by adding an excess of thyroglobulin to the system. However, this problem is of minimal importance, since antimicrosomal antibodies are present much more commonly than antithyroglobulin antibodies, whereas antithyroglobulin antibodies are rarely present in the absence of antimicrosomal antibodies. A preponderance of antimicrosomal antibodies was found by Pinchera et al. (1979) to be even more pronounced in patients with Graves' disease.

These antibodies have a close relationship to the antibodies to cell surface antigens, which have been found in a large proportion of patients with Hashimoto's thyroiditis, idiopathic myxoedema or Graves' disease either using immunofluorescence (Fagraeus and Jonson 1970) or by a mixed haemadsorption technique using monolayer cultures (Jonsson and Fagraeus 1969). Jonsson and Fagraeus (1969) have demonstrated a close relationship between the presence of elevated antimicrosomal antibody titres and elevated antibodies to the cell surface antigens. Nevertheless, this relationship is not absolute, and several discrepancies were observed. Similar results have been found by Pinchera et al. (1979) and by Noguchi (1978). It would thus appear that while there may be common antigens involved in both systems, there are also some different antigens involved in these reactions. In any event, the cell surface antigen demonstrable in this manner is separate and distinct from the antigen to which the thyroid-stimulating immunoglobulin is the antibody, which may also involve the TSH receptor on the thyroid cell membrane.

The response of these antibodies to various therapeutic modalities will be dealt with below (see Sect. 2.2.10). At this juncture, however, it may be pointed out that these antibodies do tend to fall in many, but not all, patients following antithyroid drug therapy for Graves' disease, or after severe myxoedema has occurred spontaneously in patients with Hashimoto's thyroiditis.

2.2.3.3 Antibody to a Colloid Component Other than Thyroglobulin

Sera from some patients with either Graves' or Hashimoto's disease will show a uniform immunofluorescence in the colloid or fixed sections of thyroid tissue, even after absorption with thyroglobulin (Doniach 1975). The antigen to which these antibodies are directed appears to be a non-iodide containing protein. This antibody is also found in some cases of thyroid malignancy and in subacute thyroiditis. Its significance is undetermined.

2.2.3.4 Antibodies to the Thyroid Hormones

Antibodies are occasionally directed towards the thyroid hormones thyroxine (T4) and tri-idiothyronine (T3). These are generally found in patients with Hashimoto's disease, but also in Graves' disease, and are only found when there is also a very high titre of antithyroglobulin. The titres of antibodies to T4 and T3 become important when measuring circulating levels ot these thyroid hormones (Staeheli et al. 1975; Ginsberg et al. 1978; Inada et al. 1980 a). Depending upon the extraction and separation procedures, spuriously high or low T4 or T3 concentrations may result, if these antibodies are present in sufficiently high titres.. With polyethylene glycol radio-immunoassays, the values will be spuriously low, whereas when the hormones are extracted from serum with a Sephadex G-25 column, the values are increased to their true high values (Inada et al. 1980 a). This may be particularly confusing when hypothyroid patients are treated with thyroid hormones resulting in less than expected improvement, extremely high values of serum thyroxine, but also continuing high levels of TSH (Ginsberg et al. 1978). These antibodies will not affect thyroid function if the thyroid is capable of responding to TSH normally.

2.2.3.5 Thyrotrophin (TSH) Receptor-Related Antigen and Cell Surface Antigens and Their Relationship to Thyroid-Stimulating Immunoglobulin

As mentioned above, antibodies to cell surface antigens have been identified by immunofluorescence on viable suspensions of human thyroid cells and by a mixed haemadsorption technique using monolayer cultures (Fagraeus and Jonsson 1970; Jonsson and Fagraeus 1969). However, this cell surface antigen or antigens appears to be unrelated to the antigen for thyroid-stimulating immunoglobulin (Fagraeus et al. 1970).

An antigen closely related to the thyrotrophin (TSH) receptor in the plasma membrane of follicular cells appears to be responsible for the production of thyroid-stimulating antibodies (TSI, TSAb), which are present in the sera of patients with Graves' disease (McKenzie and Zakarija 1977; McKenzie et al. 1978). These antibodies are detectable by two somewhat different principles. Firstly, the antibodies may be detected by methods based on their ability to stimulate thyroid function; this may be carried out by counting of thyroid intracellular colloid droplets (Onaya et al. 1973) or by measurement of adenylate cyclase activity (Orgiazzi et al. 1976; McKenzie et al. 1978). This stimulating activity has been given several terms, including "human thyroid stimulator" (Onaya et al. 1973), "human thyroid adenyl cyclase stimulator (HTACS)" (Orgiazzi et al. 1976), "thyroid-stimulating antibody (TSAb)", and thyroid-stimulating immunoglobulin (TSI)" (McKenzie et al. 1978). The older term, "long acting thyroid stimulator (LATS)", now refers to a particular bio-assay in the mouse (McKenzie 1968).

These antibodies may also be detected by their ability to bind to thyroid cell membranes. This may be via the LATS-protector (LATS-P) assay, or by the prevention of binding of TSH to the receptor site on the thyroid cell membrane. The LATS-P assay is positive when binding to the human thyroid prevents (protects) subsequent binding of LATS (Adams and Kennedy 1971). While the radioligand assay technique (measuring the inhibition of binding of labelled TSH to its thyroid cell membrane binding site) was first termed thyroid-stimulating immunoglobulin by Mukhtar et al. (1975), some antibodies which bind to the thyroid cell membrane and prevent TSH binding thereto do *not* stimulate, and some may even inhibit the action of TSH (see below). Thus this term cannot be considered appropriate and has given way to other more descriptive terms. Likewise, the term "thyrotropin-displacement activity assay (TDA)" (O'Donnell et al. 1978) is not quite accurate, since in fact the assay measures the *prevention of* TSH binding by the receptor site, rather than its displacement. Hence the term which will be increasingly accepted in all probability for this assay system is "thyrotrophin-binding inhibitor immunoglobulin (TBII)". In the remainder of this discussion, the term "TBII" will be applied to this assay, no matter what term was employed by the particular authors. For the assays which actually measure cell stimulation, the term "TSAb" will be utilized throughout the remainder of this discussion, again without relation to the term applied by the particular authors being cited. It is hoped that this manoeuvre will reduce some of the terminological confusion which has surrounded this field.

The precise site of binding of this antibody has not been settled. Certainly it is clear that the antibody produces its stimulation by interacting in some manner with the TSH receptor, stimulating adenyl cyclase and thus increasing cyclic AMP within the thyroid cell (Kendall-Taylor 1975). Thus participation of the TSH receptor is beyond doubt. However, these observations and the clear demonstration of the inhibition of binding of TSH by the antibody do not settle the issue as to the actual site of binding of the immunoglobulin. Smith (1980) has demonstrated that Graves' immunoglobulins appear to interact with the TSH receptors in thyroid membranes in a manner similar to TSH receptors dispersed in detergent micelles. Moreover, he found that the binding of TSH and the immunoglobulins to the detergent-dispersed receptors appears to be mutually exclusive. Consequently, he concluded that the inhibition of TSH binding to thyroid membranes by Graves' immunoglobulins appears to be due to direct binding of the immunoglobulins to the TSH receptor. He conceded, however, that the immunoglobulins and TSH may interact with different sites on the same receptor molecule.

Smith et al. (1977) have also demonstrated that TBII inhibits the binding of labelled TSH to thyroid membranes in a dose-dependent manner and that this effect is localized in the Fab part of the TBII molecule. Analysis of the binding data suggested that TBII and TSH bound to the same receptor site. These authors were able to show that the effects of TBII and unlabelled TSH on the labelled hormone-membrane interaction were only additive, and that no modification of the TSH-binding process was induced by TBII. Moreover, kinetic studies indicated that the binding of TBII to the thyroid membrane was not rate limiting in the process of stimulating cyclic AMP production.

However, Madsen and Bech (1979) studied adenyl cyclase activity in human thyroid homogenates after stimulation with TSH or thyroid-stimulating antibodies. They found that TSAb prepared from different patients with Graves' disease showed different adenylate cyclase activation patterns, and a lag phase was frequently observed. Thyroid-stimulating hormone and TSAb appeared to cause mutally inhibitory activation of thyroid adenylate cyclase. The maximum adenylate cyclase activity was higher with TSH than with TSAb, although the authors felt that this might be due to contamination of TSAb preparations with an adenylate cyclase inhibitor. They also incubated thyroid homogenates with cortisol, which then produced a dose-dependent decrease in the adenylate cyclase response to TSAb, whereas the response to TSH was either increased or unchanged. These authors felt, therefore, that TSH and TSAb might activate thyroid adenylate cyclase through different pathways in the plasma membrane.

Fenzi et al. (1980), however, have attempted to characterize the different thyroid plasma membrane antigens and to study their interactions with thyroid auto-antibodies and their relationship to the TSH receptor. They found that these membrane antigens could be freed of the TSH receptor by pre-absorption with TSH-containing polymer. The pre-absorbed thyroid plasma membrane material, however, still retained its binding to Graves' IgG, as well as to Hashimoto's IgG, indicating that antigens different from the TSH receptor and present in thyroid plasma membrane interact with Graves' IgG. These membrane antigens incidentally included thyroglobulin and other lower molecular weight components. The important point from this study is that the Graves' IgG samples did bind to the thyroid plasma membrane even when it was devoid of the TSH receptor.

However, it may be remembered that Mori and Kriss (1971) were unable to separate "antimicrosomal" antibody from LATS. One interpretation thus might be that while anti-cell membrane antibodies may occur *without* thyroid-stimulating immunoglobulin, the reverse may not be true, i.e. thyroid-stimulating immunoglobulin may always coexist with antibodies to the thyroid cell-membrane. Whether such antibodies represent two antibodies which cannot currently be separated or represent a single type of molecule acting on more than one antigenic site, remains to be clarified. However, since non-stimulating anti-cell membrane antibody may occur alone, it is the author's speculation that two currently inseparable antibodies are involved when TSAb is present.

If, indeed, the antibody does not interact directly with the TSH receptor, it is nevertheless capable of influencing the TSH receptor and activating it in a manner not yet evident. However, if there are different molecules of TSI in different patients with Graves' disease, some of which bind on one site and some on another, than this may explain some of the discrepancies which have been reported between different assay systems.

The controversy regarding the actual site of binding of thyroid-stimulating immunoglobulin may be reflected in the results of the various assays. Long-acting thyroid stimulator (as measured by the mouse bio-assay) was only detectable in about 50 % of sera from patients with active untreated Graves' disease (Major and Munro 1962) and titres of LATS bore no relationship to the degree of thyrotoxicosis (Kendall-Taylor 1975). It was for this reason that the role of LATS in the pathogenesis of Graves' disease was in doubt for some years (Volpé et al. 1972). Indeed, following the advent of human thyroid preparations in the various assay systems, there was a suggestion that LATS was only a mouse thyroid stimulator and that other, separate, Graves' immunoglobulins stimulated the human thyroid alone (Adams et al. 1975). However, it soon became clear that the same molecule was indeed a stimulator of the human thyroid gland and that the variation in response of the mouse thyroid to Graves' IgG was either a problem of variable mammalian cross-reactivity (Zakarija and McKenzie 1978 a) or sensitivity (Zakarija and McKenzie 1978 b; McKenzie and Zakarija 1979).

There is also a variation from laboratory to laboratory in the results obtained for the detection of the antibody. Even when the same techniques are employed, or modifications of the same procedure, widely differing results are obtained. For example, Mukhtar et al. (1975) have found that with the radioligand assay for TBII, virtually 100 % of the patients with active untreated Graves' disease were positive. However, O'Donnell et al. (1978) were only able to find 76% of patients positive in this assay, and Schleusener et al. (1976) found such antibodies in only 54 % of such patients with active untreated Graves' disease. Kuzuya et al. (1979) found this antibody present in 63 % of a similar group of patients in Japan. On the other hand, the use of stimulatory assays for TSAb, such as the generation of cyclic AMP, has brough a higher yield of positive results in active untreated Graves' disease. These have varied from 81 % (Sugenoya et al. 1979 b), 82 % in the study of Bech and Madsen (1979) to 95 % in the reports by McKenzie and Zakarija (1976 a, b) (see Figs. 2.3, 2.4).

Moreover, when radioligand (TBII) and stimulating (TSAb) assays are carried out in the same specimes in the same laboratories, widely divergent results between the two assay systems are still observed. In the study of Sugenoya et al. (1979 b), even in active untreated Graves' disease there was no correlation between the results of the radioligand assay (TBII) and a stimulatory assay, measuring the generation of cyclic AMP in thyroid slices (TSAb). As in the study of Smith and Hall (1974), correlation was obtained only in that subset of patients who were positive in both assay systems. Similar discrepancies were noted by Kuzuya et al. (1979) and by Pinchera et al. (1980).

The reasons for these discrepancies are not entirely clear. It is of course possible that technical problems in both assay systems may be one factor in bringing about discrepancies. This is particularly of importance when it is recollected that normal IgG will variably bind to the thyroid cell membrane and prevent TSH binding, and this occasionally can be marked (McKenzie and Zakarija 1979; McKenzie et al. 1978). However it is also possible that there may be some TSAb molecules which

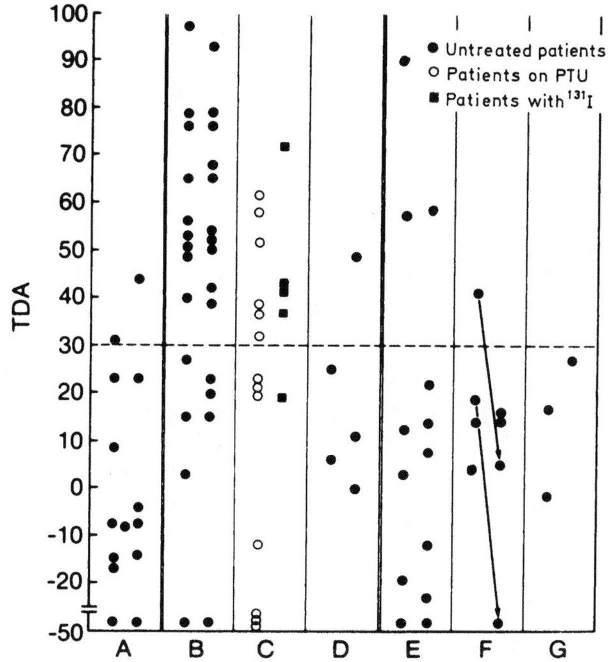

Fig. 2.3. Results of the radioligand assay for the antibody which binds to the thyroid cell membrane, thus inhibiting TSH binding (TDA, TBII). The same IgG samples were used in this figure as compared with Fig. 2.4. The TDA is expressed in TDA units, and 30 represents the 95% confidence limit for normal IgG values. *Column A*, IgG sample from blood bank (normal) contributors; *Column B*, active untreated Graves' disease; *Column C*, patients with Graves' disease treated with antithyroid drugs or radioactive iodine; *Column D*, patients in remission 1 year after the cessation of antithyroid drugs; *Column E*, Hashimoto's thyroiditis; *Column F*, subacute thyroiditis; *Column G*, non-toxic nodular goitre. It may be seen that while about 70% of patients with active untreated Graves' disease were positive in this assay, there was almost a 30% false negative result obtained in these patients. Conversely, some patients with Hashimoto's thyroiditis and subacute thyroiditis were also positive in this assay. (Sugenoya et al. 1979 b)

bind to the thyroid cell membrane, interact with the TSH receptor and thus stimulate the thyroid cells, without at the same time inhibiting the binding of TSH any more than do normal IgG samples. This suggestion might give credence to the notion that the binding of TSAb is not necessarily directly to the TSH receptor itself. However, until all technical problems are solved, and until more evidence accrues in relation to the precise site of binding of TSAb, the nature of these discrepancies will not be revealed.

In studying the radioligand and stimulating assays in thyroid disorders other than Graves' disease itself, interesting results have been obtained. Positive results in the radioligand assay have been obtained in a small proportion of patients with Hashimoto's thyroiditis, in significant numbers of patients with subacute thyroiditis and in a small proportion of patients with thyroid carcinoma (Mukhtar et al. 1975; Sugenoya et al. 1978; Smith 1976). In addition, Brown et al. (1978) found this assay to be positive in non-toxic goitres and toxic multinodular goitres, but others have not found positive results in those particular categories (O'Donnell et al. 1978; Bolk et al. 1979). There is on the other hand, general agreement about the finding of

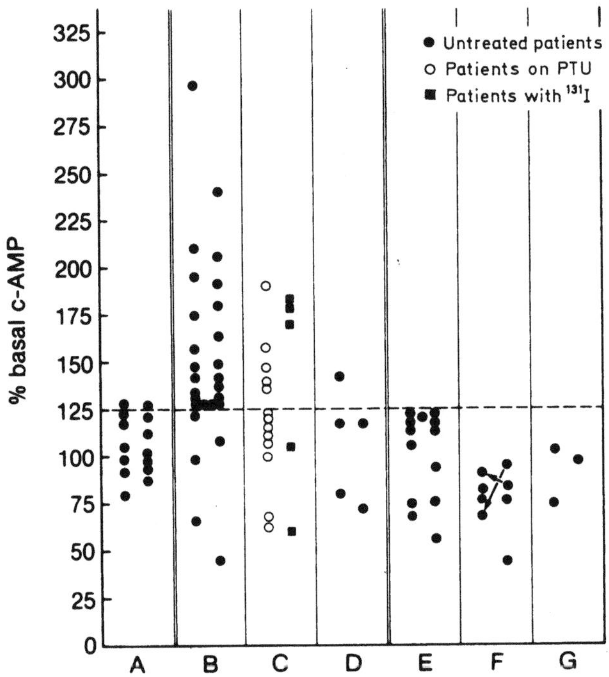

Fig. 2.4. Results using the same IgG samples as were depicted in Fig. 2.3, but with an assay measuring cyclic AMP in thyroid slices as the end point. Thus this is a stimulatory assay, rather than a binding assay. Note that the yield of positive values was greater in active, untreated Graves' disease than with the radioligand assay (about 84%). Note also that those samples from patients with Hashimoto's thyroiditis or subacute thyroiditis that were positive in the radioligand assay were now negative in the TSAb assay. (Sugenoya et al. 1979 b)

positive radioligand assays in some patients with Hashimoto's thyroiditis and subacute thyroiditis; however, when stimulatory assays are then employed, the results have been almost invariably negative (Sugenoya et al. 1979 b) (see Figs. 2.3 and 2.4). Thus it is clear that there are antibodies which are positive in the TBII assay, but which yet have no stimulatory activity. Moreover, Endo et al. (1978) and Konishi et al. (1980) have described antibodies positive in the TBII assay which block TSH activity, leading to atrophy of the thyroid gland and actual hypothyroidism. Clearly for these reasons, the radioligand assay cannot necessarily be equated with the term "thyroid-stimulating immunoglobulin or antibody".

The organ-specificity of TSAb for the thyroid cell membrane has been a subject of some study. It is known, that TSH binds to, and has effects on, other organs, such as fat cells, monocytes, testis and adrenal (Trokoudes et al. 1979). It has been shown that there is also an effect of TSAb on testis (Trokoudes et al. 1979) and fat cells (Hart and McKenzie 1971; Kishihara et al. 1979). These latter studies would lend support to those who argue that TSAb is an antibody to the TSH receptor, and thus wherever TSH receptors are found one might expect a TSAb-TSH receptor interaction.

While, therefore, it remains to be ascertained where the precise binding of TSAb on the thyroid cell membrane takes place, the author is prejudiced to the view that there is probably a direct TSAb-TSH receptor interaction, and that the antibody is directed to some part of the TSH receptor itself as well as to contiguous parts of the cell membrane.

In any event, a central role for this antibody in causing the stimulation of the thyroid cells (and thus the hyperthyroidism) of Graves' disease seems inescapable. Firstly as McKenzie and Zakarija (1976 a, b) have been able to show, TSAb can be demonstrated in 95 % of patients with active untreated Graves' disease. Moreover, the effects on the thyroid which are shared by TSAb and TSH include the uptake, discharge and release of radioactive iodine in vivo and in vitro, colloid droplet formation in follicular cells, glucose oxidation and incorporation of ^{32}P into phospholipids, adenyl cyclase activity and cyclic AMP accumulation (Kendall-Taylor 1975) (see Table 2.4). While there has not been unanimity with respect to a good correlation between the various assay systems and the severity of the hyperthyroidism, some groups have shown a fair correlation with respect to early thyroidal uptakes of ^{131}I or ^{99m}Tc (Mukhtar et al. 1975; Endo et al. 1978). More importantly, if the assay for thyroid-stimulating antibody remains positive after patients have been controlled with propylthiouracil for long intervals, then cessation of the therapy will almost bring about a recurrence (O'Donnell et al. 1978; McKenzie et al. 1978; Teng and Yeung 1980; McGregor et al. 1980 b). Moreover, neonatal Graves' disease, which is almost always a transient disorder lasting less than 3 months, has been shown to have a very good correlation with the presence of high titres of thyroid-stimulating immunoglobulin (or LATS protector) in the mothers and (by passive transfer) in the newborns (McKenzie and Zakarija 1978; Kendall-Taylor 1975; Dirmikis and Munro 1975; Dirminkis et al. 1976). It thus is contended that TSAb reflects the immune disorder which is the basis of Graves' disease and is *the cause* of the hyperthyroidism of this disorder.

The uniqueness of TSAb, an antibody which interacts with a receptor and stimulates it (i. e. acting as an agonist) has been a matter of concern among sceptics. Other antireceptor antibodies, e. g. the antibody against the acetylcholine receptor in myaesthenia gravis (Drachmann 1978), or against the insulin receptor in certain forms of diabetes mellitus (Flier et al. 1978, 1979), are generally blocking (antagonistic) antibodies. However, occasionally the anti-insulin receptor antibody can act as an agonist (resulting in hypoglycaemia), thus diminishing the uniqueness of TSAb (Flier et al. 1979).

The thyroid-stimulating antibodies have generally not been found in relatives of patients with Graves' disease who are asymptomatic (McKenzie et al. 1978). The presence of thyroid antibodies of all kinds in relation to exophthalmos, in relatives

Table 2.4. Biological effects on thyroid shared by LATS (and TSI) and TSH (Kendall-Taylor 1975)

Stimulation of:
Uptake and discharge of ^{131}in vivo
Release of ^{131}I in vitro
Colloid droplet formation in follicular cells
Glucose oxidation
Incorporation of ^{32}P into phospholipids
Adenylcyclase activity
cAMP accumulation

of patients with Graves' or Hashimoto's disease, during pregnancy, or following treatment of these disorders, will be discussed separately below.

2.2.3.6 Immune Complexes, Rheumatoid Factors and Other Antibodies

Circulating immune complexes have been detected in the sera from patients with Hashimoto's thyroiditis and Graves' disease (Calder et al. 1974a; Cano et al. 1976; Mariotti et al. 1979). (Immune complexes within the thyroid gland itself and their possible cytolytic effect have already been discussed above (Kalderon and Bogaars 1977).) Mariotti et al. (1979) have shown data suggesting that both thyroglobulin-antithyroglobulin complexes, as well as complexes unrelated to thyroglobulin, are present in sera of patients with thyroid auto-immune disorders and thyroid carcinoma. Using the Raji cell method, Mariotti et al. (1979) were able to show that immune complexes unrelated to thyroglobulin were frequently present. Since thyroglobulin immune complexes should not fix complement, this may explain why immune complex disease is not a characteristic of auto-immune thyroid disease. However, immune complex glomerulonephritis associated with auto-immune thyroid disease has been rarely reported (Jordan et al. 1981). Van der Heide et al. (1980) studied immune complexes in relation to thyroid-stimulating immunoglobulin in patients with Graves' disease before and after antithyroid drug therapy. They found that immune complexes were present in all untreated patients who had a normal or subnormal TSI index, while such complexes were absent in all patients with an abnormal TBII index. Thus there appeared to be an *inverse* correlation between TBII and immune complexes in Graves' disease. If the immune complexes included TBII (TSAb), and thus rendered it incapable of interacting with the TSH receptor, this conceivably could be an explanation for at least one type of remission. The results of antithyroid drug therapy on the immune complexes will be discussed below when the effects of therapy on the immune system are documented. Circulating immune complexes have also been studied in relation to exophthalmos (Takeda and Kriss 1977; Brohee et al. 1979; Hopf et al. 1978); while this will be discussed below, it may be appropriate to state now that no correlation exists between the presence and/or severity of exophthalmos and the presence of immune complexes.

Doniach et al. (1979) had postulated a thyroid trophic antibody (separate from TSI) which might account for the hypertrophy of the thyroid gland in goitrous Hashimoto's thyroiditis. More recently, the same group (Drexhage et al. 1980) have detected the presence of such an antibody in some patients with goitrous Hashimoto's thyroiditis. Moreover, they were able to demonstrate antibodies which *inhibited* the trophic effect of TSH in most cases of atrophic primary myxoedema. This antibody apparently did not prevent the binding of TSH to its receptor, but only its trophic effect. Thus, there appear to be antibodies in these disorders which cause atrophy or hypertrophy, and are distinct from previously demonstrated antibodies.

Antibodies to *Yersinia enterocolitica* have been found in increased frequency in Graves' disease (about 59%), compared with about 20% in control groups (Bech et al. 1977a). Indeed, Bech et al. (1977a, 1977b) also found a positive correlation between migration inhibition of thyroid and *Yersinia* antigens in the group of patients with Graves' disease, while no correlation could be demonstrated in the control population. Moreover, direct immunofluorescence techniques revealed a high frequency of thyroid cell membrane directed antibodies in sera with *Yersinia* agglutinating antibodies. This led Bech et al. (1977 b) to conclude that there was no actual *Yersinia* infection in patients with thyroid disease, but there was a cross-reaction between antigenic components of the thyroid and *Yersinia* (Bech et al. 1977a,b). Moreover, Shenkman and Bottone (1976) demonstrated that antibodies to *Yersinia* were found in populations of patients with Graves' disease in North America, despite the fact that *Yersinia* infections are much less common in North America than in Europe. This also seemed to favour the view that *Yersinia* was playing no role whatever in these patients, but that there was some crossreactivity between thyroid and *Yersinia* antigens. Thus, the detection of antibodies to *Yersinia* is almost certainly an artefact, and of no relevance to the pathogenesis of Graves' disease.

Antibodies to other organs are also found in some patients with Graves' and Hashimoto's diseases, i.e. auto-antibodies to gastric antigens, islet cell antigens, adrenal antigens and others (Irvine 1975). These will be discussed further below, under the heading "Association with other auto-immune diseases".

2.2.3.7 Production of Thyroid Antibodies and Thyroid-Stimulating Immunoglobulin In Vitro

When lymphocyte preparations from patients with Graves' disease are cultured with phytohaemagglutinin (PHA), the lymphocytes will release TSAb into the medium (McKenzie and Gordon 1965; Miyai et al. 1967; Knox et al. 1966 a; McLachlan et al. 1977). Since PHA stimulates only T-lymphocytes (Greaves et al. 1974), these studies imply that PHA stimulated thyroid-directed helper T-lymphocytes, which then interacted with thyroid-directed B-lymphocytes; the B-lymphocytes then responded by releasing thyroid-stimulating immunoglobulin into the culture medium. Lymphocytes from patients with non-immune thyroid disease, or healthy controls, generally do not produce thyroid-stimulating immunoglobulin under these circumstances (see Fig. 2.5).

In addition, Knox et al. (1976 b) have shown that lymphocytes from patients with Graves' disease stimulated by crude human normal thyroid antigen in vitro will also produce TSAb into the culture medium (see Fig. 2.6). Since the thyroid tissue employed as antigen in this study was normal, this does *not* then support the notion that thyroidal antigenic change is a prerequisite for the initiation of Graves' disease; however, this will be discussed further below.

More recently, McGregor et al. (1979 a) and McLachlan et al. (1977) have demonstrated that readily detectable amounts of thyroglobulin and microsomal antibodies could be synthesized by thyroid and peripheral blood lymphocytes from patients with Hashimoto's thyroiditis cultured for 2–3 weeks in Marbrook flasks. McGregor et al. (1979b) have also shown that if lymphocytes from patients with Hashimoto's thyroiditis were irradiated with 2000–3000 rads and then were cocultured in vitro with non-irradiated cells, strong stimulation of IgG and auto-antibody synthesis was observed. However, if the peripheral blood lymphocytes were irradiated all together before culture, this would result in a dose-dependent inhibition of IgG and thyroglobulin auto-antibody synthesis as well as cell viability. This would suggest that the suppressor T-lymphocytes were preferentially damaged by irradiation, allowing the helper T-lymphocytes to stimulate B-lymphocytes more vigorously. Moreover, this group has found that methimazole can suppress the thyroid auto-antibody production by lymphocytes in vitro, suggesting that

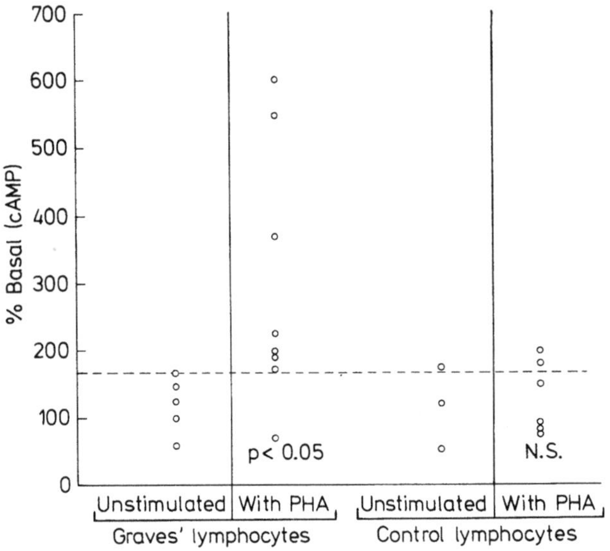

Fig. 2.5. Stimulation of lymphocytes by phytohaemagglutinin (PHA). When lymphocytes from patients with Graves' disease were cultured with phytohaemagglutinin for 6 days they released thyroid-stimulating immunoglobulin into the medium. This supernatant was tested by incubating with human thyroid slices, and the amount of thyroid-stimulating immunoglobulin was expressed as the percentage increase in cyclic AMP over baseline values. Normal lymphocytes did not produce TSI under the same culture conditions. Neither Graves' lymphocytes nor normal lymphocytes would produce TSI without PHA stimulation. (Knox et al. 1967 a)

immunosuppression is one possible mechanism of action of the antithyroid drug when it favourably influences the course of patients with Graves' disease (McGregor et al. 1979 c). Beall and Kruger (1979) and McLachlan et al. (1979, 1980) have also demonstrated antithyroglobulin production by peripheral blood leucocytes in vitro, stimulated by pokeweed mitogen and phytohaemagglutinin respectively. This, too, will be discussed in Sect. 2.2.4.5.

2.2.4 Cellular Aspects of Graves' and Hashimoto's Diseases

2.2.4.1 Thyroid Lymphocytes

Graves' disease and Hashimoto's thyroiditis have several cellular aspects in common. In both conditions the gland is infiltrated with lymphocytes, frequently organized as germinal centres (Bastenie and Ermans 1972), and the two conditions may coexist within the same thyroid gland (Fatourechi et al. 1971; Doniach 1975). As mentioned above, the clinical expression in the presence of TSAb (i.e. hyperthyroidism, euthyroidism, or hypothyroidism) will depend on the availability of thyroid follicular cells which can respond to TSAb. If there are simply too few cells to respond, the patient will, of course, be hypothyroid (Christy and Morse 1977). Totterman (1978) has recently reported the distribution of T-, B- and thyroglobulin binding lymphocytes infiltrating the thyroid gland of Graves' disease, Hashimoto's thyroiditis and DeQuervain's subacute thyroiditis. He has shown that in both Graves' and Hashimoto's diseases about 40% of the lymphocytes were T-lymphocytes, with an equal proportion of B-lymphocytes. (In DeQuervain's

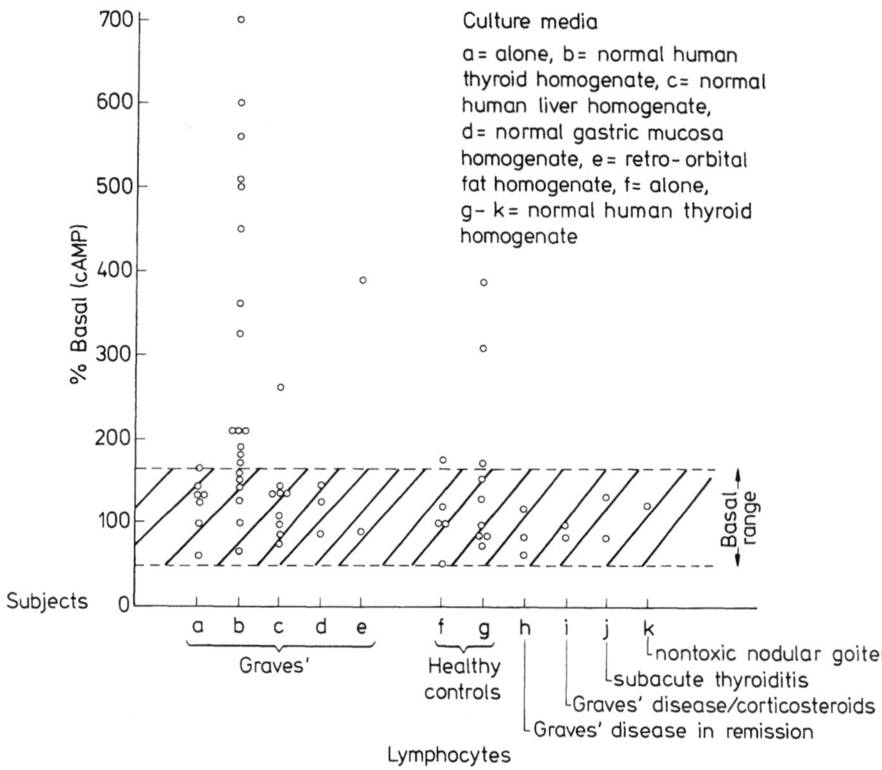

Fig. 2.6. Results of stimulating the lymphocytes with crude normal human thyroid antigen, when compared to other organ antigens. It may be seen that lymphocytes from patients with Graves' disease respond to thyroid antigenic stimulation by producing TSI into the medium. However, there was no significant TSI production by the same lymphocytes when cocultured with other organ antigens. Conversely, control lymphocytes (taken from normal persons) did not release TSI into the medium when stimulated by thyroid antigen (with two exceptions). These two exceptions were laboratory personnel who handle thyroid antigen continually, and possibly these persons may have sensitized themselves to this antigen. (Knox et al. 1976b)

thyroiditis, incidentally, the majority of thyroid infiltrating cells were T-lymphocytes, with only a few B-lymphocytes.) The frequency of thyroglobulin binding lymphocytes was also studied, and found to be high in the thyroid infiltrates of patients with both Graves' and Hashimoto's diseases. Subsequently, Totterman et al. (1979) have recently been able to shown that the infiltrating T-lymphocytes from patients with Graves' disease were sensitized against thyroid antigen (by means of a leucocyte migration inhibition test in cells obtained at fine needle aspiration biopsy). Surprisingly, they could not demonstrate that the infiltrating lymphocytes from Hashimoto's thyroiditis were positive in this test procedure, although they pointed out that this lack of reactivity could be caused by an excess of antigen.

Totterman et al. (1979) also argued that the considerably increased frequency of thyroglobulin-binding lymphocytes within the thyroid gland of both disorders argues against the possibility that the thyroid-infiltrating lymphocytes are merely "passive bystanders", secondarily trapped in the thyroid after some unknown traumatic mechanism. Moreover, the striking accumulation of thyroglobulin-binding B-lymphocytes, plus the finding of mature plasma cells in the gland of Hashimoto's patients, suggests an intrathyroidal synthesis of auto-antibodies.

Similar proportions of B-and T-lymphocytes in the thyroid gland of Graves' disease have been described by Skoldstam et al. (1978). Although the *proportion* of T-lymphocytes is not increased within the thyroid glands in these disorders, the absolute numbers are clearly vastly increased, particularly in Hashimoto's thyroiditis.

2.2.4.2 Peripheral Blood Lymphocytes

Totterman (1978) has additionally shown that patients with either Graves' or Hashimoto's disease also had about twice as many circulating thyroglobulin-binding cells as compared to healthy subjects, most of which were B-lymphocytes, althoug a few T cells binding thyroglobulin were also found in the blood and thyroid infiltrate of patients with these conditions. The finding of an increased number of thyroglobulin-binding peripheral blood lymphocytes in Hashimoto's patients was also confirmed by Richter et al. (1978), Ludwig et al. (1978) and Gordin et al. (1979). While there was a definite increase in thyroglobulin-binding lymphocytes in such patients, there was no correlation between these cells and the presence or titre of the various thyroid auto-antibodies, particularly auto-antibodies against thyroglobulin. Moreover, similar cells, although in small numbers, are found in normal healthy control persons. Similar observations to those in human auto-immune thyroid disease have been made in experimental OS chickens with auto-immune thyroiditis (Wick et al. 1974).

Several studies have been carried out attempting to determine the numbers, type and activity of peripheral blood lymphocytes circulating in patients with Graves' or Hashimoto's disease. Earlier suggestions that there might be an increased proportion of T-lymphocytes in these disorders have been ruled out (Volpé and Row 1975; Mulaisho et al 1975). In fact, recent evidence indicates that there is a slight reduction in the proportion of T-lymphocytes within the circulation of patients with Graves' disease (Wall et al. 1977; Grinblat et al. 1979). At least one study of the *number* of suppressor T-lymphocytes in Hashimoto's thyroiditis showed no alteration from normal (Canonica et al. 1981). The percent and absolute B-lymphocyte count are increased (Mori et al. 1980). It may be noted incidentally, that while there is a relative lymphocytosis in Graves' disease, the absolute lymphocyte counts may be within normal limits (Irvine et al. 1977 b), or moderately increased (Mori et al. 1980). Studies of the activity of peripheral blood lymphocytes in auto-immune thyroid disease have been carried out by various workers. Hsu et al. (1976) have shown that there are definite B-lymphocyte abnormalities associated with hyperthyroidism, manifested by the simultaneous presence of multiple IgG classes, including IgE on a single B-lymphocyte. Results of studies of incubation of the patients' plasma with lymphocytes from healthy individuals and studies of surface immunoglobulins by overnight culture of the patients' lymphocytes, with or without prior trypsinization, suggested that the surface immunoglobulin was generated endogenously by the cell on which it resided. Folb and Bank (1974, 1976) have shown that there is an increased proportion of "activated" lymphocytes in Graves' disease, demonstrated by an autographic labelling technique which facilitated the identification of those lymphocytes which were actively synthesizing nuclear deoxyribonucleic acid at the time of blood sampling. Whether these "activated" cells were T- and/or B-lymphocytes was not studied. However, Wall et al. (1977), studying peripheral blood T-lymphocytes specifically, actually found *low* to normal proportions of "activated" T-lymphocytes in Graves' disease.

The response of lymphocytes to thyroid antigen has also been a subject of great interest in these auto-immune disorders. Aoki and DeGroot (1979) have studied the blastogenic response of lymphocytes to human thyroglobulin in auto-immune thyroid disease and have reviewed past contradictory reports of the results of this procedure. These authors found that the optimal dose level for thyroglobulin for maximal blastogenesis in culture differs from patient to patient; consequently, they found it inappropriate to use a single dose level of thyroglobulin for evaluation of the blastogenic response in study groups. By using serial thyroglobulin dose levels of 0.5 through 30 µg/ml in cultures, it was found that the incidence of positive responders in Graves' disease was 69.2%, in Hashimoto's thyroiditis 71.4%, in metastatic thyroid carcinoma 59%, and in healthy controls 9.1%. All of the positive responders in the cancer group had elevated thyroglobulin levels, but no antithyroglobulin antibody in their sera.

Aside from blastogenic response of lymphocytes to thyroglobulin, other thyroid antigens have also been employed in similar procedures. Makinen et al. (1978) studied lymphocyte transformation resulting from the stimulation by thyroid cell membranes. They used the uptake of ^{125}I-labelled deoxyuridine within the cells as a reflection of lymphocyte stimulation. The stimulation index was calculated by dividing the mean counts per minute of the test cultures by those ot the control cultures. The mean lymphocyte stimulation index for ten healthy persons tested with thyroid membranes as the antigen was 1.02 ± 0.22. The stimulation was considered positive when the stimulation index was more than 1.50. When thyroid membranes were used as antigen, the mean stimulation index was 3.64 in the patients with Graves' disease, most of whom showed a positive response. However, preincubation of the thyroid membrane preparation with TSH blocked the ability of the preparation to stimulate the lymphocytes, and this was considered strong evidence consistent with the hypothesis that auto-immunization against the TSH receptor on the thyroid follicular cell membrane is the pathogenic mechanism of hyperthyroidism in Graves' disease. Indeed, work from our own laboratory (Knox et al. 1976b; Sugenoya et al. 1978) has shown that thyroid cell membrane preparations (from normal thyroid glands) can stimulate lymphocytes from patients with Graves' disease to produce thyroid-stimulating immunoglobulin. This also suggested that thyroid cell membrane antigen(s) might be the most appropriate antigen(s) in Graves' disease with which the lymphocytes in that condition interact.

Wenzel et al. (1978) and Schleusener et al. (1979) have studied the binding of peripheral blood lymphocytes from patients with Graves' disease to the solubilized TSH receptor, and were able to show that there were significantly higher numbers of antigen-binding lymphocytes in patients with Graves' disease when compared with normal volunteers. This binding could be inhibited by preincubation with unlabelled TSH, unlabelled receptor protein, or antiserum to IgG/IgM/IgA. However, it should be pointed out that lymphocytes which could bind TSH receptor were also present in very small numbers in the normal control population.

Indeed, Salabé et al. (1978) have also been able to show antigen binding lymphocytes against thyroglobulin and thyroidal microsomes in healthy subjects. However, these antigen-binding lymphocytes are primarily B-lymphocytes, so that the presence of a small number of such lymphocytes in healthy people has no real relationship to the disease entities (since it would require specific sensitization of thyroid-directed "forbidden" clones of helper T-lymphocytes to stimulate those already-present appropriate B-lymphocytes to produce the appropriate antibodies). This point has been taken up in Chap. 1 and will again be discussed in the summary of this chapter.

2.2.4.3 Cytotoxic Lymphocytes

Lymphocytes from patients with chronic lymphocytic thyroiditis have been shown to be cytotoxic to thyroid cells in tissue culture (Laryea et al. 1973), a finding similar to earlier observations using lymphocytes from animals with experimental thyroiditis. Moreover, lymphocytes from patients with Hashimoto's disease are also cytotoxic to heterologous cells coated with thyroid antigens (Podleski 1972). Furthermore, Amino and DeGroot (1975) have developed an assay for lymphocytotoxins which is positive in Hashimoto's thyroiditis. The possible role of "killer" (K) cells, already discussed with respect to animal models, will be discussed below in relation to the human disorder.

2.2.4.4 Migration Inhibition Factor Procedures

Perhaps the most common procedure for the measurement of cell-mediated immunity has been the measurement of leucocyte migration in response to crude human thyroid antigens. While whole leucocyte preparations have been employed, the response to the specific antigen has been considered an index of the sensitization of the T-lymphocytes in the preparation. Using the leucocyte migration inhibition factor (LIF) test, a number of workers have shown that the results are positive in response to thyroid antigen in both Graves' and Hashimoto's diseases, although not in other forms of hyperthyroidism or non-toxic nodular goitre (Goust et al. 1972; Lamki et al. 1973; Wartenberg et al. 1973; Helmke and Federlin 1974; Moulias et al. 1970). The leucocyte inhibition procedure was considered to be a reflection of the production of migration inhibition factor (MIF), a lymphokine secreted by T-lymphocytes when exposed to the antigen to which they have been previously sensitized. This lymphokine inhibits the migration of white blood cells from the site of an immune reaction. The test is carried out in vitro by packing capillary tubes with peripheral blood leucocytes and setting them in a planchet containing medium. If a non-specific antigen was added to the medium, the white cells would continue to freely migrate out of the capillary tubes. If, however, the medium contained an antigen to which the T-lymphocytes in the capillary tubes had been previously sensitized, cell migration from the tubes was impeded. This reduction in cell migration has been considered an index of MIF production, and evidence of sensitization of T-lymphocytes (hence a reflection of cell-mediated immunity).

The leucocyte inhibition test has been found to be positive in both Graves' and Hashimoto's diseases when various human particulate thyroid antigens have been employed (Lamki et al. 1973). On the other hand, when thyroglobulin was employed as an antigen, the MIF test was found to be negative in Graves' disease, whereas it remained positive in Hashimoto's thyroiditis (Lamki et al. 1973). In addition, these authors found that patients with non-immune thyroid disease (such as toxic nodular goitre, non-toxic nodular goitre, or thyroid carcinoma), as well as patients with other auto-immune diseases (such as systemic lupus erythematosus, or rheumatoid arthritis), did not show evidence of MIF production in response to various thyroid antigens. Moreover, in either Graves' or Hashimoto's disease, LIF responses did not correlate with the levels of various circulating thyroid antibodies.

However, this procedure was criticized on a number of points. Firstly, it was found to be less than completely organ-specific, since mitochondrial antigen (whether from human thyroid, liver, kidney, or even rat liver) was found to also elicit increased MIF production by Graves' and Hashimoto's leucocytes (Wartenberg et al. 1973). Moreover, it had been demonstrated that under certain circumstances immune complexes may also play some role in MIF production (Packalén and Wasserman 1971; Kotkes and Pick 1975; Hall 1978). Thus, there was concern that the B-lymphocytes were playing a role in the leucocyte inhibition factor procedure (Rocklin et al. 1974; Yoshida et al. 1973). However, recently, Kowalczyk and Zembala (1978) have demonstrated that isolated peripheral blood T-lymphocytes have the ability to migrate from a capillary tube both in the direct and indirect MIF test; moreover, the migration of T-lymphocytes from Mantoux-positive donors was inhibited by purified protein derivative (PPD) and/or supernatants which contained lymphokines. Additionally, Totterman et al. (1979) have shown that the MIF test in auto-immune thyroid diseases is dependent on the presence of T-lymphocytes. Accordingly, in our laboratory, Okita et al. (1980a, b) demonstrated clearly that isolated preparations of T-lymphocytes from patients with Graves' disease or Hashimoto's thyroiditis will manifest MIF production in response to human thyroid antigen (see Fig. 2.7). T-lymphocytes from normal persons would not respond in this manner when exposed to the same thyroid antigen (Okita et al. 1980a, b). Moreover, the T-lymphocytes from patients with Graves' disease or Hashimoto's thyroiditis would not produce MIF when in contact with human liver antigen or PPD. From these observations, therefore, it seems clear that there are indeed T-lymphocytes in these disorders which are sensitized specifically to the thyroid antigen. Moreover, in the studies of Okita et al. (1980a), a thyroid cell membrane preparation as antigen was more potent than a crude thyroid antigen, suggesting once again that the appropriate antigen or antigens in Graves' and Hashimoto's diseases is/are cell membrane antigen(s).

However, in order to establish beyond doubt that the results of the direct MIF test really mean that a lymphokine is being produced, it is necessary to do an indirect procedure, whereby the supernatants from lymphocyte cultures exposed to a given antigen are removed and then mixed with completely normal leucocytes. If the supernatant obtained in this manner were to inhibit normal cells from migrating (whereas neither supernatants from *normal* lymphocytes incubated with the same antigens, nor supernatants from Graves' lymphocytes incubated with other organ antigens were to do so), then this would be proof of lymphokine production.

Until recently, this proof had not been forthcoming. Indeed, Matsui et al. (1977), using normal human leucocytes as the migrating cells, were not able to detect MIF lymphokine in the supernatants of Graves' or Hashimoto's leukocytes. However, Okita et al (1981b) have now reported that, in response to crude thyroid antigens, or thyroid cell membrane antigens, lymphocytes from patients with Graves' or Hashimoto's disease will release the MIF lymphokine into the circulation, when

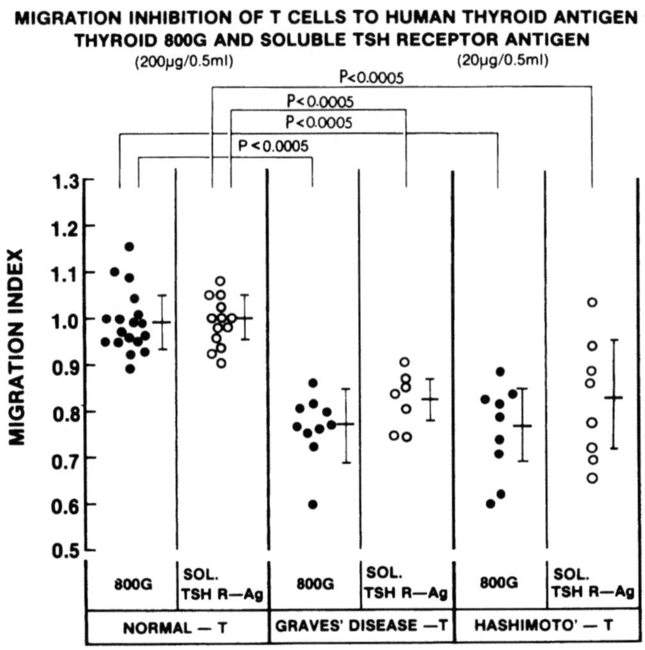

Fig. 2.7. Results of the direct migration inhibition factor (MIF) test using preparations of T-lymphocytes alone, and employing a crude 800 g antigen prepared from normal human thyroid tissue, as well as a "solubilized TSH receptor preparation" (actually a cell membrane preparation) from the same tissue. Normal T-lymphocytes when exposed to these antigens do not elaborate MIF. However, T-lymphocytes from patients with either Graves' or Hashimoto's disease do show marked MIF activity on exposure to these same antigens. This clearly indicates that there is indeed sensitization of T-lymphocytes to thyroid antigen in Graves' and Hashimoto's diseases. (Kidd et al. 1980)

normal human T-lymphocytes are used as the final migrating indicator cells in the second stage of the indirect test (see Fig. 2.8).

Since we now can conclude that there are indeed sensitized T-lymphocytes in both Graves' and Hashimoto's diseases, the question arises as to what the function of these cells might be. It may be suggested that these cells are primarily sensitized helper T-lymphocytes, which are then capable of interacting with appropriate and already present thyroid-directed (self-reactive) B-lymphocytes. It has already been mentioned that lymphocytes from patients with Graves' or Hashimoto's disease when cultured with phytohaemagglutinin (PHA) will release thyroid-stimulating immunoglobulin into the medium (Knox et al. 1976 a). Since PHA stimulates only T-lymphocytes (Greaves et al. 1974), this study implies that PHA stimulated thyroid-directed helper T-lymphocytes, which in consequence directed already present thyroid-directed B-lymphocytes to release thyroid-stimulating immunoglobulin into the medium. Lymphocytes from patients with non-immune thyroid disease or healthy controls generally do not produce TSI under these circumstances (Knox et al. 1967 a).

It has been pointed out above that self-reactive thyroglobulin-binding B-lymphocytes are present in normal persons, and it can be assumed that many others types of self-reactive B-lymphocytes are also always present. What is thus required

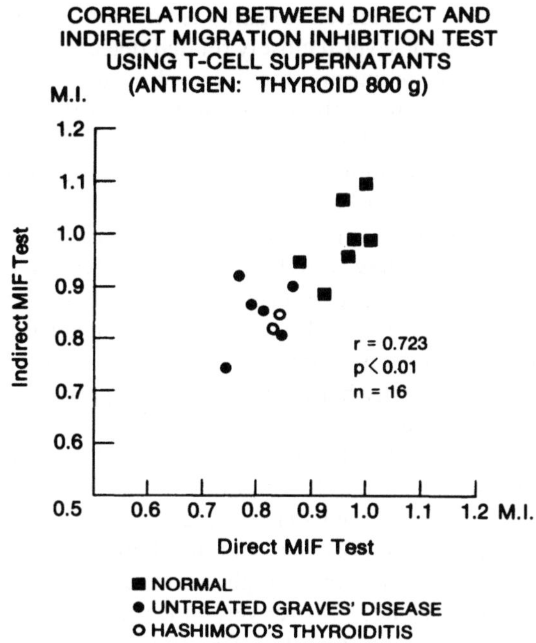

Fig. 2.8. Correlation between the direct MIF test using T-lymphocytes alone versus the indirect MIF test using supernatants from T-lymphocyte cultures added to normal T-lymphocytes as second-stage indicator cells. The excellent correlation indicates that there is indeed a soluble lymphokine produced by the sensitized Graves' or Hashimoto's T-lymphocytes in response to the thyroid antigen, which, when removed, causes inhibition of migration of normal T-lymphocytes. This production of lymphokine has been shown to be organ-specific and occurs only with the appropriate sensitized lymphocytes. (Okita et al. 1981 b)

to stimulate groups of these B-lymphocytes is the emergence of specific helper T-lymphocytes, which are then capable of mounting an auto-immune process.

2.2.4.5 *Evidence for a Defect in Suppressor T-lymphocytes*

The current author had proposed several years ago that both Graves' and Hashimoto's diseases probably represented disorders in immunoregulation (Volpé et al. 1970, 1972). However, those proposals were based on circumstantial rather than direct evidence. It seemed probable, however, that both disorders could be due to specific genetic defects in clones of suppressor T-lymphocytes. The observation that there is no increased generalized hypersensitivity in Graves' disease would argue against the possibility that there is a generalized defect in suppressor T-lymphocytes (Robinson et al. 1974). It may thus have been predicted that if there is a single defect in the immune system which is responsible for either Graves' or Hashimoto's disease, procedures which test the whole system should be normal, while, those which test for a specific defect will be abnormal. While, therefore, we might expect that each of the organ-specific auto-immune diseases is due to a single defect in immunoregulation, one would have to account for the association of more than one auto-immune disease in the same person. Since, however, these occur at different times in relation to one another, it seems likely that even in patients with multiple associated organ-specific auto-immune disorders there has been inheritance of several closely related defects in immunoregulation, i. e. several specific but separate suppressor T-lymphocytes defects may be present, but still there is evidence that there is not generalized hypersensitivity (see Chap. 5). Recently, Beall and Kruger (1979) studied lymphocyte cultures from patients with auto-immune thyroid disease, measuring antithyroglobulin antibody as a product of these lymphocytes. They showed that by varying the amount of T-lymphocytes in the mixture, they were able to influence the amount of antibody produced. They noted that helper T-lymphocytes were essential to allow the B-lymphocytes to produce thyroid antibody. However, it did not seem to matter whether the T-lymphocytes were obtained from patients with auto-immune thyroid disease or from normal persons. Moreover, if they increased the number of T-lymphocytes (whether from normal persons or from patients with auto-immune thyroid disease), these lymphocytes took on a suppressor function. Thus, Beall and Kruger reasoned that there were no defects demonstrable in either immunoregulation or in helper T-lymphocytes that were specific in auto-immune thyroid diseae.

However, these workers used a non-specific mitogen, pokeweed mitogen, in their studies. It is possible that to demonstrate an antigen-specific abnormality in immunoregulation, it might be necessary to use a specific antigenic stimulation in similar studies. Moreover, since these authors manipulated the numbers of lymphocytes in the ratio of T- and B-lymphocytes in their culture preparations, it is not clear what analogy can be drawn between these experiments and the in vivo situation.

Similar results have been obtained by McLachlan et al. (1980). These workers studied the ability of peripheral blood mononuclear cells (PBM) from patients with Hashimoto's thyroiditis and normal persons to synthesize thyroid antibodies in response to phytohaemagglutinin (PHA) under various conditions. When normal PBM were cocultured with Hashimoto's PBM (in the presence of PHA), there was no inhibition of thyroid antibody production. In addition, T-lymphocyte enriched populations from two normal donors were unable to specifically inhibit thyroid antibody synthesis by Hashimoto B-lymphocyte enriched fractions from two Hashimoto's patients. These authors were thus unable to demonstrate suppressor cell function in normal PBM by this procedure. The authors conceded, however, that specific antigen stimulation (rather than non-specific mitogenic stimulation) might be necessary for such a demonstration.

Nevertheless, despite these results and the theoretical concerns mentioned above, Aoki et al. (1979) have shown evidence that in active untreated Graves' disease there is a mild *generalized* deficiency in suppressor T-lymphocyte function. These workers utilized a procedure of stimulating the peripheral mononuclear cells with concanavalin-A or pokeweed mitogen, either at initiation of culture, or after a 24-h period of preincubation. Four days after the addition of the mitogens, the cultures were harvested and a measure of DNA synthesis was carried out. In cells from patients with Graves' disease, preincubation lessened the enhancement of subsequent concanavalin-A and pokeweed mitogen stimulation. Because suppressor cells are short-lived and adhere easily to surfaces, 24-h preincubation was supposed to effectively remove any suppressor activity that was existing at the initiation of the culture. Thus, these findings were similar to those previously reported in patients with active systemic lupus erythematosus and suggested that circulating suppressor cells may be relatively lacking in patients with Graves' disease. However, the same authors found no such defect in Hashimoto's thyroiditis. Moreover, when patients with Graves' disease were placed on propylthiouracil, the results tended to normalize. While these authors suggested that their findings were of pathogenetic significance, it could equally be argued that the excessive thyroid hormone present in active untreated Graves' disease might have acted to suppress the T-lymphocytes, as it has already been demonstrated that thyroxine may inhibit T-lymphocyte function (Sorkin and Desedovsky 1976; Wall et al. 1979 a). Thus, this interpretation would suggest that the findings of Aoki et al. (1979) were a result of the hyperthyroxinaemia, rather than the cause of the hyperthyroidism.

Similar findings were observed by Balázs et al. (1979 b), using a similar procedure. As in the report by Aoki et al. (1979) when the patients became euthyroid on methimazole, the results of Balázs et al. (1979 b) tended to move towards the normal range. Moreover, there appeared to be an inverse relationship with antithyroglobulin titres and transformation responses of lymphocytes to human thyroglobulin. Thus, once again, one might interpret these results as suggesting that hyperthyroxinaemia itself can induce a depression of suppressor T-lymphocytes.

Fragu et al. (1980) have used yet another assay system in which suppressor T-lymphocyte function can be determined by the ability of indomethacin to inhibit the ability of the suppressor cells to produce prostaglandins. These workers have reported defective suppressor cell function to be present in patients with untreated and treated Graves' disease which persists when they become euthyroid. However, only 4 of 15 patients with Hashimoto's thyroiditis showed similar findings. These authors pointed out that while abnormal suppressor cell activity may be related to auto-immunity, variation in function with this procedure was very great, and they urged caution in interpretation of these results.

Bonnyns et al. (1978) have shown that in hyperthyroidism responses of lymphocytes to phytohaemagglutinin were more responsive on the first day, and less responsive on the sixth day of incubation when compared with normal control subjects. These differences were not found with patients who were studied after 3 to 10 months of treatment with propylthiouracil. On the other hand, delayed hypersensitivity to four antigens injected intradermally in patients with active untreated Graves' disease was normal. It would seem likely that the appropriate interpretation of these data was that, once again, the hyperthyroidism itself was suppressing suppressor T-lymphocyte function; this consequently enhances helper T-lymphocyte activity, allowing the increased response of the lymphocytes to the mitogen. Balázs et al. (1980) have studied the effect of the in vitro addition of tri-iodothyronine to lymphocyte cultures. This hormone induced increased tritiated thymidine incorporation into lymphocytes stimulated by phytohaemagglutinin, again suggesting a depressing effect of tri-iodothyronine on suppressor T-lymphocytes, thus allowing the more numerous helper T-lymphocytes and B-lymphocytes to be stimulated. Jeevanram et al. (1977) studied the effect of lymphocyte stimulation by phytohaemagglutinin in patients with thyroid carcinoma who had been adequately treated by thyroidectomy and radioactive iodine. They found that when patients were finally treated with thyroxine therapy, the lymphocytes showed much more blastogenesis than they had shown prior to the commencement of such therapy, again suggesting a depressing effect of thyroid hormone on suppressor cell function.

Experimentally, Fabris (1973) demonstrated that the removal of the thyroid gland in newborn or in young adult rats causes a reduction in the number of peripheral blood lymphocytes, and depression of either the humoral immune reaction against sheep and chicken erythrocytes, or the response of spleen cells to phytohaemagglutinin. These immunological defects are fully established in perinatally thyroidectomized rats after weaning, while in an animal thyroidectomized at a young adult age, they are observable 45–65 days after the operation. In both instances, daily injections with thyroxine can completely restore the lymphoid system of thyroid-deprived animals. These data are in accord with the view that thyroxine itself will suppress suppressor T-lymphocytes, and the absence of thyroxine will thus permit excess suppressor activity, thus inhibiting helper T-lymphocytes and their effect on auto-antibody production. Thus it would appear that thyroid hormones themselves can depress suppressor T-lymphocyte function, and this might explain the findings of Aoki et al. (1979) and Balázs et al. (1979 b), in which an apparent generalized depression of suppressor T-lymphocytes was observed in active untreated patients with Graves' disease, which tended to improve with treatment (whereas generally results were negative in Hashimoto's thyroiditis).

These comments are not offered to obviate a possible role for suppressor T-lymphocytes in the pathogenesis of Graves' disease. However, the lack of generalized hypersensitivity in these patients with active untreated hyperthyroid Graves' disease, the tendency to normalize with treatment, and the negative findings in Hashimoto's disease permit reservations about a role for a *generalized* defect in suppressor T-lymphocytes in initiating these conditions. Indeed, these data do suggest an effect of excessive thyroid hormone concentrations on depressing suppressor T-lymphocyte function, and such an effect may be very important in potentiating Graves' disease and causing it to be a self-perpetuating disorder (see Sect. 2.2.12). It may also be added that Wall and Ryan (1980) and Miller et al. (1979) have been unable to confirm the findings of Aoki et al. (1979) and Balázs et al. (1979 b) using similar techniques. However, what has been required is some techniques which can detect *isolated* antigen-specific defects in immunoregulation, i. e. an *isolated* defect in suppressor T-lymphocytes. Fortunately, studies in our own laboratory have recently established that such a defect is indeed detectable.

Thus, Okita et al. (1981a) have recently demonstrated a new approach to the study of suppressor T-lymphocytes. They have employed a modification of the migration inhibition factor procedure, using preparations of T-lymphocytes alone. They have shown that T-lymphocytes from either Graves' or Hashimoto's disease will produce MIF in response to thyroid antigen. If, however, one adds *normal* T-lymphocytes to the Graves' or Hashimoto's T-lymphocytes, in ratios as low as 1:9 of normal to patient's lymphocytes, then the ability of the latter sensitized T-lymphocytes to produce MIF in response to the thyroid antigen is abolished. If, however, Graves' T-lymphocytes are added to Graves' T-lymphocytes from a second patient in similar ratios, the ability of the lymphocytes to produce MIF is retained, thus ruling out a mixed lymphocyte reaction as the cause of the original abolition of the MIF effect (see Figs. 2.9, 2.10). Conversely, if the normal T-lymphocytes are initially incubated with mitomycin C and subsequently added to the Graves' lymphocytes, the normal T-lymphocytes lose their ability to influence the Graves' T-lymphocytes (which will then produce MIF as before when in contact with the appropriate antigen). In more recent studies, our group has shown that

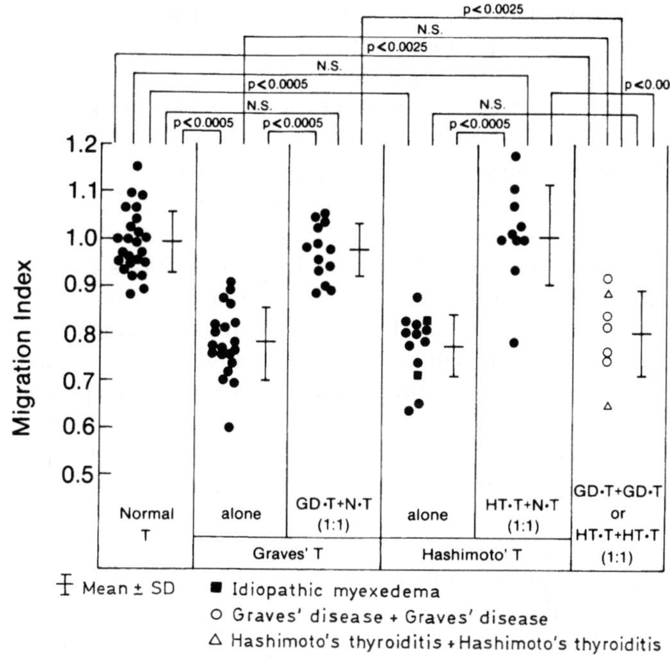

Fig. 2.9. The direct MIF test using T-lymphocytes alone. This graph depicts the effect of adding normal T-lymphocytes to the Graves' or Hashimoto's T-lymphocytes in a ratio of 1 : 1. Note that the production of MIF is abolished by the addition of the normal T-lymphocytes, thus indicating that these normal cells appear to be able to suppress the Graves' or Hashimoto's T-lymphocytes, thus preventing them from producing MIF in response to the thyroid antigen. (Okita et al. 1981 a)

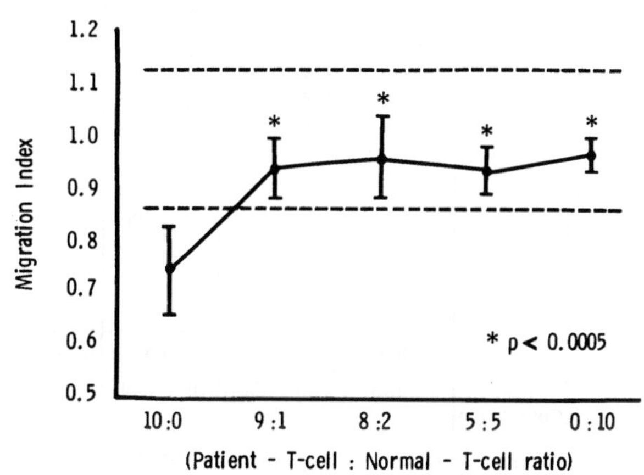

Fig. 2.10. In order to be certain that the effect of normal T-lymphocytes on sensitized T-lymphocytes in abolishing the ability of the latter to produce MIF (in response to specific antigen) was not due to a dilutional effect, the ratio of the normal T-lymphocytes versus the Hashimoto's or Graves' lymphocyte was varied. Even in as low a ratio as 1 : 9 normal: sensitized T-lymphocytes, the ability of the sensitized lymphocytes to produce MIF was abolished. Thus it does not take many normal T-lymphocytes to be able to suppress the Graves' or Hashimoto's T-lymphocytes from producing MIF in response to the antigen. This suggests the presence of a suppressor factor in the normal T-lymphocytes which is absent in the Graves' or Hashimoto's T-lymphocytes. (Okita et al. 1981 a)

irradiation of normal T-lymphocytes with 1000 rads (sufficient to inhibit suppressor T-lymphocyte function without damaging the viability of the lymphocytes or affecting helper functions) will abolish the normal suppressor T-lymphocyte activity when these cells are added to Graves' or Hashimoto's T-lymphocytes; thus, once again, the sensitized T-lymphocyte will produce MIF as before when in contact with the appropriate antigen (Okita et al. 1980 b) (see Fig. 2.11). These studies can only be interpreted as indicating that in Graves' and Hashimoto's diseases there is a loss of specific suppressor activity. i.e. there is a defect in suppressor T-lymphocyte function in both Graves' and Hashimoto's diseases. Because even the cell membrane antigen employed in these studies is not pure, there is no way to distinguish the results between Graves' disease on the one hand, and Hashimoto's thyroiditis on the other. This point will be discussed below (see Sect. 2.2.1).

In any event, it should be possible to exploit this procedure further to determine whether there are single specific defects in immunosuppression for each of the organ-specific auto-immune diseases, by mixing T-lymphocytes from other organ-specific auto-immune diseases (e. g. pernicious anaemia) with the T-lymphocytes from patients with Graves' disease. If the immunosuppressive defect is common to the two disorders, then the ability of the Graves' disease lymphocytes to produce MIF in response to thyroid antigen should remain unaffected. If the defect is not common, the lymphocytes from patients with pernicious anaemia should act like normal lymphocytes as cited in the preceding paragraph. Our laboratory is currently involved in such studies.

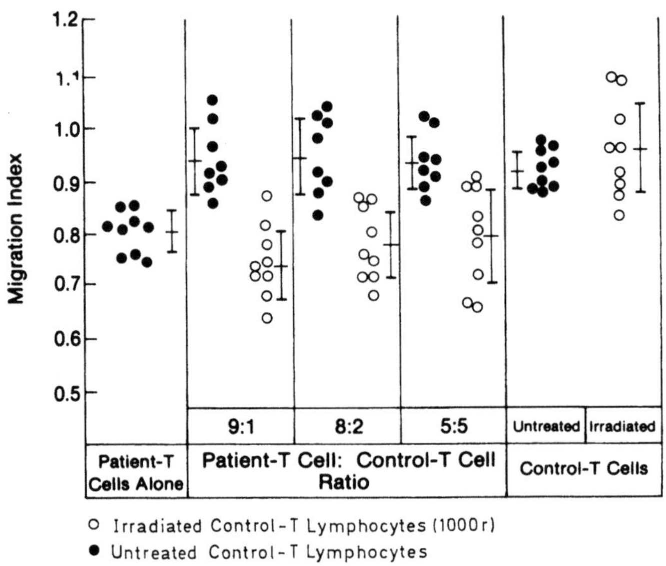

Fig. 2.11. Effect of irradiating the normal T-lymphocytes with 1000 rad prior to incubating them with the Graves' or Hashimoto's T-lymphocytes. Note that prior to irradiation the normal T-lymphocytes would abolish the ability of the Graves' or Hashimoto's T-lymphocytes to elaborate MIF in response to thyroid antigen. This capacity of the normal T-lymphocytes to suppress this activity was itself abolished by irradiation of the normal lymphocytes. The dosage of 1000 rad is known to affect suppressor T-lymphocytes without affecting their viability and without affecting "helper" T-lymphocytes. (Okita et al. 1980 b)

2.2.4.6 Other Cellular Mechanisms

Rapaport et al. (1978) and Yamamoto et al. (1978) have advanced evidence indicating that lymphocytes may produce prostaglandins when exposed to their antigens, and have proposed that this product may be a mediator in stimulating the thyroid gland in Graves' disease. However, this effect appears to be non-specific. Moreover, "killer" (K) cells also appear to play a pathophysiological role, which as yet is not well-defined, particularly in Graves' disease (Calder et al. 1974 b, 1976).

"Killer" (K) cells may be defined as antibody-dependent cytotoxic lymphoid cells. Calder et al. (1974b, 1976) have summarized the literature as well as their own observations with respect to the role of K cells in auto-immune thyroid disease. Cytotoxicity is thought to be independent of the release of soluble factors and appears to be triggered by the combination of the K cell with the activated Fc region of the antibody-antigen complex present on the target cell surface. Relatively few lymphoid cells are required to cause cell damage. Since the K cell belongs to neither the T-nor the B-lymphocyte population, it follows that a peripheral blood lymphoid cell suspension can contain a maximum of 5%–15% K cells, and therefore each K cell has the capacity to destroy several target cells (Calder et al. 1974 b, 1976). Studies in the laboratory of Calder et al. (1974 b, 1976) have indicated that lymphoid cells from the peripheral blood of patients with Hashimoto's thyroiditis have a significantly greater cytotoxic effect on antibody-coated erythrocytes than lymphoid cells from age and sex matched control populations. However, this was not so in Graves' disease. Although much information has been accumulated concerning the in vitro functional characteristics of K cells, relatively little is known about their specific role in vivo. There is evidence that this mechanism may be important in bringing about cellular damage in experimental auto-immune thyroiditis (see above). However, it is clear that antibody from the serum of patients with Hashimoto's thyroiditis, when incubated with K cells, will produce cytotoxic effects on target cells coated with thyroglobulin.

Studies of macrophages have been of interest. Silverberg et. al. (1978 a) have studied the leucocyte adherence procedure in auto-immune thyroid diseases. Leucocyte adherence to glass is inhibited when the peripheral leucocytes from patients with Graves' disease or Hashimoto's thyroiditis are incubated with thyroid antigen. The phenomenon appears to be related to the presence of circulating monocytes that bear immunoglobulin attached to their Fc receptor. When the antigen specific for that bound antibody combines with it, the previously adherent monocyte becomes non-adherent. Thus, the test may indicate circulating monocytes "armed" with antithyroid antibodies.

Sugenoya et al. (1979a) have examined lymphocytes from patients and normal control persons that have been cultured with thyroid antigen. When the donor had thyroid auto-immune disease, there was an increased number of macrophage-lymphocyte "rosettes" detectable, i.e. monocytes surrounded by lymphocytes (see Fig. 2.12). Such rosettes could reflect the initial steps of a postulated mechanism of immune activation, whereby macrophages "process" an antigen and "present" it to lymphocytes (Möller 1978).

2.2.5 The Role of the Antigen: Is There Antigenic Stimulation?

It is thus increasingly evident that there is indeed a primary defect in immunoregulation which serves as the predisposition for Graves' and Hashimoto's diseases, and

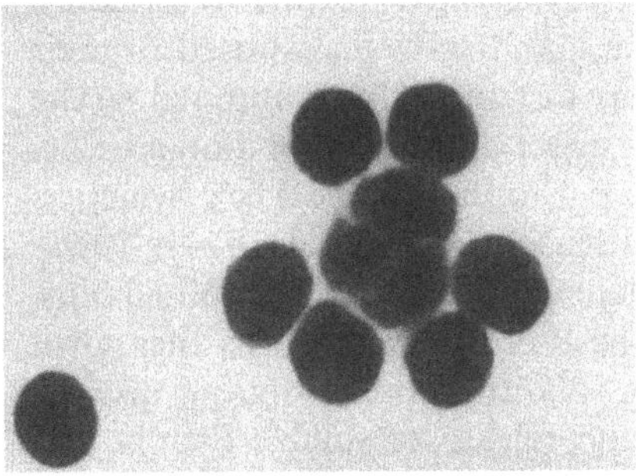

Fig. 2.12. A typical macrophage-lymphocyte rosette in a preparation of blood lymphocytes and monocytes from a patient with Graves' disease following exposure to thyroid antigen. The central cell is the monocyte (macrophage) that is seen ingesting latex particles added to the preparation for the purpose of identification. The surrounding cells are lymphocytes. (Sugenoya, et al. 1979 a) × 800

this appears to be due to a specific defect in a clone or clones of suppressor T-lymphocytes. The proposal that anti-idiotypic antibodies (Wigzell et al. 1978) may play a role in immunoregulation is within the realm of possibility, but there is no evidence for a defect in this form of immunoregulation as yet demonstrated in these disorders. Thus, accepting that there is a specific disorder in suppressor T-lymphocytes, it does not seem necessary to invoke antigenic stimulation as a necessary initiator of these conditions, merely the presence and availability of the appropriate antigen.

Nevertheless, Werner and Fierer (1972) have suggested that there might be an occult antigenic change within the thyroid (possibly viral induced) to which the immunological phenomena are secondary. Indeed, Joasoo et al. (1975) have observed an increased frequency of antibodies to influenza B in a group of thyrotoxic patients when compared to normal persons. There have also been cases of Graves' disease which have occurred following viral and bacterial infections (Alexander et al. 1968; Salisbury and Embil 1978; Ziring et al. 1975). Moreover, viral-like particles have been demonstrated in the thyroid of auto-immune thyroiditis in chickens (Wick and Graf 1972), a finding permitting the postulate that the immune disturbance in human chronic thyroiditis may be initiated by a virus, with secondary occult thyroidal antigenic change. Furthermore, similar viral-like particles have been observed in thyroid tissue in the human disease (Kahn and Dale 1973). However, they can also be demonstrated in normal thyroids as well as in other tissues (Kahn and Dale 1973). It would seem, therefore, that these particles are almost ubiquitous.

However, Werner (1979) has returned to this argument in a publication of a case report of Graves' disease following acute (subacute) thyroiditis. Indeed, Sheets (1955) and Perlof (1956) had also reported similar patients and Volpé et al. (1967) and Volpé (1976, 1979 b) have reported the rare instance of Hashimoto's thyroiditis following subacute thyroiditis. It is true that in subacute thyroiditis, there may be observed secondary immunological phenomena, such as thyroid auto-antibodies, the appearance of TBII, and the appearance of sensitized T-lymphocytes (Volpé 1979 b) (see Fig. 2.13). Thyroid auto-antibodies occur in less than half of the patients, appearing some weeks after onset, rarely reaching high titres, and then subsiding spontaneously (Volpé et al. 1967). TBII has been demonstrated during the course of subacute thyroiditis by Hashizume et al. (1977), by Strakosch et al. (1978) and by Sugenoya et al. (1979 b). However, in those instances in which it was detected, there

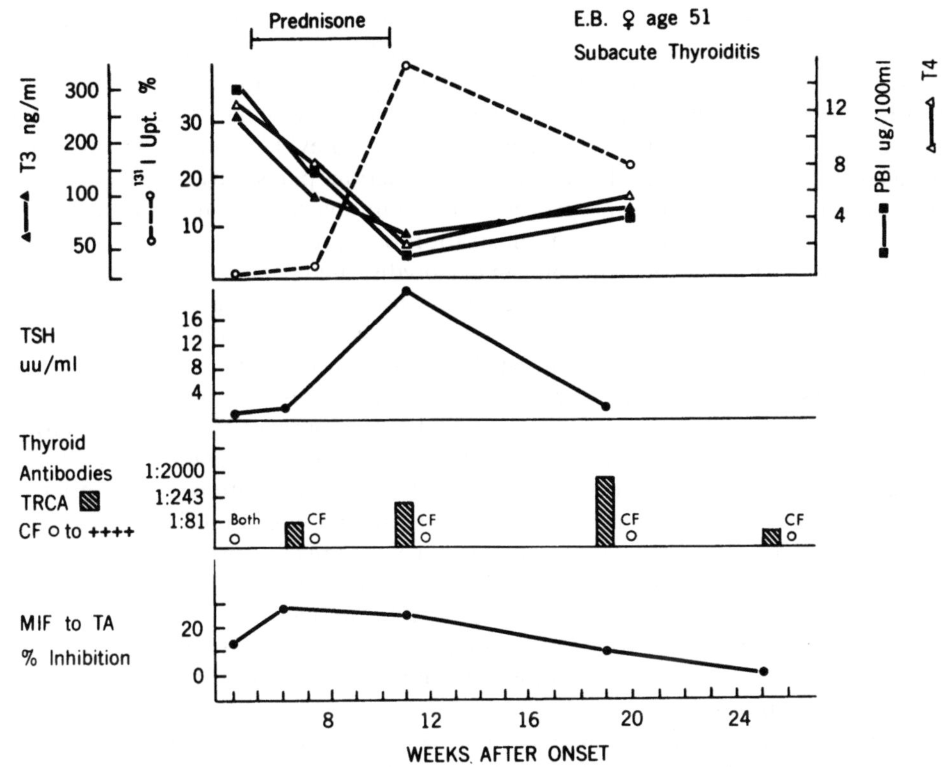

Fig. 2.13. The course of subacute thyroiditis in a 51-year-old woman. Thyroidal antigenic release in subacute thyroiditis produces only a transient, mild immune response, a point against the view that such release is a precursor in Graves' or Hashimoto's disease. *TRCA*, antithyroglobulin; *CF*, antimicrosomal antibodies; *TA*, thyroid antigen. (Volpé 1976)

was no correlation with the presence of hyperthyroidism, nor was there evidence that the TBII represented a true thyroid stimulator, i. e. it was negative in the TSAb assay (Sugenoya et al. 1979 b). Similarly, evidence of cell-mediated immunity has been shown to be transitory and secondary (Wall et al. 1976 a; Volpé 1976, 1979 b; Galluzzo et al. 1980). Moreover, Totterman et al. (1978) have shown that antigen-reactive T-lymphocytes are present in large numbers within the thyroid gland in subacute thyroiditis.

Nevertheless, it is exceedingly unlikely that this inflammatory reaction or its immune response is responsible for the hyperthyroidism that only rarely occurs thereafter. It should be pointed out that only a few cases of auto-immune thyroid disease have occurred following subacute thyroiditis, whereas over 99% go on to full recovery. Thus, clearly, auto-immune thyroid disease is only precipitated in those patients who are alredy predisposed to it, and thus the finding of the frequently positive HLA-Bw35, as is seen in subacute thyroiditis (Bech et al. 1977d; Nyulassy et al. 1977), bears no relationship whatever to the Graves' disease that occurs in Caucasians (see "HLA associations" below).

Since, on the one hand, almost all patients with subacute thyroiditis go on to recovery (and not on to auto-immune thyroid disease), whereas virtually all patients with Graves' or Hashimoto's disease arise de novo, it is much more likely that in those few cases where these disorders have followed subacute thyroiditis, or another viral infection, these inflammatory diseases have acted as a non-specific "stress" to precipitate the hyperthyroidism, as will be discussed below under "The role of stress in the precipitation of hyperthyroidism". There is no evidence that the thyroidal antigenic alteration induced by the viral infection plays any special role in precipitating the auto-immune process. Thus, any infection, acute trauma, emotional disturbance, or even the administration of thyroid hormone itself, may be sufficient to precipitate hyperthyroidism in a predisposed person, by virtue of effects *on the immunoregulatory system*, rather than on the target organ (see below).

It has already been mentioned above that in studies of lymphocyte cultures from patients with Graves' disease it can be shown that *normal* thyroid cell membrane preparations can stimulate the Graves' lymphocytes to produce thyroid-stimulating immunoglobulin (Sugenoya et al. 1978). Moreover, thyroid-stimulating immunoglobulin, whether produced in vivo or in vitro will interact with perfectly normal thyroid tissue in the various assay systems. In addition, the transfer of human lymphocytes from patients with Graves' disease into "nude" (athymic) mice has been shown to produce transient hyperthyroxinaemia, lasting for about 2 weeks (Kidd et al. 1978). These mice have no thyroid abnormality, only an immunoregulatory abnormality. These pieces of evidence indicate that there is no need for any thyroidal antigenic change which is necessary for lymphocyte-thyroid interaction in Graves' disease, and one can extrapolate from these data to postulate the same for Hashimoto's thyroiditis. In addition, von Westarp et al. (1977) were unable to demonstrate any antigenic differences between Hashimoto's and normal thyroid antigens. Knight and Adams (1980) were similarly unable to show any variation in the auto-antigen for the thyroid-stimulating auto-antibodies in a variety of thyroid tissues. These authors concluded that there was no antigenic alteration necessary to initiate Graves' disease.

In addition, Carayon et al. (1978) have shown that the thyrotrophin receptor adenylate cyclase system is unchanged in Graves' disease thyroid glands when compared to normal thyroid glands (thus contradicting previous reports by Lee et al. 1977); they have stated therefore that an antigenic abnormality has not been demonstrated in the Graves' thyroid gland and thus could not act as the initiator of this disorder. Newer techniques are being attempted to further purify and characterize the receptor (Hearn et al. 1980; von Westarp et al. 1980), but much more needs to be done before a truly "pure" TSH receptor is achieved. Such an ultimate preparation may permit more precise investigations into the role of the TSH receptor in the initiation and pathophysiology of Graves' disease.

Actually, there are several reasons for considering that it is not necessary to invoke an occult antigenic change as the initiator for Graves' or Hashimoto's disease. Firstly, this presupposes a genetically based hyperimmune response to not only the thyroid antigen, but also gastric antigen, islet cell antigen, and a few other organ-specific antigens (to account for the overlap with other organ-specific auto-immune diseases), and yet not to all the host of other possible antigens, since generalized hypersensitivity is not a feature of Graves' or Hashimoto's disease (Robinson et al. 1974). Secondly, since the immune response to what has been postulated as an occult thyroidal antigenic change is very excessive indeed, this would necessitate a defect in immunoregulation as has been discussed above.

Indeed, such a defect has now been clearly demonstrated (see: "Evidence for a defect in suppressor T-lymhocytes" above). With such a disorder in immunoregulation, there is no need for any alteration of the antigen, merely the availability of the antigen. Thirdly, as we have noted above, there is no evidence that there is any thyroidal antigenic change demonstrable. Finally, where there is severe thyroidal antigenic change, as in severe subacute thyroiditis, only very rarely is there progression to either Graves' or Hashimoto's disease. For the above reasons, there is no reason to invoke thyroidal antigenic change as a *sine qua non* in initiating either disorder.

2.2.6. The Genetics of Graves' and Hashimoto's Diseases

As noted above, it is clear that both Graves' and Hashimoto's diseases aggregate in specific families, and thus appear to be genetically induced (Friedman and Fialkow 1978). Indeed, these two disorders tend to occur in the same families, and may even coexist within the same thyroid gland (Doniach 1975; Fatourechi et al 1971). Moreover, homozygous twins have been reported where one twin has Graves' disease and the other has Hashimoto's thyroiditis (Jayson et al. 1967; Chertow et al. 1973). The increased incidence of other organ-specific auto-immune diseases both in patiens with Graves' or Hashimoto's disease, as well as in their families, is now well-known, and will be discussed below.

2.2.6.1 Observations in Twins

The occurrence of Graves' disease in both siblings of dizygotic twins is reported to be about 3%–9%, and of monozygotic twins to be about 30%–60% (Lehman 1964; Vogel 1959; Bartels 1941; Volpé et al. 1970, 1972). Numerous case reports attest to the frequency of concordance of monozygotic twins for Graves' disease (Cunningham and Kral 1959; Ehrenfeld and Levy 1972; Hassan et al. 1966; Harvald and Haug 1956; Lowenstein 1961; Neff 1932). The fact that monozygotic twins have a higher concordance rate is strong evidence for a genetic basis for Graves' disease , but genetic factors alone do not explain why some develop the disease, while others do not, i. e. the lack of concordance in 40%–70%. It is of further interest that even in highly selective case reports of twin studies of Graves' disease the ages of initiation of the disease vary greatly between the twins, even as much as ten years in siblings under 18 years of age. Thus, it would appear that influences other than purely genetic are necessary before the disease is expressed (Volpé et al. 1970, 1972; Volpé 1978 b).

2.2.6.2 Age-specific Incidence Rates in Graves' and Hashimoto's Diseases

Burch and Rowell (1963) showed mathematical evidence to support the notion that Hashimoto's thyroiditis occurs randomly in a genetically predisposed population. From the statistics obtained by Burch and Rowell, it was concluded there was no reason to suppose that Hashimoto's thyroiditis was primarily a disease of "disturbed antigen", as had been generally assumed. Rather, it appeared to be a condition due to disturbed tolerance, initiated by somatic mutations of "forbidden" clones of lymphocytes. Their data were also not in keeping with the probability of infection or any other thyroid gland injury.

Following their mathematical analysis, there was some criticism of their mathematics with respect to the proportion of the population at risk, resulting in a lively exchange of letters (Burch 1963a, b; Maynard-Smith and Maynard-Smith 1963a, b). However, even the critics conceded that the original data did indicate a random appearance of the disorder in a genetically predisposed group, as amplified by Burch (1966a, b, 1968).

Since Hashimoto's thyroiditis had relatively high incidence in females, Burch and Rowell (1963) felt that there would be a central role for the X chromosome in antibody synthesis. Since the age-specific incidence rates suggested a high penetrance (almost all of the population at risk develop the disease within the normal lifespan), it seemed probable that this subpopulation is characterized, at least in part, by functionally dominant genes on the X chromosome. On the basis of statistics cited by these authors, the most obvious interpretation was that individuals in this subpopulation inherited dominant mutant genes on the X chromosome. Thus, females had at least twice the chance of having the genetic defect. If several genetic defects are necessary for production of the disease, the ratio can be even higher. The problem with this contention, as will see later, is that it is now known that the genetic basis of these disorders lies in linkage disequilibrium with HLA genes on chromosome 6. It is possible, however, that the X chromosome exerts some modifying influence on the expression of these diseases. Moreover, Talal and Roubinian (1978) have produced evidence that oestrogen may also affect the expression of auto-immune disease, and thus may be a factor in the increased incidence of such disorders in females.

The age-specific incidence rates and sex incidence of Graves' disease and Hashimoto's thyroiditis in relation to the proportion of the general population in each decade of life have been analyzed by Volpé et al. (1970, 1972, 1973). The relative age-specific incidence rates for Graves' disease are shown on Fig. 2.14. This represents the age-specific incidence rates obtained at a University of Toronto clinic over the interval 1959–69. (The female: male ratio was approximately 4 : 1, and this was also observed in Hashimoto's thyroidits.)

In order to arrive at age-specific incidence rate for each decade interval, it was necessary to relate the cases of disease appearing in each decade of life to the total population of the same age-group. The latter was arbitrarily chosen as the population of Ontario taken from the 1966 census. The assumption was made that the age proportions of the population in the referral area were the same as the age proportions generally in the province. One thus divides the proportion of cases of Graves' disease in each decade by the proportion of people in the province in that age decade. Separate age-specific incidence rates were expressed for each sex.

It was somewhat surprising that there appeared to be a drop in the age-specific incidence rates in the male group (and to a lesser degree in the female group) in the fifth decade. These rather unexpected reductions might represent either some manner of bias unconsciously introduced into the selection of cases, so that the curves are bimodal rather than monomodal; otherwise, a bimodal curve would indicate that patients with Graves' disease arise from two genetic populations. For a variety of reasons, however, the bimodal variations between male and female groups seem improbable, and it is unlikely that Graves' disease does represent two populations. Similar data for Hashimoto's thyroiditis (but with only monomodal

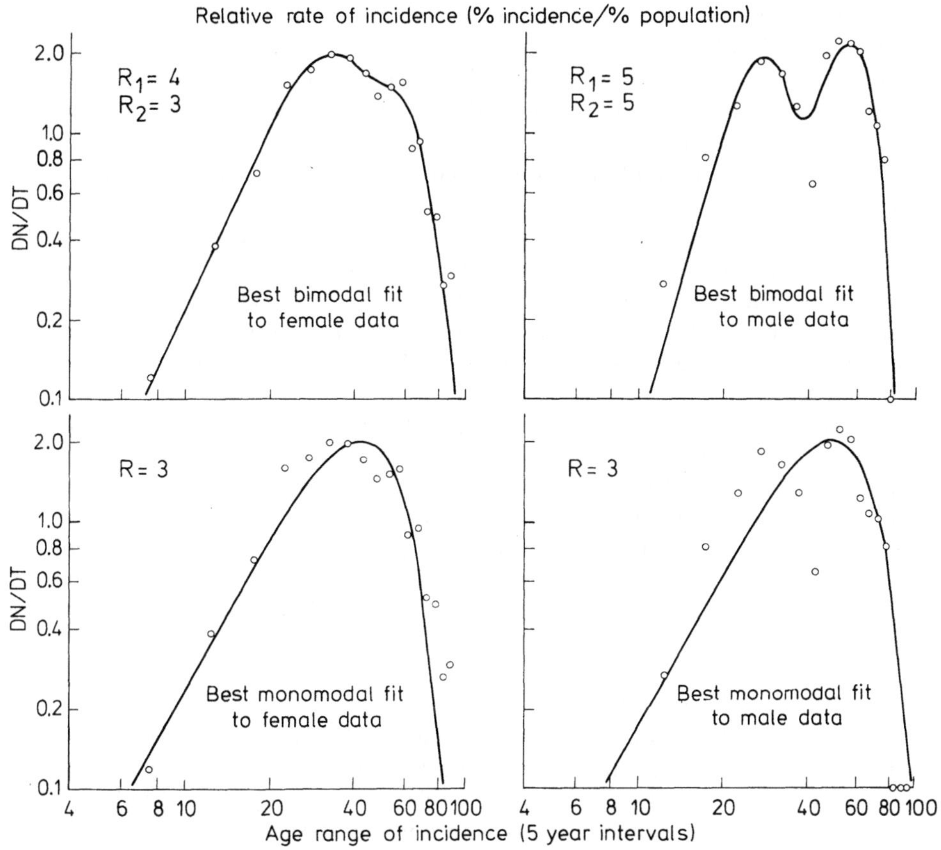

Fig. 2.14. Age-specific incidence rates of Graves' disease in 873 patients (184 males, 689 females), obtained at a University of Toronto clinic over the interval 1959–1969. In order to arrive at an age-specific incidence rate for each decade interval, it is necessary to relate the number of cases of the disease occurring in each decade of life to the total proportion of the same age group. The latter was arbitrarily chosen as the population of Ontario from the 1966 census, with the assumption that the age proportions of the population in our referral area were the same as the age proportions generally in the province. The proportion of cases of Graves' disease in that decade is divided by the proportion of people in the province in that decade (for each sex). See text for further discussion. (Volpé et al. 1972)

curves) were obtained (Volpé et al. 1973), again rather similar to the results of Burch and Rowell (1963).

In non-mathematical terms, the meaning of these data is as follows: if at birth a subpopulation is at special risk through inheritance with respect to the development of given disease, then as this subpopulation ages, more and more members of it will succumb to the disease.

If the probability of onset increases rapidly with age, then the proportion of predisposed members who have not succumbed to it will decrease rapidly with age. When this proportion becomes small enough, the age- specific incidence rate, expressed with respect to the general population, will fail to increase with age. Consequently, a peak in the age-specific incidence rate will be attained, and this will be followed by a falling incidence with increasing age. Theoretically, when every member of the predisposed population has finally been affected, the age-specifc incidence rate should fall to zero.

Burch and Rowell (1963) have suggested that the aetiology of conditions which fit the type of curve obtained for Graves' and Hashimoto's diseases would conform to the following conditions: (1) the disease is restricted to a (genetic) carrier subpopulation; (2) onset of the disease requires the accumulation in a carrier individual of at least two discrete changes; (3) these discrete changes or events are random in nature and their average probability of occurrence is constant with respect to time (somatic mutation is a perfect example of such events); (4) the penetrance of the inherited tendency to the disease aproaches unity within the normal lifespan; (5) the average age-specific mortality rates are the same in the general population and in the carrier subpopulation before the onset of the auto-immune disease.

In the view of the author, the important point to be drawn from these data is that these maladies do appear to occur at random in the genetically predisposed populations. This, coupled with the lack of concordance in approximately 50% of monozygotic twins, and the variation in those twins with respect to the age of initiation of the disease, makes it obvious that (a) there is a genetic basis for the predisposition for the disease, and (b) there is some other (random) event which initiates the clinical condition. Both the genetic basis and the "random event" will be discussed below.

2.2.6.3 Thyroid Auto-antibodies and Chromosomal Abnormalities

Graves' disease, other clinical thyroid disorders and thyroid auto-antibodies have all been observed more often than expected amongst patients with Down's syndrome (mongolism) and their maternal relatives (Friedman and Fialkow 1978; Takahashi et al. 1979). Some patients with gonadal dysgenesis and perhaps their mothers also, have increased frequency of thyroid auto-immunity (Friedman and Fialkow 1978; Chen et al. 1978). Since Down's syndrome (mongolism) and gonadal dysgenesis (Turner's syndrome) are due to different chromosomal abnormalities, it is currently unclear how these influence the expression of auto-immune thyroid disease. Whether these chromosomal abnormalities influence or modulate the basic genetic defect on chromosome 6 (see Sect. 2.2.6.4 below) or have some effect exaggerating or permitting the expression of an otherwise occult disorder, is not yet evident.

2.2.6.4 HLA Associations

The background of HLA associations in auto-immune disease is discussed in Chap. 1. In recent years, histocompatibility testing has been applied to studies of patients with Graves' and Hashimoto's diseases. In Caucasians with Graves' disease there is an increased incidence of HLA-B8 and Dw3 (Friedman and Fialkow 1978; Grumet et al. 1974; Thorsby et al. 1975; McMichael et al. 1975; Bech et al. 1977c). The relative risk of Graves' disease in such patients with HLA-B8 compared to persons lacking this antigen is 2.4. Although this relative risk is not large, the observed association between HLA-B8 and Graves' disease is very unlikely to have occurred by chance alone (Friedman and Fialkow 1978). The relative risk for having Graves' disease in individuals with HLA-Dw3 is 5.2, indicating that it is of much more significance than the HLA-B8 association. (HLA-DRw3 is also found to be increased in Graves' disease (Farid et al. 1979; McGregor et al. 1980b). However, it is clear that not all patients with HLA-Dw3 will develop Graves' disease, nor will all Caucasian patients with Graves' disease have HLA-Dw3. It thus seems more probable that linkage of defined HLA loci to disease-predisposing gene(s) is responsible for the HLA associations observed with Graves' disease. This disease susceptibility might well be due to human homologues of the murine Ir (immune response) or Is (immune suppression) genes which modulate the strength and characteristics of the immune responses to certain specific antigens (Klein 1975; Katz and Benacerraf 1976). As yet, neither Ir nor Is genes have been unequivocally demonstrated in man.

In Japanese (who lack HLA-B8), the association for Graves' disease was found to be with HLA-Bw35 and DHO (Kawa et al. 1978; Sasazuki et al. 1978). The term HLA-DHO has recently been changed to HLA-Dw12 (Farid and Bear 1981). In Chinese, only the B locus has yet been investigated, and shows an increase in HLA-Bw46. The risk for having Graves' disease with Bw46 alone was 3.74. This risk could be increased when associated with two other B locus antigens, B40 and B13 (relative risks 8.74 and 5.88 respectively). However, homozygosity in Bw46 was not associated with an increased risk of thyrotoxicosis, and the risk associated with Bw46 was reflected in the Bw46 heterozygotes (Chan et al. 1978). These results thus differ from those of Farid et al. (1976), where B8 homozygosity appeared to be associated with an increased risk when compared with B8 heterozygotes.

The relationship of these HLA antigens to the expression and course of Graves' disease has been of considerable interest. Balázs et al. (1978) detected a correlation between the presence of the B8 antigens and ophthalmopathy, as well as increased human thyroglobulin antibody titres and lymphocyte transformation indices. Moreover, the same group (Balázs et al. 1979a) have found that the activity of short-lived and concanavalin A activated suppressor T-lymphocytes in patients with B8 was lower than in those without B8. They thus felt it possible that B8 or B8 linked susceptibility genes might play a role in the control of suppressor T-lymphocyte function.

However, Bech et al. (1977b), and Schernthaner et al. (1978) were unable to show any significant influence of HLA-B8 or HLA-Dw3 on auto-antibody formation or on the presence of ophthalmopathy. Thus, this question remains to be resolved. Farid et al. (1978) have found a significant increase in the IgG heavy chain allotype marker (Gm), fnb/fb, in patients with Graves' disease compared to controls, raising the possibility of allotypic restriction of thyroid stimulating antibodies in this condition. This influence of fb on the susceptibility to Graves' disease was found to be independent of HLA-B8 status, suggesting that the immunological network operated by the histocompatibility linked genes was independent of that centred around IgG allotypes. These workers postulated that, whereas the former genes determine the level of helper T-lymphocyte function in the production of thyroid-stimulating antibodies in Graves' disease, a person who also happens to carry the Gm marker fb would be assured of the production of IgG antibodies with thyroid-stimulating activity.

As will be discussed further below, the prevalence of HLA-B8 in thyrotoxic patients who relapsed after withdrawal of antithyroid drugs was found to be much greater (69%) by Irvine et al. (1977a) when compared with the prevalence in patients who remained in remission (40%) and in healthy controls (28%). Similar results have been reported by Bech et al. (1977b) with respect to the incidence of HLA-Dw3; 65% of those with HLA-Dw3 relapsed after discontinuance of the antithyroid drug, whereas only 33% of those who remained in remission for at least 1 year were positive for HLA-Dw3. This difference was statistically significant. Similar findings have been reported by McGregor et al. (1980b). Thus, it appears that there is a genetic basis which permits remissions after antithyroid drug therapy in Graves' disease, or, conversely, prevents such remissions. This will be explored further below.

Studies of HLA associations in Hashimoto's thyroiditis have not been as successful as those in Graves' disease in illuminating an HLA association. Most studies have failed to show any association of the goitrous form of Hashimoto's thyroiditis with any HLA gene (Irvine 1978). However, the atrophic form of auto-immune thyroiditis has been shown to have an association with HLA-B8 (Irvine 1978; Moens et al. 1979), and in one study at least, the atrophic form has been shown to be associated with HLA-DRw3 (Moens and Farid 1978). Thus, the link between Graves' and Hashimoto's diseases which seems so clearly evident on family studies and clinical grounds may be via the DRw3 link. However, a recent study indicates that Hashimoto's disease in Caucasians is associated with an increase in HLA-DR5 (49%) when compared to normal persons (23%) (Weissel et al. 1980). If confirmed, this would represent a genetic difference with respect to Graves' disease.

Studies of the HLA associations in families with Graves' or Hashimoto's disesases have been of interest. Chopra et al. (1977) have shown that thyroid functional abnormalities occur as frequently in Graves' relatives without HLA-B8 as with it, suggesting that at least this marker is not an adequate marker for Graves' disease in the population predisposed to that disorder. Thyroid functional abnormalities were found to occur when HLA-B8 locus patterns were normal. Similar observations have been made by Mather et al. (1980). However, studies of the D locus in families will be awaited with interest. A further discussion of thyroid functional abnormalities will be presented below.

2.2.6.5 Studies of Relatives of Patients with Graves' and Hashimoto's Diseases

The aggregation of Hashimoto's thyroiditis, primary myxoedema and thyrotoxicosis in the same families is well-known (Doniach 1975). There are many reports of monozygotic twins with Hashimoto's disease (Irvine et al. 1961) and with Graves' disease (as noted above). Hall et. al. (1960) reported thyroid auto-antibodies in about 50% of the siblings of patients with auto-immune thyroiditis. Moreover, Hall and Stanbury (1967) found that the disease could be inherited equally from either parent. Family studies in thyrotoxicosis have shown similar results (Hall and Stanbury 1967; Chopra et al. 1977). Studies of the concordance rates in monozygotic and dizygotic twins have already been presented above.

Studies by Bartels (1941) and by Hall and Stanbury (1967) showed rather early that there was a high incidence of thyroid-related abnormalities in blood relatives of patients with Graves' and Hashimoto's diseases. Chopra et al. (1977) have investigated the frequency of thyroid-related abnormalities or their relation with HLA antigens or both, in first-degree relatives of patients with Graves' disease or Hashimoto's thyroiditis. In 92 first-degree relatives of patients with Graves' disease, and 14 first-degree relatives of patients with Hashimoto's thyroiditis, some abnormality of thyroid function and/or thyroid auto-antibodies were found in almost half of the relatives. However, as mentioned above, there was no significant difference in the occurrence of the abnormalities in HLA-B8 positive relatives, compared with the HLA-B8 negative relatives; this was also the case for goitre, non-suppressibility, antithyroid antibodies and supranormal TSH responses to TRH. These data indicate that thyroid functional abnormalities occur frequently, even when HLA patterns are normal and HLA-B8 is absent. Similar observations, as noted above, have also been made by Mather et al. (1980).

Carey et al. (1980) have studied 153 children of parents with Graves' disease, compared to 129 control children, selected on the basis of a negative history for Graves' disease among first-degree relatives. Thirty-six percent of children of parents with Graves' disease had one or more abnormality of thyroid function or thyroid auto-antibodies, as compared to 24% of control children (a surprisingly high proportion in the control group). The incidence of abnormalities increased with age, and was more common in females. The abnormalities in both groups were similar in variety and intensity, but differed mainly in frequency. Half of the minor abnormalities detected in the thyroid, including firmness, enlargement or lobulations, were accompanied by chemical abnormalities, such as high or low serum throxine level, abnormal thyroglobulin or tri-iodothyronine level, or the presence of thyroid auto-antibodies. One-quarter of the children having some minor abnormality in the thyroid had definite evidence of Hashimoto's thyroiditis. Assays for thyroid-stimulating antibodies, cell-mediated immunity to thyroid antigens and thyroglobulin immune complexes were negative.

During follow-up examinations extending over 3 years, in a significant fraction of children the original abnormality was lost or modified or new abnormalities developed; these included single cases of asymptomatic thyrotoxicosis, exophthalmos, vitiligo, and Hashimoto's thyroiditis. Carey et al. (1980) thus suggested that there might be a progressive evolution of abnormalities in thyroid function, and that these are especially common with certain families. They felt that it might be possible to determine from sequential examinations, which children are at risk of developing thyrotoxicosis. Nevertheless, they admitted that the abnormalities changed from year to year, and did not necessarily represent a progressive process. They applied the term "pre-Graves' disease" to this condition. However, this term may well be unfortunate, since Doniach et al. (1979) have studied some Hashimoto's patients for over 15 years, and made the remarkable observation that very few of the relatives with high titres of antibodies progressed to an overt clinical stage of the disease; they suggested that these disorders may remain subclinical (in a "controlled" state, as suggested at the end of Chap. 1) for many years, although perhaps not indefinitely. Gordin and Lamberg (1975) have determined that only about 10% of serologically positive persons will develop clinical symptoms. However, the observations of Carey et al. (1980) are of interest in that the findings do vary from year to year. This suggests that the immunoregulation in these persons is precarious, barely capable of preventing overt disease in these asymptomatic relatives. It would appear that at times the regulatory mechanisms are more effective than at others, and this may relate to the milieu interieure, i. e. those elements which favourably or adversely affect immunoregulation. It will be of great importance to follow such persons for several decades, since the adverse effects on immunoregulation of aging after the fifth or sixth decade may bring out these occult lesions and allow them to be clinically expressed. The role of "stress" (another possible precipitating factor) on the immune system will be discussed below.

2.2.6.6 Other Auto-immune and Neoplastic Associations

It is clear that Graves' and Hashimoto's diseases coexist with other organ-specific auto-immune disorders, both within and without the endocrine system. Even exophthalmos might be considered such a disorder, since it is the author's view that it represents a separate, very closely related, organ-specific auto-immune disease that overlaps very frequently with Graves' disease and less often with Hashimoto's thyroiditis. However, this aspect will be discussed separately below. Pernicious anaemia, or its morphological counterpart, atrophic gastritis, is a common association with auto-immune thyroid disease. In thyrotoxicosis, there is a 1.7% incidence of pernicious anaemia, as opposed to 4.2% in goitrous Hashimoto's thyroiditis and 11.4% in primary atrophic myxoedema. The incidence rises as age progresses, and it is rare for pernicious anaemia to be found before the age of 40 years. Auto-antibodies to gastric antigen are commonly found in auto-immune thyroid disease, even when the overt gastric disorder is not present. The incidence of these antibodies also rises with age, reaching 70% in Hashimoto's thyroiditis in the seventh decade, and approximately 40% in either Graves' disease or atrophic myxoedema (as opposed to about 10% of control females in this age bracket). Similarly, patients with auto-immune thyroiditis tend to give positive migration inhibition tests when crude gastric antigen is employed (Irvine 1975). Moreover, the converse is true also, i. e. there is a marked increased incidence of auto-immune thyroid disease in patients with pernicious anaemia. Thus, Doniach et. al. (1965) found 10 of 71 relatives of probands with pernicious anaemia had small goitres, with substantial thyroid antibody titres suggestive of mild thyroiditis, five had overt Hashimoto's thyroiditis, four had thyrotoxicosis, five had myxoedema.

Moreover, studies of members of the families of patients with either auto-immune thyroid disease on the one hand, or pernicious anaemia on the other, will show similar results. Antibodies specific to the thyroid were found by Doniach et al. (1965) in 50% of first-degree relatives of patients with pernicious anaemia, three times higher than in normal controls.

Isulinopenic diabetes mellitus is also found in association with auto-immune thyroid disease, either Graves' or Hashimoto's disease (Irvine 1975, 1980). The form of diabetes which is in association with auto-immune thyroid disease has now been clearly related to HLA-B8-Dw3 (Friedman and Fialkow 1980), and is discussed in Chap. 3. Perlman (1961) estimates that diabetes is three times more common with Graves' disease than in the general population, and conversely about 12% of diabetics develop hyperthyroidism. Farid et al. (1980) have found that 9 of 175 patients with Graves' disease suffered from type I (insulin-dependent) diabetes, while the same was true for 13 of 157 patients with auto-immune thyroiditis. Conversely, the incidence of thyroid auto-immune disease and thyroid auto-antibodies is significantly increased in patients with type I diabetes mellitus and in their relatives (Fialkow et al. 1975). In fact, Gray et al. (1980) have recently shown that subclinical hypothyroidism (i. e. a raised TSH value with normal circulating thyroid hormone values) may be found in 17% of females and 6.1% of males with type I diabetes, an exceedingly high incidence when compared with the general population (Tunbridge 1979).

Myaesthenia gravis is another organ-specific auto-immune disease which has been associated with auto-immune thyroid disease. Grob (1958) has estimated that as high as 3% of patients with Graves' disease also have associated myaesthenia gravis. A more realistic estimate indicates that less than 1% of patients with hyperthyroidism have myaesthenia gravis (still a much higher prevalence than in the general population), whereas the incidence of hyperthyroidism in myaesthenia gravis has ranged from 3%–6% (Millikan and Haines 1953; McEachern and Parnell 1948). Simpson (1968) has estimated that the frequency of thyroid disease in patients with myaesthenia gravis is between 10% and 20%. Judged by the small number of reported cases, thyroiditis has been considered rare in myaesthenia gravis (Ramsay 1974). However, Aarli et. al. (1978) found 3 out of 40 patients with myaesthenia gravis to have chronic thyroiditis. Of the remaining 37 patients, two had enlarged thyroid glands, a positive history of thyroid disease, and antibodies to thyroglobulin. However, the exact proportion of patients with myaesthenia gravis amongst the population with Hashimoto's thyroiditis has not been precisely calculated, and appears to be less than that seen with Graves' disease. Since there is an increased incidence of HLA-B8 and Dw3 in myaesthenia gravis (Friedman and Fialkow 1978), this again is clearly the link (or at least the marker) that connects auto-immune thyroid disease and myaesthenia gravis.

Auto-immune adrenal insufficiency (idiopathic Addison's disease) is more often associated with auto-immune thyroid disease than would be expected from its incidence in the general population (Irvine 1975). While it is difficult to determine an incidence of Addison's disease in patients with either Graves' or Hashimoto's disease, it has been possible to determine the converse relationship, i. e. the incidence of auto-immune thyroid disease in idiopathic Addison's disease. Irvine (1975) has found a 9% prevalence of auto-immune thyroiditis (either goitrous Hashimoto's thyroiditis or atrophic myxoedema) in idiopathic Addison's disease. The prevalence of Graves' disease is likewise about 9% in idiopathic Addison's disease, as opposed to 2% in tuberculous Addison's disease (Irvine 1975). Actually, the combination of Hashimoto's thyroiditis with idiopathic Addison's disease has been termed Schmidt's syndrome (Schmidt 1926), and has been reported quite frequently (Irvine 1975). Occasionally, patients with Addison's disease will be found to have subclinical reductions in thyroid function (Faber et al. 1979) that may return to normal following replacement doses of steroids (Gharib et al. 1972; Schwartz 1973; Topliss et al. 1980).

Once again, the connection between auto-immune thyroid disease and auto-immune adrenal disease is through its linkage with HLA-B8-Dw3 (Friedman and Fialkow 1978). The association with auto-immune hypoparathyroidism or hypogonadism is somewhat less than with adrenal disease; most of the latter patients will also prove to have auto-immune adrenalitis as well (Edmonds et al. 1973; Irvine 1975).

Vitiligo is now considered likely to be an auto-immune disease, and antibodies to melanocytes have been demonstrated in this disorder (McBurney 1979). McBurney (1979) has reported that approximately 20% of patients with vitiligo will also show antithyroid antibodies. Conversely, in auto-immune thyroid disease, particularly Graves' disease, about 25% of patients will be found to have vitiligo (Ochi and DeGroot 1969). A close relationship between vitiligo and auto-immune thyroid disease was reported by Cunliffe et al. (1968). Curiously, no specific HLA marker has been found in patients with vitiligo as yet (McBurney 1979).

Sjögren's syndrome has been reported much more often in association with Hashimoto's thyroiditis than with Graves' disease (Martinez-Lavin et al. 1979;

Shearn 1971; Whaley et al. 1973). Similarly, chronic active hepatitis (Elling et al. 1966) and rheumatoid arthritis (Monroe 1935) have been found more commonly with Hashimoto's thyroiditis than with Graves' disease, whereas idiopathic thrombocytopenic purpura (Dunlap et al. 1974) has been found to occur more commonly in Graves' disease. There is also a suggestion that there is an increased incidence of the polymyalgia rheumatica-giant cell arteritis syndrome in association with auto-immune thyroid disease (How and Bewsher 1980).

While there is also a relationship of hyperthyroidism to thyrotoxic periodic paralysis in Oriental patients, this relationship is on a different basis from those reported above. Patients with thyrotoxic periodic paralysis in Chinese are found to have HLA antigens A2–Bw33 and Aw19–B17, and these are not present in patients without thyrotoxic periodic paralysis. In Chinese patients with Graves' disease, the common HLA antigen is HLA–Bw46, or Bw46/B40. Thus, it would appear that when particular patients have both sets of antigens, then the development of hyperthyroidism would also permit periodic paralysis to occur, because of the appearance of two coincidental genetic abnormalities (Yeo et al. 1978 b).

While there does not appear to be any true relationship between Hashimoto's thyroiditis and carcinoma of the thyroid (Fisher and Beall 1976; Volpé 1978 c), there does appear to be a slightly increased incidence of lymphoma of the thyroid associated with Hashimoto's thyroiditis (Burke et al. 1977). The precise incidence of lymphoma of the thyroid in relation to Hashimoto's thyroiditis is unclear, as the proportion has not been systematically calculated, and it is obviously uncommon. However, conversely, the finding of chronic thyroiditis in malignant lymphoma of the thyroid is quite common (Burke et al. 1977). It thus appears that the auto-immune process of Hashimoto's thyroiditis can occasionally evolve in some manner into an immunological neoplasm.

There has been no such increase in lymphoma of the thyroid gland in association with Graves' disease. However, there has been a reported moderate increase in the incidence of leukaemia associated with Graves' disease, which is unrelated to treatment (Saenger et al. 1968). The nature of this association is unknown, but one cannot help but consider the possibility of some abnormality of immunoregulation in the initiation of the leukaemia.

2.2.7 Interrelationships Between Graves' and Hashimoto's Diseases

As pointed out at great length above, there is much in common between Graves' disease and Hashimoto's thyroiditis, to the extent that some observers have considered that these two conditions represent opposite ends of the same spectrum of a single entity (Bastenie and Ermans 1972). Indeed, depending on one's perspective of what variants a "single entity" may reasonably include, this notion may be acceptable. The evidence for at least genetic, pathogenetic and immunological overlap between the two disorders is overwhelming, and will be listed in the following paragraphs. Yet, there are elements in each condition which are clearly different, and the author's perception at present is that Graves' disease and Hashimoto's thyroiditis are two different entities, no matter how closely related they are to one another.

Evidence for common features includes the observation that both conditions may aggregate in the same families (Doniach 1975), or even coexist within the same thyroid gland (Fatourechi et al. 1971; Doniach 1975). In some identical twins, one may have Graves' disease, and the other, Hashimoto's thyroiditis (Jayson et al. 1967; Chertow et al. 1973). Lymphocytic infiltration of the thyroid is observed in both conditions (Bastenie and Ermans 1972), and various immunoglobulins may be observed in the thyroid stroma of each malady (Werner et al. 1972; Kalderon and Bogaars 1977). Thymic enlargement is common to both (Michie and Gunn 1966), and "conventional thyroid auto-antibodies" (i. e. thyroid auto-antibodies other than TSAb) are commonly found in both conditions (Mori and Kriss 1971). Studies of asymptomatic relatives of patients with each disorder yield similar functional and immunological abnormalities (see above). In addition, Graves' disease may spontaneously culminate in Hashimoto's thyroiditis (and hypothyroidism) (Wood and Maloof 1975; Wood and Ingbar 1979). Conversely, Hashimoto's thyroiditis with or without hypothyroidism may ultimately change into Graves' disease associated with hyperthyroidism (Goolden et al. 1971; James 1971; Gavras and Thomson 1972; Bremner and Griep 1976; Hochstein et al. 1977; Blackett et. al. 1978; Sung and McDougall 1978; Schatz et al. 1979). Additionally, tests of sensitized T-lymphocytes (in response to thyroid antigen (s)) and tests which demonstrate a defect in suppressor T-lymphocyte function are likewise common to both (Okita et al. 1980 a, b and 1981 a, b).

However, the differences that can be discerned between these two auto-immune diseases may be of fundamental importance. Of course, at the extremes, the clinical presentation may be quite disparate, with hyperthyroidism as the expression of Graves' disease, and hypothyroidism reflecting Hashimoto's thyroiditis (i. e. stimulation of the thyroid gland versus destruction of the gland, respectively). In terms of HLA associations, while one study has shown Hashimoto's disease in Caucasians to be associated with HLA-DRw3 (Moens and Farid 1978) (similar to the HLA-DRw3 association with Graves' disease), only in the atrophic form of Hashimoto's thyroiditis is there an association with HLA-B8 (Irvine 1978). In the goitrous form of the condition, there appears to be an association with HLA-DR5 (Weissel et al. 1980). Moreover, exophthalmos, which is commonly associated with Graves' disease, is only rarely observed in patients with Hashimoto's thyroiditis (Wyse et al. 1968). The incidence of TBII, found in most patients with active untreated Graves' disease (Mukhtar et al. 1975; O'Donnell et al. 1978), is detectable in only about 13% of patients with Hashimoto's thyroiditis. Indeed, if a stimulatory rather than a radioligand assay is performed, many of the Hashimoto's patients with a positive TBII will have a negative TSAb (Sugenoya et al. 1979 b). The incidence of various associated organ-specific auto-immune diseases seems to differ significantly between the two diseases, e. g. Sjögren's syndrome is much more commonly associated with Hashimoto's thyroiditis, rather than with Graves' disease (Martinez-Lavin et al. 1979). These discrepancies suggest that there may be subtle genetic and pathogenetic differences between these two disorders, and if this is so, would further suggest that lymphocyte populations (and thus precise antigens) are different.

However, with currently available thyroidal antigenic preparations, it is not possible to separate off the two putative antigen systems. Even with preparations labelled "solubilized TSH receptor", it is clear that this is merely a preparation rich in cell membranes (hence rich in TSH receptor protein), composed of many membrane antigens (as well as some non-membrane antigens) (Okita et al. 1980 a, b, and 1981 a, b). Hence it should come as no surprise that tests of cell-mediated immunity employing such preparations should provide similar results for the two diseases.

It is the author's current view that the two entities are separate disorders, however closely related they are to one another, and however much they may overlap. Speculatively, both conditions may involve antigens closely related on the thyroid cell membrane. Whether these antigens will yield technically to procedures to separate them, remains to be seen. The genes which cause each disorder, if indeed separate, must be very closely related to one another, with inheritance of both genes being common enough to cause frequent overlap. The concurrence of both conditions in identical twins may be explained by the inheritance of both genes in each; the subsequent random appearance of slightly different thyroid directed "forbidden" clones of helper T-lymphocytes, for which immunoregulation is genetically inadequate, might dictate which of the two entities is finally expressed (despite the identical available genetic predisposition to both diseases in each twin).

2.2.8 Relationship of Painless ("Silent") Subacute Lymphocytic Thyroiditis to Chronic Auto-immune Thyroiditis

The condition of painless thyroiditis is characterized clinically by the appearance of manifestations of mild hyperthyroidism due to the leakage of thyroxine and tri-iodothyronine from the thyroid gland; the 24-h radioactive iodine uptake, however, is depressed to almost undetectable levels. The laboratory values and course of the disease are very similar to those of subacute (DeQuervain's) painful thyroiditis (Volpé 1979 a). However, in subacute lymphocytic thyroiditis, the thyroid gland is not painful or tender, and is of normal size or only slightly enlarged. However, after the early phase has subsided, both DeQuervain's thyroiditis and painless thyroiditis are often associated with a phase of transient hypothyroidism due to depletion of the follicular contents, followed by a rebound and then a recovery phase, with spontaneous and complete resolution being the general rule.

While Nikolai (1979; Nicolai et al. 1980) has suggested that this disorder is a new form of transient hyperthyroidism, in fact painless subacute thyroiditis has been observed for many decades (Volpé 1979 a). It is nevertheless true that the number of such patients seems to have markedly increased; moreover, certain features of this variant are clearly different from the painful form of subacute thyroiditis.

The most cogent difference is in the histological picture, since in most biopsies obtained during the course of this painless disorder, lymphocytic infiltration predominates (Nikolai 1979; Nikolai et al. 1980). This has led some authors (Gluck et al. 1975) to the conclusion that this malady represents an unusual form of chronic lymphocytic thyroiditis. However, as Nikolai (1979) Nikolai et al. (1980) point out, only about one-third of the specimens show evidence of Hürthle cells, which when present were generally infrequent as well. Fibrosis was usually absent or minimal. These last two features were certainly unlike chronic lymphocytic thyroiditis, where Hürthle cells and fibrosis are common features.

Moreover, thyroid auto-antibodies are usually undetectable in this condition, using ordinary serological techniques, although such antibodies have been detected by radioassay (Dorfman et al. 1977). It has already been emphasized above, however, that the discrepancy between the serological procedures for thyroid antibodies and the findings by radioassay may be a result of interference by excessive amounts of thyroglobulin liberated during the course of the thyroiditis (Van Herle et al. 1979), which may give artefactual levels of antithyroglobulin by radioassay (Pinchera et al. 1979). Thus, there is no certainty that there are significant thyroid auto-antibodies appearing often in this entity.

Moreover, it is now known that in subacute lymphocytic (painless) thyroiditis, there is complete histological resolution upon recovery (Inada et al. 1980 b). It thus would appear that this condition does *not* represent chronic auto-immune thyroiditis, since recovery is quick and there is doubt that there are significant thyroid auto-antibodies present throughout the course of this illness. While the aetiology of this condition is not clear, it still may be a variant of subacute DeQuervain's thyroiditis or may be yet another form of thyroidal inflammatory response to viral or other aetiological agents.

It may be, however, that the form of this condition seen commonly in the post-partum period (Amino et al. 1980) could conceivably be auto-immune in nature, despite the fact that clinically and pathologically it resembles the form of painless thyroiditis referred to in the paragraph above. The possible auto-immune nature of this particular category will be discussed below, under the heading "Auto-immune thyroid disease in pregnancy and neonate". It thus may well be that painless ("silent") thyroiditis is aetiologically heterogeneous, but at least those cases which are *unrelated* to pregnancy do not have any demonstrable relationship to auto-immune processes. The author's current conception, therefore, is that while the histological appearance of these cases does seem similar to chronic auto-immune thyroiditis, there is very likely some other aetiological explanation, at least in those instances where there is no relationship to pregnancy.

2.2.9 Auto-immune Thyroid Disease in Pregnancy and the Neonate

2.2.9.1 Post-partum Auto-immune Thyroid Disease

In 1976, Amino and his colleagues found that pregnancy and delivery strikingly influenced the clinical course of auto-immune thyroid diseases. At that time, this group observed patients with transient post-partum hypothyroidism and auto-immune thyroiditis (Amino et al. 1976) and subsequently described transient post-partum hyperthyroidism in Graves' disease and in auto-immune thyroiditis (Amino et al. 1977 a, b). Subsequently, this same group studied changes of serum anti-thyroglobulin by haemagglutination during pregnancy and delivery in Graves' disease and auto-immune thyroiditis (Amino et al. 1978). Both of these antibodies decreased as pregnancy progressed, and sometimes became negative in late pregnancy. (Of course, in some patients, the thyroid auto-antibodies or TSAb persist throughout the pregnancy.) Following delivery, however, these antibodies increased again and the titres reached peaks about 3 to 4 months post-partum in more than half of the patients. In some patients, antibodies developed after delivery. Similar transient increases in antibodies were observed after spontaneous and therapeutic abortion. The authors speculated that these changes appeared to be induced by physiological and immunological changes occurring during pregnancy and after delivery. Some similar observations have been recently made by How et al. (1980).

Amino et al. (1980) have now studied the mechanisms of these changes. Ten patients with auto-immune thyroiditis were studied without treatment during and after pregnancy. Once again, they found that the titres of antithyroglobulin and antithyroid microsomal antibodies declined as pregnancy progressed. Recurrence of transient post-partum hypothyroidism was observed in all five patients who had had transient hypothyroidism following previous pregnancies. Between 1 and 2 months after delivery, three patients showed painless thyroiditis with a hyperthyroid phase, subsequently going through a transient hypothyroid phase. Goitre size increased 1 to 2 months post-partum and antithyroid antibodies also increased after delivery. Studies of peripheral blood lymphocytes in 15 healthy females and 25 patients with auto-immune thyroiditis showed that total lymphocytes and K cells decreased in pregnancy and increased after delivery. The percentage of T-lymphocytes decreased and that of B cells increased 3 to 4 months post-partum (Table 2.5). These data indicated that there were definite immunological changes throughout pregnancy which rebounded following the cessation of pregnancy, and which might account for transient post-partum exacerbation of auto-immune disease.

Walfish and Green (1980) have described three patients who have suffered painless thyroiditis repeatedly in the post-partum interval of two to three pregnancies. These patients all showed the typical features of painless thyroiditis, with a hyperthyroid phase and a very depressed radioactive iodine uptake, going on to recovery in each instance. Needle biopsy in one patient during the active stage showed lymphocytic thyroiditis. Walfish and Green have suggested that these recurrent post-partum disorders might represent an auto-immune process.

It may well be that painless ("silent") thyroiditis (subacute lymphocytic thyroiditis) may be clinically and pathologically homogeneous, but aetiologically heterogeneous. It is entirely possible that those cases that are *not* associated with pregnancy have *no* auto-immune basis, as has been propounded above ("Relationship of painless ('silent') subacute lymphocytic thyroiditis to chronic auto-immune thyroiditis"). On the other hand, it seems probable that those patients who suffer recurrent painless thyroiditis following pregnancy may belong to a different category, and may well be due to the transient rebound of auto-immune processes following cessation of pregnancy, as suggested by Amino et al. (1977 a, b, 1978, 1980). The precise aetiology of this condition remains to be precisely clarified, but it certainly seems that those patients with true Graves' disease or auto-immune thyroiditis following pregnancy fit into this sequence.

Table 2.5. Number of T-lymphocytes, B-lymphocytes and "killer" cells in normal pregnancy and during the pregnancy of patients with auto-immune thyroiditis (Amino et al. 1980)

	Controls	Auto-immune thyroiditis		
		Non-pregnancy	Pregnancy	Postpartum
Lymphocytes/mm^3	1632 ± 279	2042 ± 634	1229 ± 154^b	1920 ± 395
T cells %	79.9 ± 4.2	79.1 ± 6.7	80.6 ± 4.1	66.7 ± 8.4^b
B cells %	18.3 ± 5.6	21.2 ± 5.7	21.1 ± 2.8	27.9 ± 10.6^a
K cells %	6.0 ± 1.6	6.9 ± 2.5	3.1 ± 1.0^b	6.3 ± 1.4

Difference from controls at $P < 0.02$ ^{a} and $P < 0.001$ ^{b}

2.2.9.2 Passive Transfer of Antibodies to the Foetus

Another element to be considered is the passive transfer of thyroid auto-antibodies and thyroid-stimulating immunoglobulin to the foetus, since IgG passes the placental barrier readily. While thyroid auto-antibodies might produce transient, mild hypothyroidism in the newborn, there is no evidence that they cause permanent hypothyroidism or any long-term effects on the children born to mothers with Hashimoto's thyroiditis (Parker and Beierwaltes 1961). Similar negative findings have been observed in experimental thyroiditis (Chandler et al. 1962). On the other hand, however, the passage of thyroid-stimulating antibody across the placenta, if present in large enough titre, will certainly produce passive transfer of neonatal Graves' disease (Dirmikis and Munro 1974, 1975; McKenzie and Zakarija 1977, 1978). The higher the titre of thyroid-stimulating antibody in the mother's circulation, the more likely will the baby suffer neonatal Graves' disease. This may last several weeks while the IgG gradually disappears from the infant's circulation and it can be a hazard to life if not recognized and treated. If, on the other hand, TSAb is present in low titre in the mother's circulation, then the infants will generally be born normal.

Thus, propylthiouracil given to a hyperthyroid mother during her pregnancy will treat not only her hyperthyroidism, but may also be treating foetal Graves' disease at the same time, since this drug also crosses the placental barrier. This also creates some diagnostic difficulties following birth, since such babies may be born normal, but may develop hyperthyroidism when the drug effects wear off (Mujtaba and Burrow 1975). Conversely, mothers who have had treatment for Graves' disease years earlier may sometimes still harbour high titres of TSAb, despite the fact that they themselves are completely normal (or have hypothyroidism treated by thyroxine therapy). Thus, it is possible to have foetal or neonatal Graves' disease with a mother who is not then hyperthyroid. In other instances, mothers with high levels of TSAb may be euthyroid or hypothyroid (because of coexisiting autoimmune thyroiditis) *without* any history of hyperthyroidism (with the possible consequence of passive transfer neonatal Graves' disease) (Liddle et al. 1965; Blackett et al. 1978). This raises the question of administering thionamides in low doses to such women during the latter part of their pregnancy, not of course to treat the woman herself, but to prevent foetal and early neonatal hyperthyroidism, which may otherwise be a very severe hazard for the foetus at risk.

2.2.10 The Effect of Pharmacological Agents, Thyroidectomy and Radioactive Iodine on the Immunological Stigmata of Graves' and Hashimoto's Diseases

2.2.10.1 Excessive Iodine Intake

Beierwaltes (1969) has suggested that the marked increased incidence of Hashimoto's thyroiditis observed over the past two generations has been due, at least in part, to the increase in the intake of iodine that has occurred during the interval. Indeed, in countries where iodine deficiency exists, Hashimoto's thyroiditis is rare (Asamer et al. 1968; Headington and Tantajumroom 1967). Moreover, excessive iodide intake will precipitate spontaneous thyroiditis in a genetically predisposed strain of beagles (Evans et al. 1969). In man, there seems no doubt that iodine administration can unmask occult Hashimoto's thyroiditis, and make it clinically obvious (Braverman et al. 1971; Fisher and Beall 1976; Okamura et al.

1978). Indeed, iodide-induced goitre and myxoedema occurring in apparently normal persons has been shown to be based frequently on clinically occult auto-immune thyroid disease (Fisher and Beall 1976; Braverman et al. 1971). While Okamura et al. (1978) have suggested that the iodine might act by producing thyroidal tissue damage, leading to antigenic stimulation, the fact that the iodide-induced effects are reversible, coupled with the lack of evidence for antigenic abnormalities in auto-immune thyroid diseases (see above), makes it seem likely that the iodide exerts its effect by virtue of a prolonged Wolff-Chaikoff effect (Nagataki 1979). However, how this effect would increase lymphocytic infiltration and antibody production (Okamura et al. 1978) is unclear. Incidentally, the Wolff-Chaikoff effect is similarly very sensitive in response to an increased iodine intake in Graves' disease (Nagataki 1979).

2.2.10.2 Thyroid Hormone Therapy

Thyroid hormone therapy (generally in the form of thyroxine) for the treatment of Hashimoto's thyroiditis may have long-term effects on thyroid antibodies. Those patients with a raised TSH level generally respond most rapidly, the goitre regresses in size, and the microsomal antibody titres fall concurrently; antithyroglobulin antibody levels fall more slowly (Doniach 1975). However, in those patients who manifest partial regression or no regression of the goitre despite appropriate thyroxine therapy, the antibodies persist indefinitely (Doniach 1975). Indeed, when goitres persist and can be biopsied, no discernible histological change can be found in sequential sections during long-term thyroxine therapy (Ling et al. 1969; Vickery and Hamlin 1961). In studies by Okita et al. (1980a) of MIF production by isolated preparations of T-lymphocytes in response to thyroid antigen, the results remained positive years after the thyroid antibodies had disappeared in patients taking long-term thyroxine for Hashimoto's thyroiditis. This was also true in patients with atrophic thyroiditis, in whom about 25% lose their antibodies after long-standing disease or treatment (Doniach 1975), yet their T-lymphocytes also retain their ability to produce MIF in response to thyroid antigen (Okita et al. 1980a). Thus, there appears to be a discrepancy between the manifestations of humoral immunity (which seem to subside in some cases with time and/or thyroxine therapy) and cellular immunity (i.e. the presence of sensitized T-lymphocytes) which persists.

Incidentally, the ingestion of thyroid hormone has occasionally precipitated Graves' disease (Cooper et al. 1978; Dymling and Becker 1967). This may well be related to the effect of increased thyroid hormone concentrations on the immune system (see section on "Evidence for a defect in suppressor T-lymphocyte function" above). In any event, it will be the subject of discussion below (see: "The role of stress in the induction of Graves' disease").

2.2.10.3 Corticosteroid Therapy

Corticosteroid therapy in Hashimoto's thyroiditis will result in regression of the goitre and lowering of the antibody titre, but of course this will not outlast the treatment (Blizzard et al. 1962; Ito et al. 1968). It is thus of no practical importance as therapy, as it cannot compete with the advantages of thyroxine therapy (suppressive *and* replacement) and thus is of theoretical interest only.

Corticosteroids in large dosage will also suppress the production of TSAb and clinical manifestations in Graves' disease (Werner and Platman 1965). However, in small amounts, it not only may *not* be of value, but may even serve to *precipitate* Graves' disease (Lamberg 1964; Brown and Lowman 1964). This will be discussed below in Sect. 2.2.11.

2.2.10.4 Effects of Radioactive Iodine (^{131}I) *Therapy for Graves' Disease*

Radioactive iodine (^{131}I) has been utilized as an effective means of ablating the thyroid of Graves' disease for over three decades, and is thus one of the major treatment modalities for this disorder. Its most common complication has been that of post-^{131}I hypothyroidism, either occurring shortly after treatment, or at a much later time (Braverman 1978). Hypothyroidism that occurs quickly is clearly due to direct dose-dependent thyroid destruction by the irradiation (Lamberg 1979), while hypothyroidism that occurs later is due to more complex causes (Malone and Cullen 1976). One such mechanism may result from a delayed effect of the radiation on the ability of the thyroid cells to replicate, while another may be the effect of continuing (and even aggravated) auto-immune processes (see below). It has been noted that those hyperthyroid patients with high titres of thyroid auto-antibodies prior to ^{131}I therapy are much more prone to develop post-treatment hypothyroidism (Lundell and Jonnson 1973). Moreover, there is also a spontaneous progression to auto-immune thyroid failure even without thyroid destructive therapy (Wood and Maloof 1975; Wood and Ingbar 1979). Thus, this natural process may be aggravated and quickened by the ^{131}I treatment. Conversely, it is a common clinical experience that those patients with very high titres of LATS (and TSAb) (and with large goitres) are quite resistant to ^{131}I, and may require much larger doses for cure of the disease (McKenzie et al. 1978).

The increased concentrations of thyroid-stimulating immunoglobulins and thyroid auto-antibodies observed after ^{131}I therapy have generally been attributed to the response of already sensitized lymphocytes to components of thyroid cells (i. e. antigenic stimulation), which are released as a result of the radiation damage (Pinchera et al. 1965; Kriss et al. 1967; Mukhtar et al. 1975; Mori and Kriss 1971; Fenzi et al. 1979). (see Figs. 2.15, 2.16) Indeed, radiation therapy in the region of the thyroid for nonthyroidal malignant disease has resulted in the development of Graves' hyperthyroidism or ophthalmopathy alone (Wasnich et al. 1973; Pilepich et al. 1978; Jackson et al. 1979) or hypothyroidism (Glatstein et al. 1971; Schimpff et al. 1980). This seemed to fit with the notion that thyroidal antigenic change, induced by radiation, could not only stimulate *already* sensitized lymphocytes (and thus aggravate the pre-existing immune process) but also, in a similar fashion, initiate the disease. However, these authors had not taken into consideration the possibility that the radiation was affecting not only the thyroid parenchymal cells (or even primarily those cells), but also the lymphoid system. The external radiation may have damaged the thymus (which was in the area of treatment) and the ^{131}I could have affected lymphocytes within the thyroid gland (McGregor et al. 1979 c). These effects may have been to reduce suppressor T-lymphocyte activity, thus permitting helper T-lymphocytes to function more vigorously (hence augmenting auto-antibody production). The recent studies of McGregor et al. (1979 b) on the effects of irradiating lymphocytes (see Sect. 2.2.3.7) are in accord with this view. McGregor et al. (1979 c) in further supporting this view noted that patients with toxic nodular goitre treated with ^{131}I did not develop thyroid auto-antibodies or thyroid-stimulating immunoglobulin.

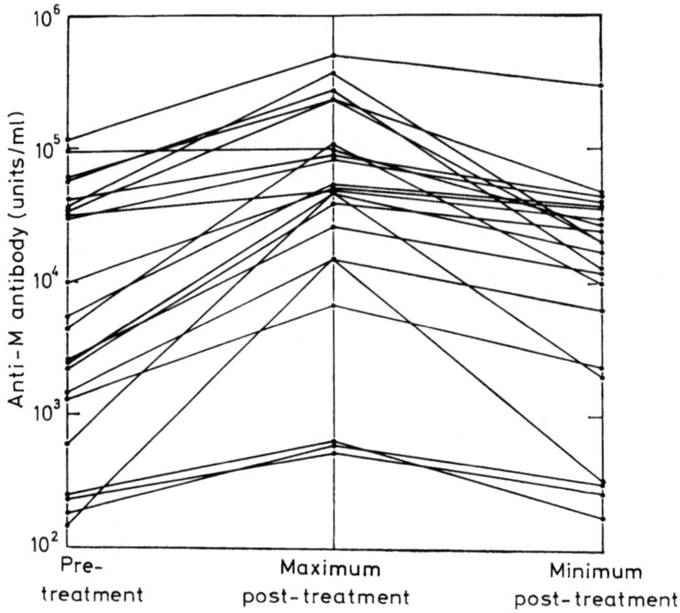

Fig. 2.15. Antimicrosomal antibodies have been shown to rise after radioactive iodine therapy, and fall thereafter. (Mori and Kriss 1971)

Often in a later period, when patients are euthyroid or hypothyroid following ^{131}I therapy, thyroid-stimulating antibodies and other thyroid auto-antibodies disappear in many, but not all, patients (McKenzie et al. 1978). The disappearance might be due to one or more of the five possible factors: (1) complete disappearance of all thyroid antigen (a difficult feat) may allow the interacting lymphocyte population to decline; (2) the effect of radiation on the suppressor T-lymphocytes may disappear and those suppressor T-lymphocytes may be gradually restored to their previous function; (3) the effect of the excessive levels of thyroid hormone on lymphocyte function should disappear when the patient reaches a euthyroid state (see Sect. 2.2.4.5); (4) the effect of "stress" on the immune system may be overcome as the initial precipitating stress fades into the background; (5) the effect of the self-perpetuating stress of the illness itself may subside as the patient achieves a euthyroid state (see Sects. 2.2.11, 2.2.12).

2.2.10.5 The Effect of Subtotal Thyroidectomy in Graves' Disease on the Immunological Disturbance

Hedley et al. (1971) suggested that the benefits derived from subtotal thyroidectomy in bringing about a cure for Graves' disease may be due, at least in part, to an amelioration of the auto-immune process. He based this proposal on the observation that LATS levels were generally much lower following thyroidectomy. Indeed, Mukhtar et al. (1975), studying the effect of various forms of management on the levels of TBII, found that TBII fell dramatically following such surgery in most of the cases. This dramatic drop in TBII levels did not occur in all instances (Hall 1980), but when present has been attributed to removal of most of the thyroid lymphocytes (which may comprise the vast majority of the sensitized lymphocytes

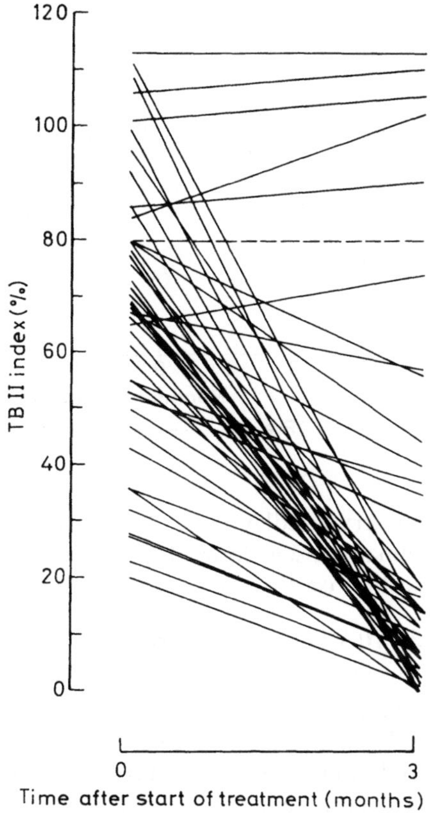

Fig. 2.16. Radioligand assay results for the antibody which binds to the thyroid cell membranes and prevents the binding of TSH (TBII activity), after ^{131}I therapy for Graves' disease. Note that the TBII activity is depicted on this graph in an opposite manner to that depicted in Fig. 2.3, i.e. positive results are *lower* than 80, negative results are greater than 80. Thus there is a rise in TBII activity in the first 3 months after radioactive iodine therapy. (McGregor et al. 1979c)

in this condition), rather than removal of most of the antigen. Antithyroglobulin antibodies also decrease rapidly post-operatively (Feldt-Rasmussen et al. 1980); the rapid decline in TBII and thyroid auto-antibodies might be due to immune complex formation, due to sudden surgically-induced release of large amounts of antigen, then complexing with the available antibody. Teng et al. (1980) have recently shown that TBII, if present just prior to surgery, often does not fall; only 5 of 12 such patients became TBII negative following surgery, and this change was not immediate (Fig. 2.17). Moreover, Wilkin et al. (1980) could not show a clear relationship between the titres of thyroid auto-antibodies with the surgical treatment, showing only wide fluctuations of antibody levels. The incidence of hypothyroidism following subtotal thyroidectomy seems to be closely related to the weight of the thyroid gland remnant (Michie et al. 1972). However, there is also evidence that post-operative hypothyroidism is additionally related to the abundance of plasma cells, lymphoid follicles and germinal centres in the thyroid tissue (Van Welsum et al. 1974) and to circulating thyroid antibodies (Lamberg 1979). The late development of hypothyroidism years after surgery (Nofal et al. 1966) may be related to such factors. In others, however, the lack of TBII (or TSI) stimulation of a small remnant may contribute to the development of hypothyroidism (Teng et al. 1980). On the other hand, the persistence or recurrence of hyperthyroidism is associated with the persistance or reappearance of thyroid-stimulating immunoglobulin; recurrent hyperthyroidism occurs in 2%–30% of patients undergoing

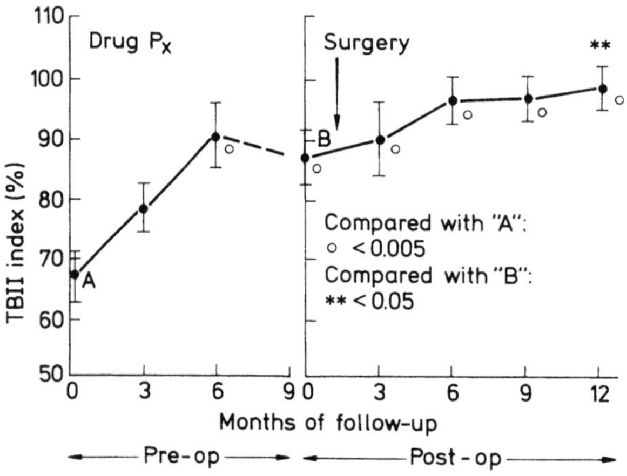

Fig. 2.17. Change in the mean ± SD TBII index with time before and after subtotal thyroidectomy. Note that these values are expressed similarly to those noted in Fig. 2.16. There was a gradual return towards normal of these values following subtotal thyroidectomy in these patients. (Teng et al. 1980b)

surgery (Hedley et al. 1971). On the other hand, if all immunological stigmata remain absent long after the thyroidectomy, the factors noted at the end of the section on ^{131}I may be invoked.

2.2.10.6 Antithyroid Drug Therapy: Effects on Immune System

The pharmacological effects of antithyroid drugs (particularly propylthiouracil and methimazole) have been the subject of recent reviews (Greer 1980; Marchant et al. 1979; Braverman 1978). Put simply, both agents block the organification of iodide, and interfere with iodotyrosine coupling. Propylthiouracil additionally interferes with peripheral conversion of thyroxine to tri-iodothyronine. Thus, the direct effect of these drugs is to reduce thyroid function in hyperthyroidism.

However, antithyroid drugs also bring about effects on the immune manifestations which are both direct and indirect. Long-term antithyroid drug therapy will cause the lymphocytes within the thyroid gland to decline in number, or to disappear altogether (Beck, to be published). Furthermore, Pinchera et al. (1969, 1979) have noted a decline in LATS activity and in the thyroid auto-antibodies in many patients with Graves' disease during the course of antithyroid drug therapy (Fig. 2.18). Using TBII or TSAb assays, similar results have been recently reported by Mukhtar et al. 1975; Hall et al. 1975; Davies et al. 1977; O'Donnell et al. 1978; McKenzie et al. 1978; Sugenoya et al. 1979b; Fenzi et al. 1979; Teng and Yeung 1980; Docter et al. 1980; Kuzuya et al. 1979 (Fig. 2.19). In these various series, there was a trend towards normalization of the results beginning as early as 1 month after the initiation of therapy. However, in all series there were many patients who were resistant to any significant decline in their values, although this proportion varied from 16% (Teng and Yeung 1980) to 50% (McKenzie et al. 1978). Similar observations have been made with respect to evidence of cell-mediated immunity, using the MIF procedure (Farid et al. 1973; Okita et al. 1980a, b).

Since there is evidence that the antithyroid drugs are weakly immunosuppressive (Wall et al. 1976b; McGregor et al. 1980a; Hallengren et al. 1980), McGregor et al. (1980a) have suggested that this effect might account for the decline in TSAb and thyroid auto-antibody titres. However, such an explanation would not cover those patients who manifest no such decline, although their thyroid hyperactivity may be

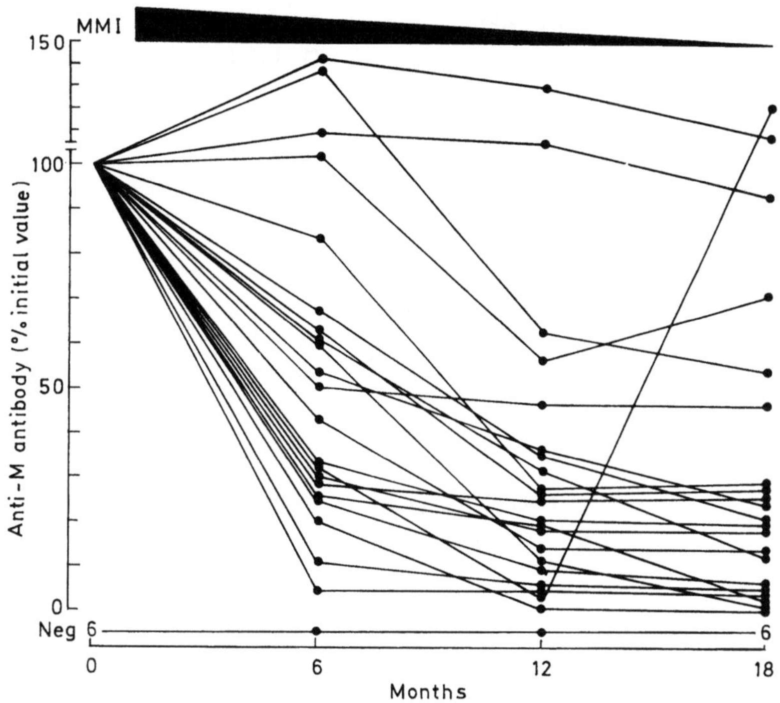

Fig. 2.18. Effect of antithyroid drug therapy on circulating antimicrosomal antibodies in 27 patients with Graves' disease. The measurement of antimicrosomal antibodies was performed by radioassay, and results are expressed as a percent of the initial value. For convenience, the six patients who had initially low (less than 75 units/ml) or undetectable antibody levels were grouped together and considered separately as "negative" (Neg). *MMI*, methimazole

similarly well-controlled. Moreover, it would not suffice to explain the long-term remissions which may persist following cessation of such therapy, since the pharmacological and immunological effects would not persist after the drug was discontinued. While not ruling out such an effect, the author feels that it is more likely that normalization of the thyroid status is a more important element in favourably influencing the immunological disturbance in appropriately susceptible patients. The effects of excessive thyroid hormone concentrations on the immune system have been dealt with above (see Sect. 2.2.4.5), and the reversal of that direct influence, as well as of indirect effects on the immune system of hyperthyroid-induced adrenocortical alterations, will be discussed below (see Sects. 2.2.11, 2.2.12)

In most of the above reported series, the experience was that if a patient was still TBII or TSAb positive after prolonged antithyroid drug therapy (despite a euthyroid state while on the medication), then cessation of the drug was virtually always associated with almost immediate recurrence (O'Donnell et al. 1978; McKenzie et al. 1978; Teng and Yeung 1980; McGregor et al. 1980b). When TSAb remained in the normal range, remissions were usually maintained, although some patients in this group will relapse (Teng and Yeung 1980). Certainly if a TSAb-negative patient subsequently converts to positive, relapse will follow (Teng and Yeung 1980). Thus, these tests are of some value for predicting remission, but the

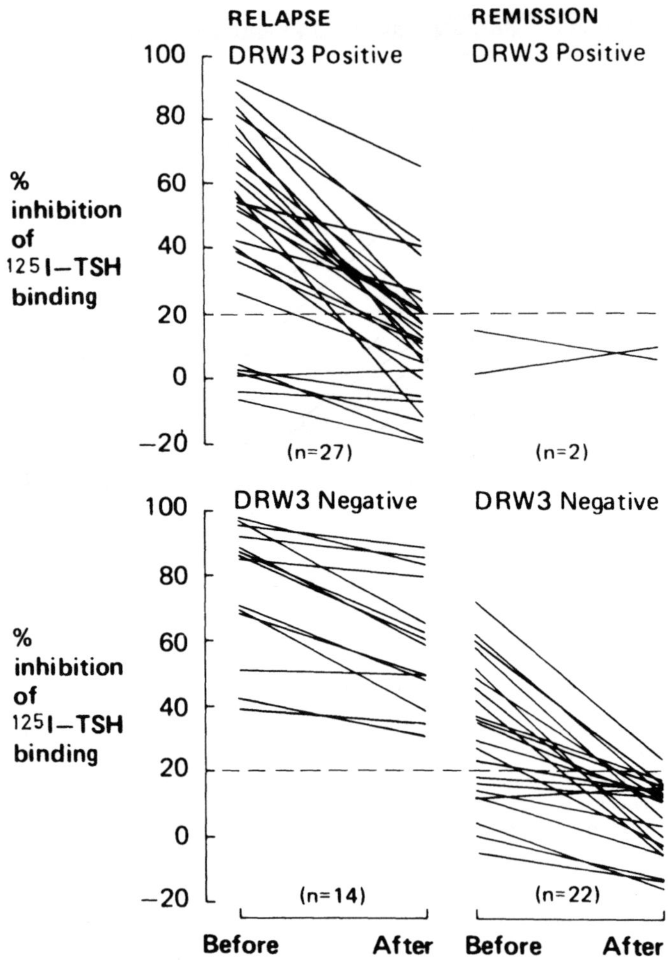

Fig. 2.19. TBII activity immediately prior to and immediately after commencement of antithyroid drug therapy in 40 patients treated with antithyroid drug therapy for hyperthyroid Graves' disease. Values depicted in the same manner as in Figs. 2.16 and 2.17. (McGregor et al. 1979 c)

value of the procedure seems to vary from laboratory to laboratory. (A notable exception was the study of Docter et al. (1980), which did not find the TBII to be of predictive value.)

Van der Heide et al (1980) have recently reported that when TBII declines during the course of antithyroid drug therapy, immune complexes rise (i. e. there is an inverse relationship between TBII and immune complexes). They have thus suggested that the immune complexes may involve thyroid-stimulating immunoglobulin, which may be rendered biologically ineffective by virtue of its complexed state, and thus may contribute to the remission. While this suggestion might account for some of the remissions, in others all evidence of humoral and cell-mediated immunity clears, and these appear to represent a true immunological remission, as will be discussed below.

McGregor et al. (1980 b) have confirmed the observation of Bech et al. (1977 c) that those patients with Graves' disease with HLA-DRw3 are very much more likely to relapse after cessation of antithyroid drug therapy, when compared to those who are negative for this gene (Table 2.6). Of their patients in remission following such treatment (13 out of 40 patients), none was positive for HLA-DRw3, and all showed a fall in TBII. Of the 27 patients in their study who relapsed, 22 (81%) were HLA-DRw3 positive, and the remaining five had persistent elevation of TBII activity at cessation of therapy. This group concluded that analysis of these two indices allowed prediction of relapse.

The relationships of remissions to the HLA-B and D genes will be further discussed below (see Sect. 2.2.12).

2.2.10.7 Propranolol or Other Beta Adrenergic-Blocking Agents

The role of such blocking agents has been amply reviewed by Levey (1979). Suffice it here to say that propranolol only relieves those clinical manifestations of thyrotoxicosis which have a beta adrenergic component, and has no direct effect on intrathyroidal iodine metabolism. There is some evidence, however, that the conversion of thyroxine to tri-iodothyronine is partially blocked (Verhoeven et al. 1974). However, most observers do not note any effect on thyroid function tests with this agent (Levey 1979). Nevertheless, the use of this agent can bring about remissions of thyrotoxicosis in about 20% of such patients (McLarty et al. 1973). Since this effect is not derived either from the metabolic control of the hyperthyroidism, or from any immunosuppressive effect, then clearly the remission must occur as the result of other factors. Since there is usually symptomatic benefit from such agents (Levey 1979), it may well be that the non-specific effect of controlling some of the manifestations of hyperthyroidism may be sufficient to induce remission in appropriate patients. Such induction may be very analogous to the type of remission which may occur spontaneously, and will be the subject of further discussion below.

2.2.11 The Role of Stress in the Induction of Graves' Disease

It is the impression of many experienced clinicians that emotional or physical stress can precipitate Graves' disease (Lidz and Cohn 1971). Actually, the second patient described by Parry (1825) (observed in 1816, but reported in 1825) was a clear example of psychological stress precipitating hyperthyroidism. Charcot and

Table 2.6. The association between HLA-B8 and Dw3 and remissions and relapses after antithyroid drug therapy in patients with Graves' disease (Bech et al. 1977 b)

Patients or controls	HLA-B8		HLA-Dw3		Numbers
	Present	Absent	Present	Absent	
Normals	23.7%	76.3%	21%	79%	
Untreated Graves' disease	40 (47%)	46 (53%)	44 (51%)	42 (49%)	86
Patients with relapse after antithyroid drugs	26 (54%)	22 (46%)	31 (65%)	17 (35%)	48
Patients without relapse	5 (27%)	13 (73%)	6 (33%)	12 (66%)	18

Trousseau also believed the disorder to be a "neurosis of the vegetative nervous system" (quoted by Sattler 1952). Every textbook of endocrinology comments on this point (Werner and Ingbar 1978) and in the author's experience there have been so many patients with Graves' disease who have had their disorder precipitated by specific acute stresses that the conclusion seems almost inescapable, i.e. that in some patients there is a cause and effect relationship between such stresses and the subsequent development of hyperthyroidism. Nevertheless, the evidence for this remains largely anecdotal, and it has not yet been possible to design an impeccable study to prove this association. An apparent epidemic of Graves' disease occurred in Denmark during the Nazi occupation (Iversen 1948). On the other hand, a recent study of Graves' disease during the period of unrest in Northern Ireland compared per capita rates of antithyroid drugs utilized before and after the civil disorders developed in 1968 (Hadder and McDevitt 1974); this study failed to show any increase in the use of antithyroid drug medication following the development of the conflict. Moreover, normal persons studied under stressful situations have generally failed to show any change in thyroid status (Volpé et al. 1960). The problem with all of these observations probably relates to the resistance (in terms of thyroid status) of normal persons to be influenced by such stresses. The appropriate study should be carried out on the population which is genetically predisposed, namely, in families of patients with Graves' disease; such a population should then be compared to an unselected population in response to equivalent stresses.

The mechanism by which stress might precipitate hyperthyroidism is, of course, unknown. One speculation that this effect might be mediated through the hypothalamic-pituitary-thyroid axis (i.e. TRH-TSH) has not been verified. Indeed, TSH in untreated Graves' disease is almost invariably low, with flat responses to TRH (Hershman and Pittman 1971) and florid Graves' disease has occurred in persons following apparent complete hypophysectomy (Furth et al. 1962). Thus, in the hyperthyroidism of Graves' disease, pituitary secretion of TSH is inhibited. When patients become hypothyroid following treatment of hyperthyroidism, TSH becomes increased, i.e. pituitary function seems normal in Graves' disease.

Another alternative and more attractive possibility is that stress may mediate its effect by depressing the lymphoid system (Amkraut and Solomon 1974; Bartrop et al. 1977); this may occur by stimulating the CRH-ACTH-cortisol axis, with its ultimate effects on suppressor T-lymphocytes and immune regulation. The well-known effects of corticosteroids in reducing T-lymphocyte function are in accord with this possibility (Claman 1972; Saxon et al. 1978; Munck et al. 1979). In this context, then, any event which has the capacity to further depress an already partially defective clone of suppressor T-lymphocytes should be able to initiate Graves' disease once the appropriate thyroid-directed clone of helper T-lymphocytes is available and in a state of partial suppression or regulation. The number of possible events which could lead to this situation seems legion. Some patients provide histories of specific physical or psychic trauma, and rigorous dieting is often found as a precipitating factor. Many other patients with Graves' disease give a history of a recent upper respiratory infection, a bout of gastroenteritis, or may have had a specific viral or bacterial infection (Alexander et al. 1968). The few cases of subacute thyroiditis which have gone on subsequently to Graves' disease or auto-immune thyroiditis would also fit into this category (Volpé 1979a; Werner 1979). Indeed, with patients who have developed hyperthyroidism following irradiation to the head and neck region (Wasnich et al. 1973; Wenzel et al. 1974; Pilepich et al. 1978), this sequence may have resulted from irradiation to the thymus (rather than irradiation to the thyroid). Even the administration of excessive amounts of thyroid hormone, which has been reported to induce hyperthyroidism (Dymling and Becker 1967), may have done so through the effect of excessive thyroid hormone concentration on the immunoregulatory mechanisms (see Sect. 2.2.4.5).

In all of these circumstances, the effect of either a slight increase in cortisol, or the direct effect of thyroid hormones or other possible mechanisms, might be to further reduce the regulatory capacity of the already defective specific suppressor T-lymphocytes. Thus, the defect which had been only minimal or partial would be temporarily converted to a complete (but still isolated) defect, rendering it impossible for the particular clone of thyroid-directed helper T-lymphocytes to be suppressed. The latter "forbidden" clone of T-lymphocytes would then initiate the disease in the manner already suggested.

In relation to this possible mechanism, it is of interest that Graves' disease has been initiated in patients taking corticosteroid or immunosuppressive therapy (Brown and Lowman 1964; McDougall et al. 1971). Moreover, one patient with Cushing's syndrome was reported who developed Graves' disease (Lamberg, 1964). (Indeed, there is a case report of a patient with Cushing's syndrome and autoimmune thyroiditis (Peillon et al. 1974).) As corticosteroid therapy in high dosage may suppress Graves' disease (Werner and Platman 1965), it may be difficult to comprehend how it could also precipitate the condition. It may well be that levels of cortisol or immunosuppressive drugs which are required to inhibit the sensitized thyroid-directed helper T-lymphocytes which are basically responsible for producing the lesions and the immunoglobulin production by B-lymphocytes (i.e. doses which would suppress the disease itself) may prove to be much larger than those necessary to suppress those suppressor T-lymphocytes with a partial defect in their functional capacity to begin with. Excessive concentrations of thyroid hormone may act directly on the immunoregulatory mechanisms, or indirectly by means of affecting adrenocortical metabolism.

Thus, once the hyperthyroidism has been initiated, it may well be that it perpetuates itself, only remitting when interrupted by specific or non-specific therapy. Thus, excessive thyroid hormone concentration may be seen by the organism as a "stress"; indeed, in hyperthyroidism there are increased cortisol secretion rates and increased adrenocortical size (Gallagher et al. 1972; Ferrari et al. 1974; Komaromi 1965; Kenny et al. 1967). Such effects may serve to continue to reduce suppressor T-lymphocyte function and perpetuate the disease, as previously discussed. Moreover, evidence has been presented at length above with respect to the possible effect of excessive concentrations of thyroid hormone on reducing suppressor T-lymphocyte function, although whether this is a direct or indirect effect is not clear. Nevertheless, the net effect is to allow the disease to continue.

2.2.12 The Nature of the Remissions

Even in early accounts of Graves' (Basedow's) disease, it was recognized that the disorder was one of remissions and exacerbations (Sattler 1952). Indeed, remissions also occur in Hashimoto's thyroiditis not uncommonly (Rallison et al. 1975;

Yamamoto and Sakamoto 1978). However, the nature of such remissions has been unclear heretofore and only recently has it been possible to at least formulate an hypothesis.

It is clear that in Graves' disease there may be several forms of clinical remission (Buerklin et al. 1976). One may be due to ^{131}I ablation or surgical removal of sufficient tissue to prevent recurrence by virtue of an insufficient thyroid remnant. However, even without such destructive therapy, continuing spontaneous thyroid damage may bring about remission, probably a result of a continuing immunological process (Wood and Maloff 1975; Wood and Ingbar 1979). Other possibilities, in the context of continuing immune processes, include the alteration of a TSAb to another, non-stimulating form of TBII, even with TSH blocking propensities as described by Endo et al. (1978) and Konishi et al. (1980). This sequence of events has not been proven as yet, so that there is little point in further speculation. Another possibility, suggested by Van der Heide et al. (1980) and Feldt-Rassmussen et al. (1980), is that immune complexes may arise which interfere with the ability of the antibody to produce its effects.

Another important form of remission is one in which all immunological stigmata of the disease disappear, including thyroid antibodies (Pinchera et al. 1979), TBII (Mukhtar et al. 1975; Fenzi et al. 1979; Teng and Yeung 1980; O'Donnell et al. 1978; McGregor et al. 1979 c, 1980 b), TSAb (McKenzie et al. 1978) and evidence of sensitization of T-lymphocytes (Okita et al. 1980 a and 1981 a, b). It seems possible that this form of remission can only occur in those patients with a *partial* defect in immunoregulation, i.e. a defect susceptible to further depression by "stress" (presumably by mechanisms described above) and which is therefore reversible when that circumstance is overcome. The restoration of a euthyroid state by whatever means (antithyroid drugs, ^{131}I, or surgery) should relieve this situation, since the effects of excessive thyroid hormones themselves directly on the immune system (see Sects. 2.2.4.5, 2.2.11), as well as the indirect effects on the adrenocortical system (see above), would be reversed under these circumstances. As well, social factors, rest, the passage of time, the clearing of infection, sedation and other non-specific measures, such as propranolol, would each serve to reduce "stress", thus allowing the partially defective immunoregulatory system to be restored to its previous functional capacity; thus, the thyroid-directed "forbidden" clone of helper T-lymphocytes would again be suppressed, and the disease would go into immunological remission. Such mechanisms could also account for the spontaneous remissions which were observed long before any specific therapy became available (Sattler 1952). Of course, such patients would be prone to recurrence if similar "stressful" events were experienced later. Stress in this sense is used in a biological (immunological) sense, rather than an emotional sense. What is required to prove this is some sensitive means of measuring suppressor function in response to such events in the appropriate genetically predisposed persons.

Those persons with a presumed *complete* defect would not be expected to go into *immunological* remission, no matter how long his/her antithyroid drug was continued, or no matter what form of therapy was employed. Only those remissions associated with continuing immunological activity directed to the thyroid and/or thyroid destruction would occur in this group. This would be in accord with the continuing evidence of humoral and cell-mediated immunity in some patients following antithyroid or other forms of therapy.

There is some genetic evidence, already mentioned above, which is consistent with this concept. Irvine et al. (1977 a) have shown that those patients with Graves' disease who lack HLA-B8 are more likely to go into remission, whereas those patients positive for HLA-B8 are likely to relapse. Similarly, Bech et al. (1977 c) have shown that the presence of HLA-Dw3 is found in significantly higher numbers in those who relapse, and conversely is much lower in incidence in those who remit (see Fig. 2.7). This finding has been confirmed by McGregor et al. (1980 b). Thus, there appears to be a genetic basis for the ability to remit (or relapse), which is also consistent with the hypothesis for remission advanced above. Those with the presumed complete defect in immunoregulation are more closely linked to HLA-Dw3, when compared to those who have only a partial defect and hence the possibility to have an immunological remission.

2.2.13 The Pathogenesis of Ophthalmopathy

The ophthalmopathy of Graves' disease is a curious disorder which is still of unknown aetiology. This condition has been extensively reviewed by Gorman (1978), and by Wall et al. (1981). It may precede, accompany, or follow hyperthyroidism (Bartels and Irie 1961), but the vast majority of patients with exophthalmos will manifest hyperthyroidism sooner or later (Schultz et al. 1960) (see Table 2.7). About 5% of patients with definite "Graves' ophthalmopathy" have no such past or present history of hyperthyroidism (Mornex et al. 1975). Ophthalmopathy has also occurred in association with Hashimoto's thyroiditis (Cathelineau and Fribourg-Desi 1974; Wyse et al. 1968) and with primary hypothyroidism (Brownlie et al. 1975). It has also occurred following irradiation of the neck region (Wenzel et al. 1974; Wasnick et al. 1973; Jackson et al. 1979). However, there may be no *clinical* evidence of thyroid disease in some patients with "euthyroid ophthalmic Graves' disease" (or "endocrine exophthalmos"); in these, careful laboratory testing may reveal some thyroid abnormality, such as lack of thyroid suppressibility to exogenous tri-iodothyronine (the T3 suppression test), lack of adequate TSH response to TRH (or conversely high basal TSH levels), lack of adequate thyroidal response to TSH, or the presence of thyroid antibodies (Gorman 1978). Finally, there is still a small group with exopthalmos with no clinical *or laboratory* evidence of thyroid disease whatsoever (Hall et al. 1970; Munro et al. 1973; Mornex et al. 1975; Solomon et al. 1977). Any theory for the pathogenesis of exophthalmos must take into account this latter group (see below).

Table 2.7. Relationship of onset of exophthalmos to the presence of hyperthyroidism. (Bartels and Irie 1961)

Temporal relationship	No. of patients
Before hyperthyroidism	9
Simultaneously with hyperthyroidism	48
After hyperthyroidism established	32
After hyperthyroidism treated	23
Unassociated with hyperthyroidism	5
	117 Total

Conversely, it should be noted that not all patients with Graves' disease develop exophthalmos. Although this statement may be obvious from clinical observation, the advent of computerized axial tomographic (C.A.T.) scanning and ultrasound examinations has indicated the condition may often be present despite lack of clinical findings (Gorman 1978). In an ultrasonograph study by Forrester et al. (1977), 63% of patients with Graves' disease without clinical eye signs had ultrasound evidence of ocular muscle involvement. Nevertheless, even this study leaves a residual 37% of such patients who do not appear to have any evidence whatsoever of exophthalmos. Thus, any theory will also have to account for the *absence* of exophthalmos in some patients with Graves' disease, as well as the temporal variation in the onset of exophthalmos in relation to the hyperthyroidism itself. It will thus be necessary to explain how exophthalmos can either predate or postdate the hyperthyroidism by months or years (see Table 2.7).

The pathology of the orbits in Graves' ophthalmopathy has been carefully studied, and reviewed by Gorman (1978). The average volume of the orbital cavity is 26 mm and in normals 70% of this is occupied by retrobulbar and peribulbar structures. The average weight of these structures is 18.9 grams, which is made up of 2.2 grams of eye muscles, 0.65 grams of lacrimal gland, and 15 grams of fibro-fatty residue. Of the last named, about 12 grams is recognizable as fat, 2.5 grams as Tenon's capsule, and 0.6 grams as nerves and blood vessels (Rundle and Pochin 1944). The degree of proptosis is simply determined by the amount of orbital tissues and the extent to which they fill the orbital cavity. Rundle and Pochin have shown that the fat content of extraocular muscles was increased absolutely in patients with exophthalmos. Doniach and Florin Christensen (1975) have shown that the extraocular muscles are involved with an inflammatory process, including lymphocytic infiltration, and muscle necrosis, followed by fibrosis in the late stages. As with Rundle and Ponchin (1944), Doniach and Florin Christensen also demonstrated proliferation of retro-orbital fat and connective tissues. However, the muscle volume may be increased eight to ten times that of normal (McDougall and Kriss 1979).

Kroll and Kuwabara (1966) have demonstrated a marked inflammatory infiltrate in the extraocular muscles consisting of not only large numbers of lymphocytes, but plasma cells, mast cells and macrophages. The inflammatory collections are perivascular and in some situations are like lymph follicles with germinal centres. Occasionally, the chronic inflammatory cells are distributed diffusely throughout the extraocular muscles. Histological examination of the muscle cells may reveal no abnormalities, even on electron-microscopy, but in severe cases, there may be disruption of the myofibrillar striations and prominent cellular vacuolations. Riley (1972) has shown an increase in the concentration of hydrophylic intercellular mucopolysaccharides, which probably contributes to some of the local oedema (Kroll and Kuwabara 1966; Riley 1972). These lesions when combined yield the clinical manifestations of proptosis, periorbital oedema and diplopia.

Despite the apparently immune nature of the lesions of exophthalmos, the precise pathogenesis of exophthalmos remains controversial and unclear. The most interesting group of patients to study in this respect are those patients with "euthyroid endocrine exophthalmos", who have no clinical evidence of overt thyroid disease. These patients are usually termed euthyroid ophthalmic Graves' disease. Immunological testing of thyroid gland function in many of these patients may show evidence of some minimal thyroid dysfunction (see above). TBII or TSAb may be present or absent in patients with ophthalmopathy who are clinically euthyroid; if present, this is clear evidence of auto-immune thyroid disease, and may be accompanied by other evidence, such as antithyroglobulin or antimicrosomal antibodies, non-suppressibility of thyroid function with T3, or an abnormal TSH response to thyrotropin-releasing hormone (TRH) (O'Donnell et al. 1978; Teng et al. 1977; Solomon et al. 1977; Wall et al. 1979 b). Patients who are negative for TBII or TSAb may have clinical Hashimoto's thyroiditis (with or without hypothyroidism), may have occult auto-immune thyroid disease with thyroid antibodies, *or may lack all evidence of a thyroid disorder, no matter how tested.*

Studies of cell-mediated immunity in exophthalmos are of interest. Whole leucocyte preparations from patients with both ocular and thyroidal auto-immune disease will exhibit MIF activity in response to retro-orbital muscle antigen and thyroid antigen. Those patients with thyroid disease alone usually have a positive test with thyroid antigen, but negative with retro-orbital muscle antigen. Conversely, if the patient with ophthalmopathy is devoid of any evidence of thyroid disease, MIF will be found only for retro-orbital muscle antigen (Munro et al. 1973) (see Figs. 2.20 and 2.21).

Moreover, there is some evidence that immunoglobulins have a role in exophthalmos; the serum of some patients with exophthalmos can cause the lesion experimentally (Etienne et al. 1976). Others have shown co-operation between antibodies and lymphocytes in the production of exophthalmos (Fakhri and Hobbs 1972). Most recently, plasmapheresis has been used to successfully treat one patient with rapidly progressive exophthalmos and coincident dermopathy improved as well (Dandona et al. 1979). Early reports that total removal of thyroid tissue (i. e. thyroid antigen) would result in improvement of the Graves' oculopathy (Catz and Persik 1965) have not been confirmed (Volpé et al. 1969; Gorman 1978).

Wall et al. (1978) have shown the presence of peripheral blood lymphocyte transformation in response to human lacrimal extract or to a membrane fraction of human lacrimal extract in many patients with Graves' ophthalmopathy. They have therefore speculated about a possible significance of lacrimal gland inflammation and a role for the lacrimal gland in the pathogenesis of Graves' ophthalmopathy, suggesting that immune reactions against orbital antigens may emanate from the lacrimal and salivary tissues via lymphocytes selectively attracted by antigenic or non-antigenic mechanisms. It should be conceded that Wall et al. (1979 b) were unable to show significant titres of serum antibodies against human eye muscle extract or subcellular fractions or macrophage inhibitory factor production in response to human orbital tissue in patients with eye disease.

From these studies of cell-mediated and humoral immunity (although clearly there are some discrepancies), it seems likely that Graves' disease and endocrine ophthalmopathy are closely related, but distinct and separable, organ-specific auto-immune diseases, as proposed by our group (Munro et al. 1973). There does not appear to be a separate HLA marker for this disorder (Bech et al. 1977 c).

Other theories for the pathogenesis of exophthalmos have been proposed. Kohn and Winand (1971) have suggested that TSH or fragments of TSH may be important aetiological factors. Although TSH has been shown to be exophthalmogenic in animal studies (Kohn and Winand 1971), there is really no evidence to suggest an aetiological role in man. On the contrary, TSH is reduced (Hershman

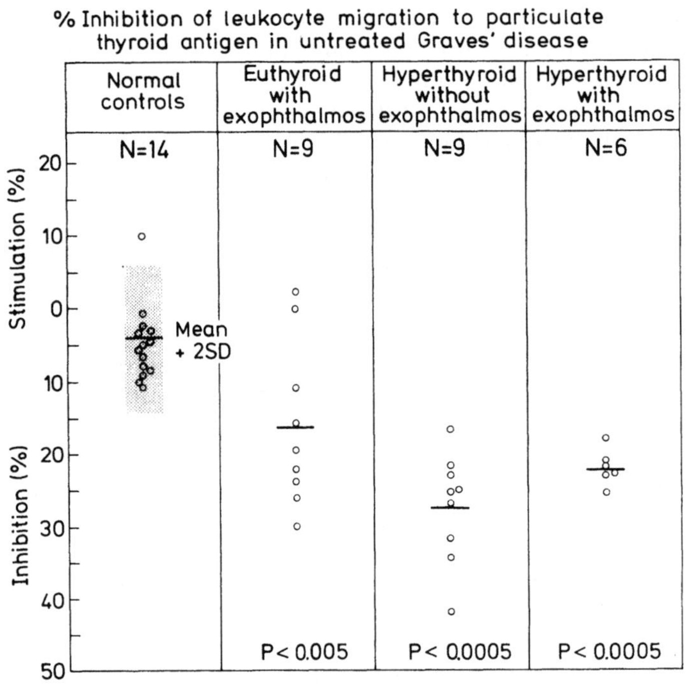

Fig. 2.20. Leucocyte inhibition factor (LIF) test in patients with Graves' disease with or without exophthalmos and in patients with "euthyroid ophthalmic Graves' disease", i. e. patients with endocrine exophthalmos, but no evidence of clinical thyroid disease; in this graph are depicted results using a crude human thyroid antigen. Note that in response to this antigen there was a positive LIF test in patients who had hyperthyroid Graves' disease, whether or not they had exophthalmos. Conversely, in those patients who had "euthyroid ophthalmic Graves' disease", only those patients were positive in this test who had some other evidence of thyroid dysfunction, e. g. thyroid antibodies, non-suppressibility with tri-iodothyronine, inadequate stimulability with TSH. Those patients who had no evidence of thyroid dysfunction whatever showed no LIF in response to the thyroid antigen. The leucocytes used in this study were also used in the study noted in Fig. 2.21. (Munro et al. 1973)

and Pittman 1971) and its alpha and beta subunits are suppressed in Graves' disease (Kourides et al. 1975). Moreover, severe exophthalmos has been reported after an apparently total hypophysectomy (Furth et al. 1962). Finally, in the MIF studies of Munro et al. (1973), TSH was ineffective as both antigen and enhancer of migration inhibition.

Two groups of investigators have been able to demonstrate that retro-orbital muscle has an affinity for thyroglobulin and thyroglobulin antibody – antibody immune complexes (Konishi et al. 1974; Mullin et al. 1977). Moreover, Kriss and Mehdi (1979) have recently shown that lymphocytes from patients with exophthalmos will injure cell membrane from extraocular muscle when the muscle is first exposed to thyroglobulin. In addition, lymphatic connections between the thyroid region and the retro-orbital area have been demonstrated (Kriss 1970). These authors have postulated that thyroglobulin, immune complexes and lymphocytes from the thyroid reach the eyes via the lymphatics and there set up an immune reaction in the retroorbital muscles. However, Takeda and Kriss (1977), studying

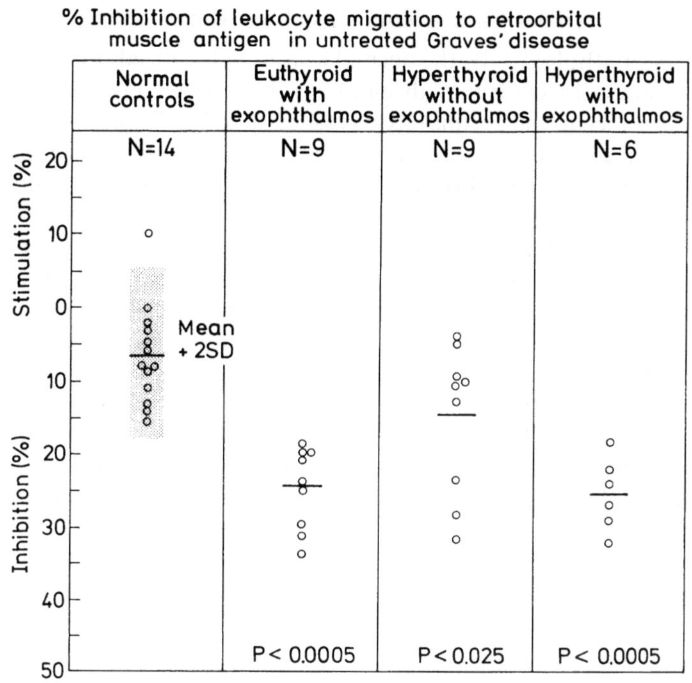

Fig. 2.21. Results from the LIF test using a crude normal retro-orbital muscle antigen. The same leucocyte preparations were employed as those depicted in Fig. 2.20. It may be noted that patients with exophthalmos were positive in this assay system, whether or not they were hyperthyroid. Conversely, in those patients with hyperthyroid Graves' disease who had no evidence of exophthalmos, many were negative in this procedure. However, there were a few who showed no clinical evidence of exophthalmos, but who showed positive LIF responses to the retro-orbital muscle antigen. It would thus appear that the antigens responsible for the ocular manifestations are different from those responsible for the thyroid manifestations, and thus the lymphocytes which subserve the ocular disease would appear to be different from those which subserve the thyroid disorder. This is in keeping with the view that exophthalmos and hyperthyroidism of Graves' disease represent two closely related, but actually separate, overlapping organ-specific auto-immune diseases. (Munro et al. 1973)

immune complexes in the circulation of patients with Graves' disease, with or without exophthalmos, have been unable to find any correlation between the presence of immune complexes and either the presence or the severity of the exophthalmos. This discrepancy has also been found by Hopf et al. (1978) and Brohee et al. (1979). Moreover, this hypothesis fails to explain the poor temporal relationship between the onset of exophthalmos and that of hyperthyroidism, or the presence of exophthalmos in the absence of thyroid disease. While, therefore, this explanation might account for some of the patients with exophthalmos, it could not be an explanation for all of these patients, and thus suffers as a unitary hypothesis.

It thus remains the view of the author that exophthalmos likely represents a very closely related, but separate, overlapping organ-specific auto-immune disease. It is felt that this proposal best fits the clinical and immunological observations, but much more investigation is required before one can have confidence that this field has been illuminated.

2.2.14 Pretibial Myxoedema (Localized Dermopathy)

Histopathologically, the dermal lesions of localized pretibial myxoedema (localized dermopathy of Graves' disease) are characterized by an accumulation of mucinous substance in the dermis (Kobayasi et al. 1976). Excess content of hyaluronic acid in the mucinous areas has been demonstrated by mucicarmine, colloidal iron, alcian blue and by metachromasia with toluidine blue. The staining is prevented if the section is influenced by hyaluronidase. Studying biopsies of this lesion by electron-microscopy has shown an overwhelming accumulation of microfibrils with Knobs (acid glycosamino glycans) in the dermis, with an amorphous material containing glycoprotein. Moreover, evidence of degradation without new formation of collagen fibrils was found. Considerable numbers of mast cells with various types of granules, fibroblasts with dilated granular endoplasmic reticulum and macrophages were seen in the mucinous areas.

Yeo et al. (1978 a) have studied six patients with this disorder with respect to immunofluorescent antibody studies. However, there was no difference in the deposition of immunoglobulin G in the dermal lesions themselves when they were compared to normal skin adjacent to the lesion, or indeed when they were compared to the normal dermal regions of thyrotoxic control patients without pretibial myxoedema or the dermal areas of normal control subjects. These studies gave no support to the hypothesis that pretibial myxoedema results from local antigen-antibody tissue reaction.

It is certainly known that levels of LATS and TSI are usually exceedingly high in patients with this lesion, suggesting some kind of association between the very high immunological activity and the presence of the lesions. LATS has also been demonstrated from homogenates of biopsy materials from involved areas by some workers (Pimstone et al. 1964; Kingery 1965). However, other workers have been unable to confirm this finding (Schermer et al. 1970; Pinchera et al. 1965; Benoit and Greenspan 1967). The data from the latter studies as well as those of Yeo et al. (1978 a) do not support the hypothesis that pretibial myxoedema results from a local antigen-antibody tissue reaction.

Cheung et al. (1978) have studied skin fibroblasts from the shoulder and lower extremity of normal persons, as well as from patients with pretibial myxoedema in tissue culture. When the cells reached the monolayer stage, they were labelled with tritiated glycosamine, and tested for hyaluronic acid synthesis in the presence of either serum from patients with pretibial myxoedema or normal human serum. All the fibroblasts from the pretibial area synthesized two to three times more hyaluronic acid when incubated with the serum from patients with pretibial myxoedema than when incubated with normal human serum. Fibroblasts cultured from other areas of the skin did not respond to these sera. This heat stable, protease sensitive and dialyzable fibroblast stimulating factor is not a 7S gammaglobulin. The enhanced sensitivity to the abnormal sera exhibited by fibroblasts from the lower extremities may explain why the lesions in this disorder are restricted generally to that area.

It may thus be seen that no final answer is currently available with respect to the pathogenesis of the dermopathy of Graves' disease, although there is now some early evidence that there is indeed a serum factor which may well be responsible. The question of the nature of this mysterious element of Graves disease will clearly exist for many long years before an acceptable answer emerges.

2.3 Summary

The author views Graves' hyperthyroidism, exophthalmos and Hashimoto's thyroiditis as very closely related but separate auto-immune diseases. These disorders, as well as other closely related organ-specific auto-immune disorders may each be attributable to separate, albeit closely related inherited isolated defects in immunoregulation. Evidence presented in this chapter would indicate that there is an antigen-specific defect in a population of suppressor T-lymphocytes (which would ordinarily suppress a clone of thyroid-directed autoreactive helper T-lymphocytes) in the patients predisposed to have either Graves or Hashimoto's disease. The defects which are present in the specific clones of suppressor T-lymphocytes are presumed to be present, perhaps from birth forward. However, there has been no investigation yet performed to establish this point, although such studies are now in progress. If one had such a defect, however, this would permit a normally, randomly mutating "forbidden" clone of thyroid-directed helper T-lymphocytes, arising at random, to survive, then to interact with its complementary antigen on the thyroid cell membrance and then to set up a localized cell-mediated immune response. This would not require any alteration of the antigen, only the mere availability of the specific antigen. The clone of self-reactive T-lymphocytes, so arising and escaping immunoregulation, would presumably then expand upon interaction with this antigen and consequently direct and co-operate with groups of (already present) B-lymphocytes, which, in turn, would produce specific immunoglobulins that appear necessary for the full expression of these disorders (see Fig. 2.22).

There appear to be slight genetic differences between Graves' and Hashimoto's disease. The gene responsible for Graves' disease may lie in close linkage

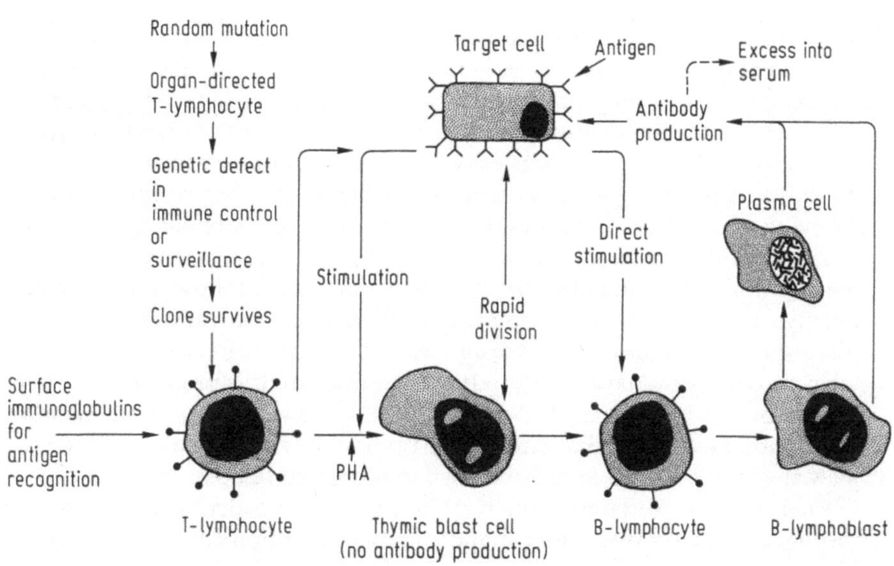

Fig. 2.22. Proposed hypothesis for the pathogenesis of Graves' disease (see Sect. 2.3). (Volpé 1977)

disequilibrium with HLA-Dw3 on chromosome 6 in Caucasians. Recent evidence suggests that in Hashimoto's thyroiditis there is an association with HLA-DR5. While it is true that the results of cell-mediated immunity and abnormalities in suppressor T-lymphocytes presented in this chapter have been common for both Graves' and Hashimoto's diseases, this may well be because it has been impossible to separate the putative antigens on the thyroid cell membrane for the two disorders. There are enough differences between the two conditions to at least suggest that they do not represent the opposite ends of a spectrum of a single entity but rather represent differing entities. It will take purification of specific antigens to prove this suggestion.

The role of anti-idiotypic antibodies in these conditions is as yet quite speculative as there are no data yet reported. Adjunctive roles for immune complexes, non-specific cells (macrophages, "killer" cells) and chemical mediators are undoubtedly important. The role of thyroid-stimulating antibody in the induction of the hyperthyroidism of Graves' disease is of considerable interest and importance; precisely how it interacts with the TSH receptor (either directly or indirectly) is not yet entirely clear. This antibody acts as an agonist, which is very unusual for anti-receptor antibodies which usually act as antagonists. Some antibodies which have the ability to prevent the binding of TSH to their receptors have been shown to be antagonistic to the effects of TSH and thus produce some confusion in assessing the results of the radio-ligand assay for Graves' immunoglobulins.

The role of stress in the induction of hyperthyroidism may be by means of its effect in further reducing immunosuppression in those persons with only a partial isolated defect. In such persons, it is entirely possible that there is a clone of suppressor T-lymphocytes which is partially defective but which is ordinarily capable of suppressing the "forbidden" clone of thyroid-directed auto-reactive helper T-lymphocytes under optimal conditions. However, if the conditions are not optimal for those suppressor T-lymphocytes, then their occult defect would become overt. Such a situation may occur with a slight increase in cortisol (resulting from stress) or other chemical mediators could be implicated. Once the disease has been initiated, it might remain self-perpetuating by virtue of the effect of the disease itself on the immune system, i.e. through an indirect effect of hyperthyroidism on the adrenal cortex, or a direct effect of thyroid hormones on suppressor T-lymphocytes. On the other hand, remissions may be brought about by restoring immunoregulation to its previous state, by means of normalizing the hyperthyroidism and/or relieving the "stress". Those persons having an isolated complete defect in immunoregulation would not be expected to achieve remissions except by destruction of thyroid parenchyma. It is of interest that those patients who retain a positive test for thyroid-stimulating antibody can be expected to relapse after discontinuance of anti-thyroid drug therapy, whereas the relapse rate is much lower when thyroid-stimulating antibody has disappeared. Moreover, there is evidence that there is an increase in HLA-Dw3 (or HLA-DRw3) in those patients who relapse when compared to those who remain in remission. This would be consistent with the view that there is a genetic basis for the ability to relapse or remit.

Finally, it is considered likely that there is one defect (therefore one gene) responsible for Graves' disease and one defect responsible for each of the other organ-specific auto-immune diseases. Since it seems evident that each gene lies close to the other, it is altogether possible that a person could inherit one, two or more such genes and therefore have a predisposition to more than one of these closely related auto-immune conditions.

2.4 References

Aarli JA, Thunold S, Heimann P (1978) Thyroiditis in myaesthenia gravis. Acta Neurol Scand 58:121–127

Adams DD, Kennedy TH (1971) Evidence to suggest that LATS protector stimulates the human thyroid gland. J Clin Endocrinol Metab 33:47–51

Adams DD, Purves HD (1956) Abnormal responses in the assay of thyrotrophin. Univ Otaga Med School Proc 34:11–12

Adams DD, Dirmikis S, Doniach D, El Kabir DJ, Hall R, Ibbertson HK, Irvine WJ, Kendall-Taylor P, Manley SW, Mehdi SQ, Munro DS, Purves HD, Smith BR, Stewart RDH (1975) Nomenclature of thyroid stimulating antibodies. Lancet 1:1201

Adlkofer F, Schleusener H, Uher L, Ananos A (1973) Heterogenity of long-acting thyroid stimulating (LATS) activity, thyroglobulin antibodies and thyroid microsomal antibodies. Acta Endocrinol (Copenh) 73:483–488

Alexander WD, Harden R McG, Shimmins J (1968) Emotion and non-specific infection as possible aetiological factors in Graves' disease. Their relation to thyroid suppressibility. Lancet 2:196–197

Allison AC (1976) Self-tolerance and autoimmunity in the thyroid. N Engl J Med 295:821–827

Amino N, DeGroot LJ (1975) Insoluble particulate antigens in cell-mediated immunity of autoimmune thyroid disease. Metabolism 24:45–46

Amino N, Miyai K, Onishi T, Hashimoto T, Arai K, Ishibashi K, Kumahara Y (1976) Transient hypothyroidism after delivery in autoimmune thyroiditis. J Clin Endocrinol Metab 42:296–301

Amino N, Miyai K, Kuro R, Tanizawa O, Azukizawa M, Takai S, Tanaka F, Nishi K, Kawashima M, Kumahara Y (1977 a) Transient post-partum hypothyroidism: fourteen cases with autoimmune thyroiditis. Ann Intern Med 87:155–159

Amino N, Miyai K, Yamamoto T, Kuro R, Tanaka F, Tanizawa O, Kumahara Y (1977 b) Transient recurrence of hyperthyroidism after delivery in Graves' disease. J Clin Endocrinol Metab 44:130–136

Amino N, Kuro R, Tanizawa F, Tanaka F, Hayashi C, Kotani K, Kwashima M, Miyai K, Kumahara Y (1978) Changes of serum anti-thyroid antibodies during and after pregnancy in autoimmune thyroid diseases. Clin Exp Immunol 31:30–37

Amino N, Mori H, Yabu Y, Kuro R, Yamada T, Hisa Y, Tanizawa O, Miyai (1980) Mechanisms of occurrence of transient post-partum hypothyroidism in autoimmune thyroiditis. In: Stockigt JR, Nagataki S (eds) Thyroid research VIII. Austral Acad Sci Canberra, pp 551–554

Amkraut A, Solomon GF (1974) From the symbolic stimulus to the pathophysiologic response immune mechanisms. Int J Psychiatry Med 5:541–563

Aoki N, DeGroot LJ (1979) Lymphocyte blastogenic response to human thyroglobulin in Graves' disease, Hashimoto's thyroiditis, and metastatic thyroid cancer. Clin Exp Immunol 38:523–530

Aoki N. Pinnamaneni KM, DeGroot LJ (1979) Studies on suppressor cell function in thyroid diseases. J. Clin Endocrinol Metab 48:803–810

Asamer H, Riccabona G, Holthaus N, Gabl F (1968) Immunohistologic findings in thyroid disease in an endemic goiter area. Arch Klin Med 215:270–272

Bacon LD, Kite RH Jr, Rose NR (1973) Immunogenetic detection of B locus genotypes in chickens with autoimmune thyroiditis. Transplantation 16:591–598

Balázs CS, Stenszky V, Kozma L, Leövey A (1978) The possible influence of HLA-1, B8 antigens on the course of Graves' disease. Biomedicine 29:263–264

Balázs CS, Stenszky V, Kozma L, Szerze P, Leövey A (1979 a) Connection between HLA B8 antigen and suppressor T cell activity in Graves' disease. Transplant Proc 11:1314

Balázs CS, Leövey A, Borden L (1979 b) Decrease of concanavalin-A activated and short-lived suppressor T cell function in thyrotoxicosis. Biomedicine 30:143–147

Balázs CS, Leövey A, Szabo M, Bako G (1980) Stimulating effect of triiodothyronine on cell-mediated immunity. Eur J Clin Pharmacol 17:19–24

Bartels EC (1941) Twin examinations: heredity in Graves' disease. Munksgaard, Copenhagen, pp 32–36

Bartels EC, Irie M (1961) Thyroid function in patients with progressive exophthalmos; study of 117 cases requiring orbital decompression. In: Pitt-Rivers R (ed) Advances in thyroid research. Pergamon, New York, pp 163–170

Bartrop RW, Luckhurst E, Lazarus L, Kiloh LG, Penny R (1977) Depressed lymphocyte function after bereavement. Lancet 1:834–836

Bastenie PA, Ermans AM (1972) Thyroiditis and thyroid function: clinical, morphological and physiopathological studies. Pergamon, Oxford (International series of monographs on pure and applied biology, modern trends in physiological sciences, Vol 36)

Bastenie PA, Neve P, Bonnyns M, Van Haelst L, Chailly M (1967) Clinical and pathological significance of asymptomatic atrophic thyroiditis; a condition of latent hypothyroidism. Lancet 1: 915–919

Bayer MF, Kriss JP (1979a) Immunoradiometric assay for serum thyroglobulin: semiquantitative measurement of thyroglobulin in antithyroglobulin-positive sera. J Clin Endocrinol Metab 49:557–564

Bayer MF, Kriss JP (1979b) A solid phase sandwich type radioimmunoassay for antithyroglobulin elimination of false positive results and semiquantitative measurement of antithyroglobulin in the presence of elevated thyroglobulin. J. Clin Endocrinol Metab 49: 565–571

Beall GN, Kruger SR (1979) Antithyroglobulin (ATG) production by peripheral blood leukocytes in vitro. J Clin Endocrinol Metab 48:712–714

Bech K, Madsen SN (1979) Thyroid adenylate cyclase stimulating immunoglobulin in thyroid diseases. Clin Endocrinol (Oxf) 11:47–58

Bech K, Nerup J, Larsen JH (1977a) *Yersinia enterocolitica* infection and thyroid diseases. Acta Endocrinol (Copenh) 84: 87–92

Bech K, Clemmensen O, Larsen JH, Bendixen G (1977b) Thyroid disease and *Yersinia*. Lancet 1:1060–1061

Bech K, Lumholtz B, Nerup J, Thomsen M, Platz P, Ryder LP, Svejgaard A, Siersbaek-Nielsen K, Hansen JM, Larsen JH (1977c) HLA antigens in Graves' disease. Acta Endocrinol (Copenh) 86:510–516

Bech K, Nerup J, Thomsen M, Platz P, Ryder LP, Svejgaard A, Siersbaek-Neilsen K, Molholm Hansen JE (1977d) Subacute thyroiditis DeQervain: a disease associated with an HLA-B antigen. Acta Endocrinol (Copenh) 86:504–509

Beck JS (to be published) Pathology of Graves' disease and the effect of treatment. Ann Coll Phys Surg Canada

Beierwaltes WH (1969) Iodine and lymphocytic thyroiditis. Bull All-India Inst Med Sci 3:145–152

Beierwaltes WH, Nishiyama RH (1968) Dog thyroiditis. Occurrence and similarity to Hashimoto's struma. Endocrinology 83:501–508

Benoit FL, Greenspan FS (1967) Corticosteroid therapy for pretibial myxoedema, observations on the long-acting thyroid stimulator. Ann Intern Med 66:711–720

Blackett PR, Seely JR, Altmiller DH (1978) Neonatal thyrotoxicosis following maternal hypothyroidism. J Pediatr 92:159–160

Blizzard RM, Hung W, Chandler RW, Aceto T Jr, Kyle M, Winship T (1962) Hashimoto's thyroiditis. Clinical and laboratory response to prolonged cortisone therapy. N Engl J Med 267:1015–1020

Bolk JH, Elte JWF, Bussemaker JK, Haak A, Van der Heide D (1979) Thyroid stimulating immunoglobulins do not cause non-autonomous, autonomous or toxic multinodular goitres. Lancet 2:61–63

Bonnyns M, Cano P, Osterland CK, and McKenzie JM (1978) Immune reactions in patients with Graves' disease. Am J Med 65:971–977

Braley-Mullen H, Sharp GC, Kyriakos M, Jepsen P (1978) Cellular and genetic control of susceptibility to experimental autoimmune thyroiditis in guinea pigs. In: Rose NR, Bigazzi PE, Warner NL (eds) Genetic control of autoimmune disease. Elsevier/North Holland, New York, pp 401–413

Braverman LE (1978) Therapeutic considerations. Clin Endocrinol Metab 7:221–240

Braverman LE, Ingbar SH, Vagenakis AG, Adams L, Maloof F (1971) Enhanced susceptibility to iodide myxedema in patients with Hashimoto's disease. J Clin Endocrinol Metab 32:515–521

Bremner WJ, Griep RJ (1976) Graves' thyrotoxicosis following primary thyroid failure. JAMA 235:1361

Brohee D, Delespesse G, Debisschop MJ, Bonnyns M (1979) Detection of circulating immune complexes in thyroid disease. Clin Exp Immunol 36:379–383

Brown DM, Lowman JT (1964) Thyrotoxicosis occurring in two patients on prolonged high doses of steroids. N Engl J Med 270:278–281

Brown RS, Jackson IMB, Pohl SL, Reichlin S (1978) Do thyroid stimulating immunoglobulins cause non-toxic and toxic multinodular goitres? Lancet 1:904–906

Brownlie BEW, Newton OAG, Singh SP (1975) Ophthalmopathy associated with primary hypothyroidism. Acta Endocrinol (Copenh) 79:691–699

Buerklin EM, Schimmel M, Utiger RD (1976) Pituitary-thyroid regulation in euthyroid patients with Graves' disease previously treated with antithyroid drugs. J Clin Endocrinol Metab 43:419–427

Burch PRJ (1963 a) A genetic theory of inflammatory polyarthritis. Lancet 2:636–637

Burch PRJ (1963 b) A genetic theory of inflammatory polyarthritis. Lancet 2:836–837

Burch PRJ (1966 a) Spontaneous auto-immunity: equation for age-specific prevalence and initiation rates. J Theor Biol 12:397–409

Burch PRJ (1966 b) Age and sex distributions from some idiographic non-malignant conditions in man. Some possible implications for growth control and natural and radiation induced ageing. In: Lindop PJ, Sacher GA (eds) Radiation and ageing. Taylor & Francis, London, pp 117–155

Burch PRJ (1968) An inquiry concerning growth, disease and ageing. The sex and age distribution of autoaggressive disease. Oliver & Boyd, Edinburgh, pp 34–69

Burch PRJ, Rowell NR (1963) Autoimmunity: aetiological aspects of chronic discoid and systemic lupus erythematosus, systemic sclerosis and Hashimoto's thyroiditis: some immunological complications. Lancet 2:507–515

Burke JS, Butler JJ, Fuller LM (1977) Malignant lymphoma of the thyroid. A clinical pathological study of 35 patients including ultrastructural observations. Cancer 39:1587–1602

Calder EA, Penhale WJ, Barnes EW, Irvine WJ (1974 a) Evidence for circulating immune complexes in thyroid disease. Br Med J 2:30–31

Calder EA, Urbaniak SJ, Penhale WJ, Irvine WJ (1974 b) Characterization of human lymphoid cell-mediated antibody-dependent cytotoxicity (LDAC). Clin Exp Immunol 18:597–593

Calder EA, Irvine WJ, Davidson NM, Wu F (1976) T, B and K cells in autoimmune thyroid disease. Clin Exp Immunol 25:17–22

Cano PO, Chertman MM, Jerry LM, and McKenzie JM (1976) Circulating immune complexes in Graves' disease. Endocr Res Commun 3:307–317

Canonica G, Bagnasco M, Moretta L, Cocco R, Ferrini O, Giordano G (1981) Human T lymphocyte subpopulations in Hashimoto's disease. J Clin Endocrinol Metab 52: 553–556

Carayon P, Guibou TM, Lissitzsky S (1978) Thyrotropin receptor adenylate cyclase system in plasma membranes from normal and diseased human thyroid glands. J Endocrinol Invest 1:321–328

Carey C, Skosey C, Pinnamaneni KM, Barsano CP, DeGroot LJ (1980) Thyroid abnormalities in children of parents who have Graves' disease – possible pre-Graves' disease. Metabolism 29:369–376

Cathelineau G, Fribourg-Desi M (1974) Ophtalmopathie de type basedowien et hypothyroidie primitive. Nouv Presse Med 3 32:1995–1998

Catz B, Perzik SL (1965) Subtotal vs. total surgical ablation of the thyroid, malignant exophthalmos and its relation to remnant thyroid. In: Cassano C, Andreoli M (eds) Current topics in thyroid research. Academic Press, New York, pp 1183–1199

Chan SH, Yeo PPB, Lui, KF, Wee GB, Woo KT, Lim P, Cheah JS (1978) HLA and thyrotoxicosis (Graves' disease) in Chinese. Tissue Antigens 12:109–114

Chandler RW, Kyle MA, Hung W, Blizzard RM (1962) Experimentally induced autoimmunization disease of the thyroid. I. The failure of transplacental transfer of anti-thyroid antibodies to produce cretinism. Paediatrics 29:961–967

Chen H, Hoffman WH, Chang CH, Hart Z, Kaplan J (1978) Lymphocytic thyroiditis, myasthenia gravis, and Turner syndrome. Birth Defects 14/6A:137–147

Chertow BS, Fidler WJ, Fariss BL (1973 Graves' disease and Hashimoto's thyroiditis in monozygous twins. Acta Endocrinol (Copenh) 72:18–24

Cheung HS, Nicoloff JT, Kamiel MB, Spolter L, Nimni ME (1978) Stimulation of fibroblast biosynthetic activity by serum of patients with pretibial myxedema. J Invest Dermatol 71:12–17

Chopra IJ, Solomon DH, Chopra U, Yoshihara E, Terasaki PI, Smith F (1977) Abnormalities in thyroid function in relatives of patients with Graves' disease and Hashimoto's thyroiditis. J Clin Endocrinol Metab 45:45–54

Christadoss P, Kong YCM, Elrehewy M, Rose NR, David GS (1978) Genetic control of T lymphocyte proliferative autoimmune response to thyroglobulin in mice. In: Rose NR, Bigazzi PE, Warner EL (eds) Genetic control of autoimmune disease. Elsevier/North Holland, New York, pp 445–454

Christy JH, Morse RS (1977) Hypothyroid Graves' disease. Am J Med 62:291–296

Claman HN (1972) Corticosteroids and lymphoid cells. N Engl J Med 287:388–397

Clinton BA, Weigle WO (1972) Cellular events during the induction of experimental thyroiditis in the rabbit. J Exp Med 136:1605–1615

Cole RK, Kite JH Jr, Witebsky E (1968) Hereditary autoimmune thyroiditis in the fowl. Science 160:1357–1358

Cooper DS, Ridgway EC, Maloof F (1978) Unusual types of hyperthyroidism. Clin Endocrinol Metab 7:199–220

Cunliffe WJ, Hall R, Newell DJ, Stevenson CJ (1968) Vitiligo, thyroid disease and autoimmunity. Br J Dermatol 80:135–139

Cunningham JAK, Kral F (1959) Thyrotoxicosis in identical twins. NZ Med J 58:600–603

Dandona P, Marshall MJ, Bidey SP, Nathan A, Harvard CWH (1979) Successful treatment of exophthalmos and pretibial myxoedema with plasmapheresis. Br Med J 1:374–376

Davies TF, Yeo PPB, Evered DC, Clark F, Smith BR, Hall R (1977) Value of thyroid stimulating antibody determinations in predicting short-term thyrotoxic relapse in Graves' disease. Lancet 1:1181–1182

Dirmikis SM, Munro DS, Hiller EJ, Crawford MJ, Wynn EJ, Purcell M (1974) Placental transmission of LATS-protector. Lancet 2:1579–1580

Dirmikis SM, Munro DS (1975) Placental transmission of thyroid stimulating immunoglobulin. Br Med J 2:665–666

Dirmikis SM, Kendall-Taylor P, Munro DS (1976) The nature and significance of LATS-protector. In: Robbins J, Braverman LE (eds) Thyroid research. Excerpta Medica, Amsterdam, pp 403–406

Docter R, Bos G, Visser TJ, Hennemann G (1980) Thyrotrophin binding inhibiting immunoglobulins in Graves' disease before, during and after therapy, and its relation to long-acting thyroid stimulator. Clin Endocrinol (Oxf) 12:143–153

Doniach D (1975) Humoral and genetic aspects of thyroid autoimmunity. Clin Endocrinol Metab 4:267–285

Doniach D, Florin-Christensen A (1975) Autoimmunity in the pathogenesis of endocrine exophthalmos. Clin Endocrinol Metab 4:341–350

Doniach D, Roitt IM, Taylor KB (1965) Autoimmunity in pernicious anemia and thyroiditis: a family study. Ann NY Acad Sci 124: 605–625

Doniach D, Botazzo GF, Russell RCG (1979) Goitrous autoimmune thyroiditis (Hashimoto's thyroiditis). Clin Endocrinol Metab 8:63–80

Dorfman SG, Cooperman MT, Nelson RL, Depuy H, Peake RL, Young RL (1977) Painless thyroiditis and transient hyperthyroidism without goiter. Ann Intern Med 86:24–28

Drachman DB (1978) Myaesthenia gravis. N Engl J Med 298: 136–142, 186–193

Drexhage HA, Bottazzo GF, Bitemsky L, Chayen J, Doniach D (1980) Evidence for thyroid growth stimulating immunoglobulins in some goitrous thyroid diseases. Lancet 2: 281–292, 62 nd Meeting, Endocrinol Soc, Washington, DC, June 18–20, 1980, Abstract 514

Dunlap DB, McFarland KF, Lutcher CL (1974) Graves' disease and idiopathic thrombocytopenic purpura. Am J Med Sci 268:107–111

Dymling JF, Becker DV (1967) Occurrence of hyperthyroidism in patients receiving thyroid hormone. J Clin Endocrinol Metab 27:1487–1491

Edmonds M, Lamki L, Killinger DW, Volpé R (1973) Autoimmune thyroiditis, adrenalitis and cophoritis. Am J Med 54:782–787

Ehrenfeld EN, Levy M (1972) Thyrotoxicosis in identical twins and in their mother. Isr J Med Sci 8:620–622

Elling P, Ranlov P, Bildsoe P (1966) A genetic approach to the pathogenesis of hepatic cirrhosis – a clinical and serological study. Acta Med Scand 179:527–533

Endo K, Kasagi T, Konishi J, Ikekubo K, Okuno T, Takeda Y, Mori T, Torizuka K (1978) Detection and properties of TSH binding inhibitor immunoglobulins in patients with Graves' disease and Hashimoto's thyroiditis. J Clin Endocrinol Metab 46:734–739

Etienne J, Kohn LD, Winand RJ (1976) Studies on the mechanism of experimental exophthalmos. In: Robbins J, Braverman LE (eds) Thyroid research. Excerpta Medica, Amsterdam, pp 380–382

Evans TC, Beierwaltes WH, Nishiyama RH (1969) Experimental canine Hashimoto's thyroiditis. Endocrinology 84:641–646

Faber J, Cohn D, Kirkegaard C, Christy M, Siersbaek-Nielsen K, Friis T, Nerup J (1979) Subclinical hypothyroidism in Addison's disease. Acta Endocrinol (Copenh) 91:674–679

Fabris N (1973) Immunodepression in thyroid-deprived animals. Clin Immunol 15:601–611

Fagraeus A, Jonsson J (1970) Distribution of organ antigens over the surface of thyroid cells as examined by the immunofluorescence test. Immunology 18:413–416
Fagraeus A, Jonsson J, El Kabir DJ (1970) What is the antibody specificity of LATS? J. Clin Endocrinol Metab 31:445–447
Fahey JL, Goodman H (1964) Antibody activity in six classes of human immunoglobulin. Science 143:588–590
Fakhri O, Hobbs JR (1972) Detection of antibodies which can cooperate with lymphocytes. Lancet 2:403–406
Farid NR, Bear JC (1981) The human major histocompatibility complex and endocrine disease. Endocrine Rev 2:50–86
Farid NR, Munro RE, Row VV, Volpé R (1973) Rosette inhibition test for the demonstration of thymus-dependent lymphocyte sensitization in Graves' disease and Hashimoto's thyroiditis. N Engl J Med 289:1111–1117
Farid NR, Barnard JM, Marshall WH (1976) The association of HLA with autoimmune thyroid disease in Newfoundland. The influence of HLA homozygosity in Graves' disease. Tissue Antigens 8:181–190
Farid NR, Newton RM, Noel EP, Barnard JM, Marshall WH (1978) The operation of immunological networks in Graves' disease. Tissue Antigens 12:205–211
Farid NR, Sampson J, Noel EP, Barnard JM, Mandeville R, Larsen B, Marshall WH (1979) A study of human leukocyte D locus-related antigens in Graves' disease. J Clin Invest 63:108–113
Farid NR, Larsen B, Payne R, Noel EP, Sampson L Immunogenetics of polyglandular autoimmune disease. 62nd Meeting, Endocrinol Soc, Washington, DC, June 18–20, 1980, Abstract 82 (to be published)
Fatourechi V, McConahey WM, Woolner LB (1971) Hyperthyroidism associated with histologic Hashimoto's thyroiditis. Mayo Clin Proc 46:682–689
Feldt-Rasmussen U, Hyltoft Petersen P, Date J, Madsen CM (1980) Sequential changes in serum thyroglobulin (Tg) and its autoantibodies (TgAb) following subtotal thyroidectomy of patients with preoperatively detectable TgAb. Clin Endocrinol (Oxf) 12:29–38
Fenzi GF, Hashizume K, Roudebush CB, DeGroot LJ (1979) Changes in thyroid stimulating immunoglobulin during antithyroid therapy. J. Clin Endocrinol Metab 48:572–576
Fenzi GF, Pinchera A, Bartalena I, Monzani F, Macchia E, Mammoli C, Baschieri L (1980) Thyroid plasma membrane antigens and TSH receptor. In: Stockigt JR, Nagataki S (eds) Thyroid research VIII. Austral Acad Sci Canberra, pp 703–706
Ferrari E, Bossolo P, Vailati A (1974) The ACTH-secreting system in hyperthyroid patients: chronoregulation and dynamic behavior. Chronobiologia 1:179–192
Fialkow PJ, Zavala C, Nielsen R (1975) Thyroid autoimmunity: increased frequency in relatives of insulin-dependent diabetes patients. Ann Intern Med 83:170–176
Fisher D, Beall GN (1976) Hashimoto's thyroiditis. Pharmacol Ther. [C] 1:445–458
Flier JS, Bar RS, Muggeo M, Kahn CR, Roth J, Gorden P (1978) The evolving clinical course of patients with insulin receptor antibodies: spontaneous remission or receptor proliferation with hypoglycemia. J Clin Endocrinol Metab 47:985–995
Flier JS, Kahn CR, Roth J (1979) Receptors, antireceptor antibodies and mechanisms of insulin resistance. N Engl J Med 300:413–419
Folb PI, Bank H (1974) Activated lymphocytes in the peripheral blood in acute hyperthyroidism (Graves' disease). Isr J Med Sci 10:785–877
Folb PI, Bank H (1976) Evidence for an active immune response in acute hyperthyroidism (Graves' disease). Am J Med Sci 272:269–276
Forrester JV, Sutherland GR, McDougall IR (1977) Dysthyroid ophthalmopathy: orbital evaluation with B-scan ultrasonography. J Clin Endocrinol Metab 45:221–224
Fragu P, Mariotti S, Lucero Y, DeGroot LJ (to be published) Indomethacin inhibited suppressor cells in thyroid disease. 62nd Meeting, Endocrinol Soc, Washington, DC, June 8–10, 1980 Abstract 14
Friedman JM, Fialkow PJ (1978) The genetics of Graves' disease. Clin Endocrinol (Oxf) 7:47–65
Fritz TE, Norris WP, Kretz ND (1970) Influence of lymphocytic thyroiditis on iodine metabolism in the beagle. Proc Soc Exp Biol Med 134:450–458
Fujita K, Yamada N, Sanbe T, Yudo T, Tsuchiya K, Shimabukuru K, Ito K, Saito M (1970) Haemagglutination test using antigen from thyroid epithelial cells. Clin Pathol (Jap) 18:213–217
Furth ED, Becker DV, Ray BS, Kane JW (1962) Appearance of unilateral infiltrative exophthalmos of

Graves' disease after the successful treatment of the same process in the contralateral eye by apparently total surgical hypophysectomy. J Clin Endocrinol Metab 22:518–524
Gallagher TF, Hellman L, Finkelstein J, Yoshida K, Weitzman ED, Roffwarg H, Fukushima DK (1972) Hyperthyroidism and cortisol secretion in man. J Clin Endocrinol Metab 34:919–927
Galluzzo A, Giordano C, Andronico F, Filardo C, Andronico G, Bompiano G (1980) Leukocyte migration test in subacute thyroiditis: hypothetical role of cell-mediated immunity. J Clin Endocrinol Metab 50:1038–1041
Gavras I, Thomson JA (1972) Late thyrotoxicosis complicating autoimmune thyroiditis. Acta Endocrinol (Copenh) 69:41–46
Gharib H, Hodgson SF, Gastineau CF, Scholz PA, Smith LA (1972) Reversible hypothyroidism in Addison's disease. Lancet 2:734–737
Ginsberg J, Segal D, Ehrlich RM, Walfish PG (1978) Inappropriate triiodothyronine (T3) and thyroxine (T4) radioimmunoassay levels secondary to circulating thyroid hormone autoantibodies. Clin Endocrinol (Oxf) 8:133–139
Glatstein E, McHardy-Young S, Brast N, Eltringham JR, Kriss JP (1971) Alterations in serum thyrotropin (TSH) and thyroid function following radiotherapy in patients with malignant lymphoma. J Clin Endocrinol Metab 32:833–841
Glover EL, Rueber MD (1968) Chronic thyroiditis in buffalo strain rats ingesting methylcholanthrene. Arch Pathol 86:542–544
Gluck FB, Nusynowitz ML, Plymate S (1975) Chronic lymphocytic thyroiditis, thyrotoxicrosis and low radioactive iodine uptake; report of four cases. N Engl J Med 293:624–628
Goolden AWG, Davidson M, Hoffenberg R (1971) Myxoedema preceding hyperthyroidism. Lancet 2:268
Gordin A, Lamberg BA (1975) Natural course of symptomless autoimmune thyroiditis.Lancet 2:1234–1238
Gordin A, Maenpaa J, Makinen T, Totterman TH, Tiilikainen A (1979) Immunological and genetic markers in a family with Hashimoto's disease. Clin Endocrinol (Oxf) 11:425–435
Gorman GA (1978) Endocrine ophthalmopathy. Clin Endocrinol Metab 7:67–96
Goust JM, Moulias R, Reinert P, Devillechabrolle A, Berthaux P (1972) L'immunité cellulaire envers les antigens d'organe au cours des affections endocriniennes étude par le test de migration des leucocytes. Rev Fr Endocrinol Clin 13:401–411
Grabar P (1974) "Self" and "not self" in immunology. Lancet 1:1320–1322
Graves RJ (1835) Clinical lectures. London Med Surg 7:516–517
Gray RS, Borsey DQ, Seth J, Herd R, Brown NS, Clarke BF (1980) Prevalence of subclinical thyroid failure in insulin-dependent diabetes. J. Clin Endocrinol Metab 50:1034–1037
Greaves M, Janossy G, Doenhoff M (1974) Selective triggering of human T and B lymphocytes in vitro by polyclonal mitogens. J Exp Med 140:1–18
Greer M (1980) Antithyroid drugs in the treatment of thyrotoxicosis. In: Oppenheimer JH (ed) Thyroid today, vol 3, no 1. Travenol, Deerfield, pp 1–5
Grinblatt J, Shohat B, Lewitus Z, Joshua H (1979) Quantitative and functional assessment of peripheral T lymphocytes in thyroid disease. Acta Endocrinol (Copenh) 90:52–61
Grob D (1958) Myaesthenia gravis: current status of pathogenesis, clinical manifestations and management. J Chronic Dis 8:536–566
Grumet FC, Payne RO, Konishi J, Kriss JP (1974) HL-A antigens as markers for disease susceptibility and autoimmunity in Graves' disease. J Clin Endocrinol Metab 39:1115–1119
Grumet FC, Konishi J, Payne RO, Kriss, JP (1976) Association in Japanese of Graves' disease with the HLA specificity W5. In: Robbins J, Braverman LE (eds) Thyroid research. Excerpta Medica, Amsterdam, pp 376–379
Hadden DR, McDevitt DG (1974) Environmental stress and thyrotoxicosis: absence of association. Lancet 2:577–578
Hahn HB, Hayles AB, Woolner LB (1965) Lymphocytic thyroiditis in children. J Pediatr 66:73–78
Hall ND (1978) Leukocyte migration inhibition with IgG-IgG complexes and rabbit IgG fragments in patients with rheumatoid arthritis. Clin Exp Immunol 34:219–225
Hall R (1980) Thyroid stimulators. In: Cumming IA, Funden JW, Mendelsohn FAO (eds) Endocrinology. Austral Acad Sci Canberra; Elsevier/North Holland, Amsterdam, New York, pp 9–12
Hall R, Stanbury JB (1967) Family studies of autoimmune thyroiditis. Clin Exp Immunol [Suppl] 2:719–725

Hall R, Owen SG, Smart GA (1960) Evidence for genetic predisposition to formation of thyroid antibodies. Lancet 2:187–188

Hall R, Doniach D, Kirkham K, El Kabir D (1970) Ophthalmic Graves' disease: diagnosis and pathogenesis. Lancet 1:375–378

Hall R, Smith BR, Mukhtar ED (1975) Thyroid stimulators in health and disease. Clin Endocrinol (Oxf) 4:213–230

Hallengren B, Forsgren A, Melander A (1980) Immunologic effects of methimazole and propylthiouracil in vitro. In: Stockigt JR, Nagataki S (eds) Thyroid research VIII. Austral Acad Sci Canberra, pp 625–628

Hart IR, McKenzie JM (1971) Comparison of the effects of thyrotrophin and long acting thyroid stimulator on guinea pig adipose tissue. Endocrinology 88:26–30

Harvald B, Hauge M (1956) A catamnestic investigation of Danish twins: a preliminary report. Dan Med Bull 3:150–158

Hashimoto H (1912) Zur Kenntnis der lymphomatosen Veränderung der Schilddrüse (Struma lymphomatosa). Arch Klin Chir 97:219–248

Hashizume K, Roudebush C, Fenzi G, DeGroot LJ (1977) The effect of antithyroid therapy on thyroid stimulating immunoglobulin (TSI) in Graves' disease. 53rd Meeting, Am Thyroid Assoc, Cleveland, Ohio, September 7–10, 1980, Abstract p. T-7 (to be published)

Hassan THA, Greig WR, Boyle JA, Boyle IT, Wallace TJ (1966) Toxic diffuse goitre in monozygotic twins. Lancet 2:306–308

Hay FC, Torrigiani G (1973) The distribution of antithyroglobulin antibodies in the immunoglobulin G subclasses. Clin Exp Immunol 15:517–521

Hazard JB (1955) Thyroiditis: a review. Am J Clin Pathol 25:289–298, 399–426

Headington JT, Tantajumroom T (1967) Surgical thyroid disease in Northern Thailand; a study in geographic pathology. Arch Surg 95:157–161

Hearn MTW, Stanton P, Adams DD, Prestidge RL (1980) The application of several new methods for the isolation of glycoprotein antigens involved in thyroid autoimmunity. 6th Internat Congr Endocrinol, Melbourne, Australia, February 10–16, 1980, Abstract 531 (to be published)

Hedley AJ, Ross IP, Beck JS, Donald D, Albert-Recht F, Michie W, Crooks J (1971) Recurrent thyrotoxicosis after subtotal thyroidectomy. Br Med J 4:258–261

Helmke J, Federlin K (1974) Humorale Antikörper und cellulare Immunmechanismen bei verschiedenen Schilddrüsenerkrankungen sowie ihre Beziehungen zum klinischen Erscheinungsbild. Klin Wochenschr 52:578–588

Hershman JM, Pittman JA (1971) Utility of the radioimmunoassay of serum thyrotrophin in man. Ann Intern Med 74:481–490

Hochstein MA, Nair V, Nevins M (1977) Hypothyroidism followed by hyperthyroidism: occurrence in a patient with elevated antithyroid antibody titer. JAMA 237:2222

Hopf U, Hutteroth TH, Meyer zum Büschenfelde KH (1978) Detection of circulating immune complexes in patients with Graves' disease (Abstract 34). Ann Endocrinol (Paris) t 39:20A

How J, Bewsher PD (1980) Autoimmune thyroid disease and the polymyalgia rheumatica-giant cell arteritis syndrome. Clin Endocrinol (Oxf) 12:209–210

How J, Khir ASM, Bewsher PD (1980) Some observations on the natural history of autoimmune (Hashimoto's) thyroiditis. Scott Med J 25:80

Hsu CCS, Chen Y, Patterson R (1976) Peripheral blood B-lymphocyte abnormalities associated with hyperthyroidism of Graves' disease. Clin Exp Immunol 26:431–440

Hung W, Chandra R, August GP, Altman PR (1973) Clinical, laboratory and histologic observations in euthyroid children and adolescents with goiters. J Pediatr 82:10–16

Inada M, Nishikawa M, Naito K, Oishi M, Kurata S, Imura H (1980a) Triiodothyronine-binding immunoglobulin in a patient with Graves' disease and its effect on metabolism and radioimmunoassay of triiodothyronine. Am J Med 68: 787–792

Inada M, Nishikawa M, Naito K, Ishii H, Tanaka K, Imura H (1980b) Correlation of the histological abnormalities of the thyroid with the stage of transient thyrotoxicosis associated with painless thyroiditis. In: Stockigt JR, Nagataki S (eds) Thyroid research VIII. Austral Acad Sci Canberra, pp 563–566

Irvine WJ (1975) Autoimmunity in endocrine disease. Clin Endocrinol Metab 4:227–499

Irvine WJ (1978) The immunology and genetics of autoimmune endocrine disease. In: Rose NR, Bigazzi PE, Warner NL (eds) Genetic control of autoimmune disease. Elsevier/North Holland, New York, pp 77–100

Irvine WJ (1980) Polyglandular autoimmune diseases. In: Cumming IA, Funden JW, Mendelsohn FAO (eds) Endocrinology. Austral Acad Sci Canberra; Elsevier/North Holland, Amsterdam, New York pp 100–105

Irvine WJ, MacGregor AG, Stuart AE, Hall GH (1961) Hashimoto's disease in uniovular twins. Lancet 2:850–853

Irvine WJ, Gray RS, Morris PJ, Ting A (1977 a) Correlation of HLA and thyroid antibodies with the clinical course of thyrotoxicosis treated with antithyroid drugs. Lancet 2:898–900

Irvine WJ, Wu FCW, Urbaniak SJ, Toolis F (1977 b) Peripheral blood leucocytes in thyrotoxicosis (Graves' disease) as studied by conventional light microscopy. Clin Exp Immunol 27:216–221

Ito S, Tamura T, Nishikawa M (1968) Effects of desiscated thyroid, prednisolone and chloroquine on goiter and antibody titer in chronic thyroiditis. Metabolism 17:317–325

Iverson K (1948) Temporary rise in the frequency of thyrotoxicosis in Denmark, 1941–1945. Rosenhilde & Bagger, Copenhagen

Jackson R, Rosenberg C, Kleinmann R, Vagenakis AG, Braverman LE (1979) Ophthalmopathy after neck irradiation therapy for Hodgkin's disease. Cancer Treat Rep 63:1392–1395

James KW (1971) Myxodema preceding hyperthyroidism. Lancet 2:156

Jayson MIV, Doniach D, Benhamou-Glynn N, Roitt IM, El Kabir DJ (1967) Thyrotoxicosis and Hashimoto goitre in a pair of monozygotic twins with serum long acting thyroid stimulator. Lancet 2:15–18

Jeevanram RK, Narkar AA, Shah DH, Ganatra RD (1977) Effect of thyroxine on lymphocyte stimulation. Indian J Cancer 14:361–363

Jepson PL, Kyriakos M, Sharp GD, Braley-Muller H (1979) Effect of neonatal thyroidectomy on experimental autoimmune thyroiditis in guinea pigs. Cell Immunol 45:356–363

Joasoo A, Robertson P, Murray IPC (1975) Viral antibodies in thyrotoxicosis. Lancet 2:125

Jonsson J, Fagraeus A (1969) On the mechanism of the ring zone effect obtained with the mixed haemadsorption technique: studies with human antithyroid sera reacting with thyroid monolayer culture. Immunology 17:387–411

Jordan SC, Buckingham B, Sakai R, Olson D (1981) Studies of immune complex glomerulonephritis mediated by human thyroglobulin. New Engl J Med 304:1212–1215

Kahn LD, Dale J (1973) Virus-like particles in Hashimoto's disease and a variety of other tissues. Lab Invest 29:350–351

Kalderon AE, Bogaars HA (1977) Immune complex deposits in Graves' disease and Hashimoto's thyroiditis. Am J Med 63:729–734

Katz DH, Benacerraf B (1976) The Role of products of the histocompatibility gene complex in immune responses. Academic Press, New York

Kawa A, Nakamura S, Nakazawa M, Sakaguchi S, Kawabata T, Maeda Y, Kanehisa T (1978) HLA Bw35 and B5 in Japanese patients with Graves' disease. Acta Endocrinol (Copenh) 86:754–757

Kendall-Taylor P (1975) LATS and human specific thyroid stimulator; their relation to Graves' disease. Clin Endocrinol Metab 4:319–339

Kenny FM, Iturzaeta N, Preeyasombat C, Taylor FH, Migeon CJ (1967) Cortisol production rate. VII. Hypothyroidism and hyperthyroidism in infants and children. J Clin Endocrinol Metab 27:1616–1622

Kidd A, Silverberg J, Sugenoya A, Row VV, Volpé R (1978) Attempted experimental production of Graves' disease (Abstract 40). Ann Endocrinol (Paris) t 38:23A

Kidd A, Okita N, Row VV, Volpé R (1980) Immunologic aspects of Graves' and Hashimoto's diseases. Metabolism 29:80–99

Kingery FAJ (1965) Myxedema in hyperthyroidism. JAMA 194:663

Kishihara M, Nakao Y, Baba Y, Matsukura S, Kuma K, Fujita T (1979) Interaction between thyroid stimulating immunoglobulins and thyrotropin receptors in fat cell membrane. J Clin Endocrinol Metab 49:706–711

Klein J (1975) Biology of the mouse histocompatibility-2 complex: principles of immunogenetics applied to a single system. Springer, Berlin Heidelberg New York

Knight A, Adams DD (1980) Lack of allotypic variation in the autoantigen for the thyroid stimulating antibodies. 6th Internat Congr Endocrinol, Melbourne, Australia, February 10–16, 1980, Abstract 536 (to be published)

Knox AJS, von Westarp C, Row VV, Volpé R (1976 a) Demonstration of the production of human thyroid stimulating immunoglobulins (HTSI) by Graves' lymphocytes cultured in vitro with phytohaemagglutinin (PHA). Metabolism 25:1217–1223

Knox WJS, von Westarp C, Row VV, Volpé R (1976b) Thyroid antigen stimulates lymphocytes from patients with Graves' disease to produce thyroid stimulating immunoglobulin (TSI). J Clin Endocrinol Metab 43:330–337

Kobayasi T, Danielsen L, Asboe-Hensen G (1976) Ultrastructure of localized myxoedema. Acta Derm Venerol (Stockh) 56:173–185

Kohn LD, Winand RJ (1971) Relationship of thyrotrophin to exophthalmos-producing substance. Formation of an exophthalmos-producing substance by pepsin digestion of pituitary glycoprotein containing both thyrotropic and exophthalmogenic activity. J Biol Chem 246:6570–6575

Kojima A, Tanaka-Kojima Y, Sakakura T, Nishizuka Y (1976a) Spontaneous development of autoimmune thyroiditis in neonatally thymectomized mice. Lab Invest 34:550–557

Kojima A, Tanaka-Kojima Y, Sakakura T, Nishizuka Y (1976b) Prevention of post-thymectomy autoimmune thyroiditis in mice. Lab Invest 34:601–605

Kolsch E, Heuer J (1979) Tolerance and autoimmunity – an introductory survey. In: Klein E, Horster FA (eds) Autoimmunity in thyroid diseases. Schattauer, Stuttgart, pp 3–16

Komaromi I (1965) The effect of thyroxine derivatives on oxygen consumption and adrenal weight in the rat. Acta Physiol Acad Sci Hung 27:213–219

Kong YCM, David SC, Giraldo AA, Elrehewy M, Rose NR (1978) Fine structure of genetic control of autoimmune response to mouse thyroglobulin. In: Rose NR, Bigazzi PE, Warner NL (eds) Genetic control of autoimmune disease. Elsevier/North Holland, New York, pp 433–444

Konishi J, Herman MM, Kriss JP (1974) Binding of thyroglobulin and thyroglobulin-antihyroglobulin immune complex to extraocular muscle membrane. Endocrinology 95:434–446

Konishi J, Kasagi K, Endo K, Mori T, Torizuka K, Yamada Y, Nohara Y, Matsuura N, Kajiama H (1980) TSH binding inhibitor immunoglobulins in Hashimoto's disease and neonatal transient hypothyroidism. In: Stockigt JR, Nagataki S (eds) Thyroid research VIII. Austral Acad Sci Canberra, pp 555–558

Kotkes P, Pick E (1975) Studies of the inhibition of macrophage migration induced by soluble antigen-antibody complexes. Clin Exp Immunol 19:105–120

Kourides IA, Weintraub BD, Ridgway EC, Maloof F (1975) Pituitary secretion of free alpha and beta subunits of human thyrotropin in patients with thyroid disorders. J Clin Endocrinol Metab 40:872–885

Kowalczyk D, Zembala M (1978) Migration inhibition of T lymphocytes from human peripheral blood by specific antigen and lymphokines. Clin Exp Immunol 32:333–338

Kriss JP (1968) Inactivation of long acting thyroid stimulator (LATS) by anti-kappa and anti-lambda antisera. J Clin Endocrinol Metab 28:1440–1444

Kriss JP (1970) Radioisotopic thyroidolymphography in patients which Graves' disease. J Clin Endocrinol Metab 31:315–324

Kriss JP, Mehdi SQ (1979) Cell-mediated lysis of lipid vesicles containing eye muscle protein. Implications regarding pathogenesis of Graves' opthalmopathy. Proc Natl Acad Sci USA. 76:2003–2007

Kriss JP, Pleshakov V, Chien JR (1964) Isolation and identification of the long acting thyroid stimulator and its relation to hyperthyroidism and circumscribed pretibial myxoedema. J Clin Endocrinol Metab 24:1005–1028

Kriss JP, Pleshakov V, Rosenblum AL, Holderness M, Sharp G, Utiger R (1967) Studies on the pathogenesis of the ophthalmopathy of Graves' disease. J Clin Endocrinol Metab 27:582–594

Kroll AJ, Kuwabara T (1966) Dysthyroid ocular myopathy. Anatomy, histology and electronmicroscopy. Arch Ophthalmol 76:244–257

Kuzuya N, Chiu SC, Ikeda H, Uchimura H, Ito K, Nagataki S (1979) Correlation between thyroid stimulators and 3,5,3′-triiodothyronine suppressibility in patients during treatment for hyperthyroidism with thionamide drugs. Comparison of assays by thyroid-stimulating and thyrotropin-displacement activities. J Clin Endocrinol Metab 48:706–711

Lamberg BA (1964) Cushing's syndrome co-existing with hyperthyroidism. Report of a case and some metabolic observations. Acta Med Scand [Suppl 412] 175:159–171

Lamberg BA (1979) Aetiology of hypothyroidism. Clin Endocrinol Metab 8:3–19

Lamki L, Row VV, Volpé R (1973) Cell-mediated immunity in Graves' disease and in Hashimoto's thyroiditis as shown by the demonstration of migration inhibition factor (MIF). J Clin Endocrinol Metab 36:358–364

Laryea E, Row VV, Volpé R (1973) The effect of blood leukocytes from patients with Hashimoto's thyroiditis on human thyroid cells in monolayer culture. Clin Endocrinol (Oxf) 2:23–35

Lee G, Grollman EF, Aloj SM, Kohn LD, Winand RJ (1977) Abnormal adenylate cyclase activity and altered membrane gangliosides in thyroid cells from patients with Graves' disease. Biochem Biophys Res Commun 77:139–146

Lehmann W (1964) Zwillings- und Familienuntersuchungen zur Erbpathologie der Hyperthyreose. In: Becker PE (ed) Humangenetik: Ein kurzes Handbuch in fünf Bänden, volume 3, part 1. Thieme, Stuttgart, pp 182–223

Levey GS (1979) The adrenergic nervous system in hyperthyroidism: therapeutic role of beta adrenergic blocking drugs. In: Hershman JM, Bray GA (eds) The thyroid, physiology and treatment of disease. Pergamon, New York (International encyclopaedia of pharmacology and therapeutics, sect 101, pp 193–208)

Liddle GW, Heyssel RM, McKenzie JM (1965) Graves' disease without hyperthyroidism. Am J Med 39:845–848

Lidz R, Cohn GL (1971) Emotional factors. In: Werner SC, Ingbar SH (eds) The thyroid, 3rd ed. Harper & Row, New York, pp 511–514

Ling SM, Kaplan SA, Weitzman JJ, Reed GB, Costin G, Landing BH (1969) Euthyroid goiters in children: correlation of needle biopsy with other clinical and laboratory findings in chronic lymphocytic thyroiditis and simple goiter. Pediatrics 44:695–708

Loeb PB, Drash AL, Kenny FM (1973) Prevalence of low titer and "negative" antithyroglobulin antibodies in biopsy-proved juvenile Hashimoto's thyroiditis. J Pediatr 82:17–21

Lowenstein JM (1961) Hyperthyroidism in identical twins: report of cases, one treated by surgery, the other by I^{131}. JAMA 176:377–378

Ludwig H, Schernthaner G, Richter E, Zambelis N, Wick G (1978) Thyroglobulin binding cells – a diagnostic marker for Hashimoto's thyroiditis. Acta Endocrinol [Suppl 215] (Copenh) 87 78–79

Lundell G, Jonsson J (1973) Thyroid antibodies and hypothyroidism in ^{131}I therapy for hyperthyroidism. Acta Radiol (Stockh) 12:443–453

Madsen SN, Bech K (1979) TSH and thyroid stimulating antibodies (TSAb) activate thyroid adenylate cyclase through different pathways. Acta Med Scand [Suppl] 624:35–42

Major PW, Munro DS (1962) Observations on the stimulation of thyroid function in mice by the injection of serum from normal subjects and from patients with thyroid disorders. Clin Sci 23:463–475

Makinen T, Wagar G, Apter L, Von Willebrand E, Pekonen F (1978) Evidence that the TSH receptor acts as a mitogenic antigen in Graves' disease. Nature 275:314–315

Malone JF, Cullen MJ (1976) Two mechanisms for hypothyroidism after ^{131}I therapy. Lancet 2:73–75

Marchant B, Lees JFH, Alexander WD (1979) Antithyroid drugs. In: Hershman JM, Bray GA (eds) The thyroid, physiology and treatment of disease. Pergamon, New York (International encyclopaedia of pharmacology and therapeutics, sect 101, pp 209–252)

Mariotti S, DeGroot LJ, Scarborough, D, Medof ME (1979) Study of circulating immune complexes in thyroid diseases: comparison of the Raji cell radioimmunoassay and specific thyroglobulin-antithyroglobulin radioassay. J Clin Endocrinol Metab 49:679–686

Martinez-Lavin M, Vaghan JH, Tan EM (1979) Autoantibodies and the spectrum of Sjögren's syndrome. Ann Intern Med 91:185–190

Mather BA, Roberts DF, Scanlon MF, Mukhtar ED, Davies TF, Smith BR, Hall R (1980) HLA antigens and thyroid autoantibodies in patients with Graves' disease and their first-degree relatives. Clin Endocrinol (Oxf) 12:155–163

Matsui Y, Beall GN, Chopra IJ, Solomon DH, Kruger S, Beall M (1977) Assay for antigen-stimulated lymphocyte-derived migration enhancement and inhibition factors from patients with thyroid disease and their relatives. Acta Endocrinol (Copenh) 86:733–741

Maynard-Smith J, Maynard-Smith S (1963 a) A genetic theory of inflammatory polyarthritis. Lancet 2:357–359

Maynard-Smith S, Maynard-Smith J (1963 b) A genetic theory of inflammatory polyarthritis. Lancet 2:738

McBurney EI (1979) Vitiligo: clinical picture and pathogenesis. Arch Intern Med 139:1295–1297

McConahey WM, Keating FR Jr, Butt HR, Owen CA Jr (1961) Comparison of certain laboratory tests in the diagnosis of Hashimoto's thyroiditis. J Clin Endocrinol Metab 21:879–886

McDougall IR, Kriss JP (1979) Management of the eye manifestations of thyroid disease. In: Hershman JM, Bray GA (eds) The thyroid, physiology and treatment of disease. Pergamon, New York (Internat encyclopaed pharmacol therapeut, sect 101, pp 309–328

McDougall IR, Grieg WR, Gray WH, Smith JFB (1971) Thyrotoxicosis developing during cyclophosphamide therapy. Br Med J 4:275–276

McEachern D, Parnell JL (1948) Relationship of hyperthyroidism to myaesthenia gravis. J Clin Endocrinol Metab 8:842–850

McGregor A, McLachlan S, Clark F, Rees Smith B, Hall R (1979 a) Thyroglobulin and microsomal autoantibody production by cultures of Hashimoto peripheral blood lymphocytes. Immunology 36:81–85

McGregor AM, McLachlan SM, Rees Smith B, Hall R (1979 b) Effect of irradiation on thyroid autoantibody production. Lancet 2:442–444

McGregor AM, Petersen MM, Capiferri R, Evered DC, Rees Smith B, Hall R (1979 c) Effects of radioiodine on thyrotrophin binding inhibiting immunoglobulins in Graves' disease. Clin Endocrinol (Oxf) 11:437–444

McGregor AM, McLachlan SM, Brook EP, Rees Smith B, Hall R (1980 a) The influence of methimazole on the thyroidal autoimmune response in vitro. In: Stockigt JR, Nagataki S (eds) Thyroid research VIII. Austral Acad Sci Canberra, pp 629–632

McGregor AM, Dewar PJ, Petersen MM, Miller M, Rees Smith B, Hall R (1980 b) Prediction of relapse in hyperthyroid Graves' disease. Lancet 2:1101–1103

McKenzie JM (1960) Further evidence for a thyroid activator in hyperthyroidism. J Clin Endocrinol Metab 20:380–388

McKenzie JM (1968) Humoral factors in the pathogenesis of Graves' disease. Physiol Rev 48:252–310

McKenzie JM, Gordon J (1965) The origin of the long-acting thyroid stimulator. In: Cassano C, Andreoli M (eds) Current topics in thyroid research. Academic Press, New York, pp 445–454

McKenzie JM, Zakarija M (1976 a) The role of the immune system in Graves' disease. In: James VHT (ed) Proc Vth Internat Congr, Endocrinol, vol II. Excerpta Medica, Amsterdam, pp 474–478

McKenzie JM, Zakarija M (1976 b) A reconsideration of the thyroid stimulating immunoglobulin as the cause of hyperthyroidism in Graves' disease. J Clin Endocrinol Metab 42:778–784

McKenzie JM, Zakarija M (1977) LATS in Graves' disease. Recent Prog Horm Res 33:29–57

McKenzie JM, Zakarija M (1978) The pathogenesis of neonatal Graves' disease. J Endocrinol Invest 2:183–189

McKenzie JM, Zakarija M (1979) Factors and concepts in autoimmune stimulation of the thyroid. In: Klein E, Horster FA (eds) Autoimmunity in thyroid disease. Schattauer, Stuttgart, pp 107–115

McKenzie JM, Zakarija M, Sato A (1978) Humoral immunity in Graves' disease. Clin Endocrinol Metab 7:31–45

McLachlan SM, Rees Smith B, Petersen VB, Davies TF, Hall R (1977) Thyroid-stimulating autoantibody production in vitro. Nature 270:447–449

McLachlan SM, McGregor A, Rees Smith B, Hall R (1979) Thyroid autoantibody synthesis by Hashimoto thyroid lymphocytes. Lancet 1:162–163

McLachlan SM, Wee SL, McGregor AM, Rees Smith B, Hall R (1980) In vitro studies on the control of thyroid autoantibody synthesis. J Clin Lab Immunol 3:15–21

McLarty DG, Brownlie BEW, Alexander WD, Papapetrou PD, Horton P (1973) Remission of thyrotoxicosis during treatment with propranolol. Br Med J 2:332–334

McMaster PRB, Lerner EM (1967) The transfer of allergic thyroiditis in histocompatible guinea pigs by lymph node cells. J Immunol 99:208–213

McMichael A, Sazuki R, Payne RO, Grumet FC, McDevitt H, Kriss J (1975) An HLA associated LD antigen in patients with Graves' disease. In: Dausset J, Svejgaard A (eds) Histocompatibility testing. Munksgaard, Copenhagen, pp 769–772

Michie W, Gunn A (1966) The thyroid, the thymus and autoimmunity. Br J Clin Pract 20:9–13

Michie W, Pegg CAS, Bewsher PD (1972) Prediction of hypothyroidism after partial thyroidectomy for thyrotoxicosis. Br Med J 1:13–14

Milgrom F, Witebsky E (1962) Autoantibodies and autoimmune diseases. JAMA 181:706–716

Miller K, MacLean D, Brown R (1979) Suppressor cell function in autoimmune thyroid disease. 61st Annual Meeting, Endocrinol Soc, June 13–14, 1979, Anaheim, California, Abstract 494 (to be published)

Millikan CH, Haines SF (1953) Thyroid gland in relation to neuromuscular disease. Arch Intern Med 92:5–39

Miyai K, Fukuchi M, Kumahara Y, Abe H (1967) LATS production by lymphocyte culture in patients with Graves' disease. J Clin Endocrinol Metab 27:855–860

Moens H, Farid NR (1978) Hashimoto's thyroiditis is associated with HLA-DRw3. N Engl J Med 299:133–135

Moens H, Barnard JM, Bear J, Farid NR (1979) The association of HLA B8 with atrophic thyroiditis. Tissue Antigens 13:342–348

Möller G (1978) Role of macrophages in the immune response. Immunol Rev 30:1–255

Monroe RT (1935) Chronic arthritis in hyperthyroidism and myxedema. N Engl J Med 212:1074–1077

Mori T, Kriss JP (1971) Measurements by competitive binding radioassay of serum anti-microsomal and anti-thyroglobulin antibodies in Graves' disease and other thyroid disorders. J Clin Endocrinol Metab 33:688–698

Mori H, Amino N, Iwatani Y, Kabutomori O, Asari S, Motoi S, Miyai K, Kumahara Y (1980) Increase of peripheral B lymphocytes in Graves' disease. Clin Exp Immunol 41:33–40

Mornex R, Fournier G, Berthezene F (1975) Ophthalmic Graves' disease. Mod Probl Ophthalmol 14:426–431

Moulias R, Goust JM, Devillechabrolle A, Buffet C, Muller-Berat CN (1970). Le test de migration des leucocytes du sang périphérique (TML) un nouveau test d'hypersensibilité retardée "in vitro" chez l'homme. II. Utilisation dans les affections autoimmunes humaines. Resultats préliminaires et interprétation. Presse Med 78:2315–2318

Mujtaba Q, Burrow GN (1975) Treatment of hyperthyroidism in pregnancy with propylthiouracil and methimazole. Obstet Gynecol 46:282–286

Mukhtar ED, Smith BR, Pyle GA, Hall R, Vice R (1975) Relationship of thyroid stimulating immunoglobulins to thyroid function and effects of surgery, radioiodine and antithyroid drugs. Lancet 1:713–715

Mulaisho C, Abdou NI, Utiger RD (1975) Lack of T-cell immune abnormalities in peripheral blood lymphocytes in patients with Graves' disease or hypothyroidism. J Clin Endocrinol Metab 41:266–270

Mullin BR, Levinson RE, Friedman A, Henson DE, Winand RJ, Cohn LD (1977) Delayed hypersensitivity in Graves' disease and exophthalmos: identification of thyroglobulin in normal human orbital muscle. Endocrinology 100:351–366

Munck A, Crabtree GR, Smith KA (1979) Glucocorticoid receptors and actions in rat thymocytes and immunologically stimulated human peripheral lymphocytes. In: Baxter JD, Rousseau GG (eds) Glucocorticoid hormone action. Springer, Berlin Heidelberg New York (Monographs on endocrinology, vol 12, pp 341–355)

Munro RE, Lamki L, Row VV, Volpé R (1973) Cell-mediated immunity in the exophthalmos of Graves' disease as demonstrated by the migration inhibition factor (MIF) test. J Clin Endocrinol Metab 37:286–292

Nagataki S (1979) Iodine induced goiter: effects of high iodine intake on thyroid function. In: Hershman JM, Bray GA (eds) The thyroid, physiology and treatment of disease. Pergamon, Oxford, pp 453–464

Nakamura RM, Weigle WO (1967) Passive transfer of experimental autoimmune thyroiditis from donor rabbits injected with soluble thyroglobulin without adjuvant. Int Arch Allergy Appl Immunol 32:506–520

Neff FC (1932) Exophthalmic goiter in identical twin girls. J Pediatr 1:239–243

Nikolai TF (1979) Lymphocytic thyroiditis with spontaneously resolving hyperthyroidism. In: Oppenheimer JH (ed) Thyroid today, vol 2, no 5. Travenol, Deerfield pp 1–51

Nikolai TF, Brosseau J, Kettrick MA, Roberts R, Beltaos E (1980) Lymphocytic thyroiditis with spontaneously resolving hyperthyroidism (silent thyroiditis).). Arch Intern Med 140:478–482

Nofal MM, Beierwaltes WH, Patuo ME (1966) Treatment of hyperthyroidism with sodium iodide I^{131}; a 16 year experience. JAMA 197:605–610

Noguchi S (1978) Autoantibodies to thyroid plasma membrane. 6th Asia and Oceania Congr Endocrinol, Singapore, January 25–27, 1978, Abstract 213 (to be published)

Nyulassy S, Hnilica P, Buc M, Buman M, Hirschova V, Stefanovic J (1977) Subacute (deQuervain's) thyroiditis: association with HLA-Bw35 antigen and abnormalities of the complement system, immunoglobulins and other serum proteins. J Clin Endocrinol Metab 45:270–274

Ochi Y, DeGroot LJ (1969) Vitiligo in Graves' disease. Ann Intern Med 71:935–940

O'Donnell J, Trokoudes K, Silverberg J, Row VV, Volpé R (1978) Thyrotropin displacement activity (TDA) of serum immunoglobulins from patients with Graves' disease. J Clin Endocrinol Metab 46:770–777

Okamura K, Inoue K, Omae T (1978) A case of Hashimoto's thyroiditis with thyroid immunological abnormality manifested after habitual ingestion of seaweed. Acta Endocrinol (Copenh) 88:703–712

Okita N, Kidd A, Row VV, Volpé R (1980 a) Sensitization of T lymphocytes in Graves' and Hashimoto's diseases. J Clin Endocrinol Metab 51: 316–320

Okita N, Topliss D, Lewis M, Row VV, Volpé R (1980b) Studies of allosuppressor effect on the immunopathology of Graves' disease and Hashimoto's thyroiditis (Abstr). Meeting Canadian Soc Clin Invest, Ottawa, Ontario, October 3–5, 1980 Clin Res 28: 674 A

Okita N, Kidd A, Row VV, Volpé R (1981a) Suppressor T lymphocyte deficiency in Graves' disease and Hashimoto's thyroiditis. J Clin Endocrinol Metab 52: 528–533

Okita N, Kidd A, Row VV, Volpé R (1981b) T lymphocyte sensitization in Graves' and Hashimoto's diseases confirmed by an indirect migration inhibition factor (MIF) test using normal T lymphocytes as indicator cells. J Clin Endocrinol Metab 52: 523–527

Onaya T, Kotani M, Yamada T, Ochi Y (1973) New in vitro tests to detect the thyroid stimulator in sera from hyperthyroid patients by measuring colloid droplet formation and cyclic AMP in human thyroid slices. J Clin Endocrinol Metab 36:859–866

Ong M, Malkin DG, Tay SK, Malkin A (1976) Activation of thyroid adenyl cyclase by antisera to thyroid plasma membrane preaprations. Endocrinology 98:880–885

Orgiazzi JDE, Chopra IJ, Solomon DH (1976) Human thyroid adenyl cyclase stimulator in immunoglobulin G (IgG) in patients with Graves' disease. In: Robbins J, Braverman LE (eds) Thyroid research. Excerpta Medica, Amsterdam, pp 407–410

Osband M, Parkman R (1978) The control of autoreactivity. I. Lack of autoreactivity in murine spleens is due to concomitant presence of suppressor and autocytotoxic lymphocytes. J Immunol 121:179–185

Owen CA Jr (1958) A review of auto-immunization in Hashimoto's disease. J Clin Endocrinol Metab 18:1015–1023

Packalén T, Wasserman J (1971) Inhibition of migration of normal guinea pig blood leukocytes by homologous immune gammaglobulin in the presence of specific antigen. Int Arch Allergy Appl Immunol 41:790–796

Paget SA, McMaster PRB, Van Boxel JA (1976) Experimental autoimmune thyroiditis in the guinea pig: characterization of infiltrating lymphocyte populations. J Immunol 117:2267–2269

Parker RH, Beierwaltes WH (1961) Thyroid antibodies during pregnancy and in the newborn. J Clin Endocrinol 21:792–798

Parry CH (1825) Collections from the unpublished medical writings of the late Caleb Hillier Parry, vol 2. Underwood, London, pp 111–128

Peake RL, Willis DB, Asimakis GK Jr, Deiss WP Jr (1974) Radioimmunologic assay for anti-thyroglobulin antibodies. J Lab Clin Med 84:907–919

Peillon F, Metzger J, Garnier H, Gilbert-Dreyfus R (1974) Cushing's syndrome due to primary adrenal tumor with hypothyroidism of autoimmune origin. Ann Med Intern (Paris) 125:169–175

Penhale WJ, Irvine WJ, Inglis JR, Farmer A (1976) Thyroiditis in T cell depleted rats: suppression of the autoallergic response by reconsitution with normal lymphoid cells. Clin Exp Immunol 25:6–16

Perlman LV (1961) Familial incidence of diabetes in hyperthyroidism. Ann Intern Med 55:796–799

Perloff WH (1956) Thyrotoxicosis following acute thyroiditis: a report of five cases. J Clin Endocrinol Metab 16:542–546

Pilepich MV, Jackson I, Munzenrider JE, Brown RS (1978) Graves' disease following irradiation for Hodgkin's disease. JAMA 240:1381–1382

Pimstone BL, Hoffenberg R, Black E (1964) Parallel assay of thyrotrophin, long-acting thyroid stimulator and exophthalmos producing substance in endocrine exophthalmos and pretibial myxoedema. J Clin Endocrinol Metab 24:976–982

Pinchera A, Pinchera MG, Stanbury JB (1965) Thyrotropin and long-acting thyroid stimulator assays in thyroid disease. J Clin Endocrinol Metab 25:189–208

Pinchera A, Liberti P, Martino E, Fenzi GF, Grasso L, Rovis L, Baschieri L (1969) Effect of antithyroid drug therapy on the long-acting thyroid stimulator and the antithyroglobulin antibodies. J Clin Endocrinol Metab 29:231–238

Pinchera A, Fenzi GF, Bartalena L, Chiovato L, Marcocci C, Pacini F (1979) Thyroid antigens involved in autoimmune thyroid disorders. In: Klein E, Horster FA (eds) Autoimmunity in thyroid diseases. Schattauer, Stuttgart New York, pp 49–67

Pinchera A, Fenzi GF, Bartalena L, Chiovato L, Marcocci C, Toccafondi R, Rotella ACM, Zonefrati R (1980) Thyroid cell surface and thyroid stimulating antibody in patients with thyroid autoimmune disease. In: Stockigt JR, Nagataki S (eds) Thyroid research VIII. Austral Acad Sci Canberra, pp 707–710

Podleski WK (1972) Cytotoxic lymphocytes in Hashimoto's thyroiditis. Clin Exp Immunol 11:543–548

Pulvertaft RJV, Doniach D, Roitt IM (1959) Cytotoxic effects of Hashimoto serum on human thyroid cells in tissue culture. Lancet 2:214–216

Rallison ML, Dobyns BM, Keating FR, Rall JE, Tyler FH (1975) Occurrence and natural history of chronic lymphocytic thyroiditis in childhood. J Pediatr 86:675–682

Ramsay I (1974) Thyroid disease and muscle dysfunction. Heinemann, London

Rapaport B, Pillarisetty RJ, Herman EA, Clark OH, Conga EG (1978) Production of a non-immunoglobulin thyroid stimulator by human lymphocytes during mixed culture with human thyroid cells. J Biol Chem 253:631–640

Richter E, Wick G, Zambelis N, Ludwig H, Schernthaner G (1978) Demonstration and characterization of thyroglobulin binding peripheral blood cells in Hashimoto patients by fluoroimmunocytoadherence. Clin Immunol Immunopathol 11:178–189

Riley FC (1972) Orbital pathology in Graves' disease. Mayo Clin Proc 47:975–979

Roberts IM, Whittingham S, MacKay IR (1973) Tolerance to an autoantigen – thyroglobulin. Antigen binding lymphocytes in thymus and blood in health and autoimmune disease. Lancet 2:936–940

Robinson RG, Guttler RB, Rhea TH, Nicoloff JT (1974) Delayed hypersensitivity in Graves' disease. J Clin Endocrinol Metab 38:322–324

Rocklin RE, McDermott RP, Coress L, Schlossman SP, David JR (1974) Studies on mediator production by highly purified human T and B lymphocytes. J Exp Med 140:1303–1316

Roitt IM, Torrigiani G (1967) Identification and estimation of undegraded thyroglobulin in human serum. Endocrinology 81:421–429

Roitt IM, Doniach D, Campbell RN, Hudson RV (1956) Auto-antibodies in Hashimoto's disease (lymphadenoid goitre). Lancet 2:820–821

Roitt IM, Ling NR, Doniach D, Couchman KG (1964) The cytoplasmic auto-antigen of the human thyroid. I. Immunological and biochemical characteristics. Immunology 7:375–393

Rose NR, Witebsky E (1956) Studies on organ specificity. V. Changes in the thyroid glands of rabbits following active immunization with rabbit thyroid extracts. J Immunol 76:417–427

Rose NR, Witebsky E (1971) Experimental thyroiditis. In: Samter M, Talmage DW, Rose B, Sherman WB, Vaughan JH (eds) Immunological diseases. Little Brown, Boston, pp 1179–1197

Rundle FF, Pochin EE (1944) The orbital tissues in thyrotoxicosis: a quantitative analysis relating to exophthalmos. Clin Sci 5:51–74

Saenger EL, Thoma GE, Tompkins EA (1968) Incidence of leukaemia following treatment of hyperthyroidism. JAMA 205:855–862

Salabe GB, Salabe H, Dominici R, Daroli C, Andreoli M (1974) Radioimmunoassay for human antithyroglobulin antibodies. II. Determination of antigen-binding capacity. J Clin Endocrinol Metab 39:1125–1132

Salabe GB, Salabe H, Accinni L, Dominici R (1978) Receptors for fluoresceinated human thyroglobulin in peripheral blood lymphocytes. Clin Exp Immunol 32:159–168

Salisbury S, Embril JA (1978) Graves' disease following congenital cytomegalovirus infection. J Pediatr 92:954–955

Sasazuki P, Kohno Y, Iwamoto I, Kosaka K, Okimoto K, Maruyama H, Ishiba S, Konishi J, Takeda Y, Naito S (1978) HLA and Graves' disease or diabetes mellitus in Japan. N Engl J Med 298:630–631

Sattler H (1952) Basedow's disease. Grune & Stratton, New York

Saxon A, Stevens RH, Ramer SJ, Clements PJ, Yu DTY (1978) Clucocorticoids administered in vivo inhibit human suppressor T lymphocyte function and diminish B lymphocyte responsiveness in in vitro immunoglobulin synthesis. J Clin Invest 61:922–930

Schatz DL, Volpé R, Higgins HP, Steiner G (1979) Primary thyroid failure followed by thyrotoxicosis. Program of the 61st Annual Meeting, Endocrinol Soc, June 13–15, 1979, Anaheim, California, Abstract 889 (to be published)

Scherbaum W, Rosenau KO, Seif FJ (1978) Rheumatoid factors and thyroid antibodies in Graves'-Basedow disease. Acta Endocrinol [Suppl 215] (Copenh) 89:77–78

Schermer DR, Roenigk HH, Schumacher OP, McKenzie JM (1970) Relation of long-acting thyroid stimulator to pretibial myxedema. Arch Dermatol 102:62–67

Schernthaner G, Schleusener H, Fink ER, Kotulla P, Ludwig H, Mayr WR (1978) Thyroid stimulating immunoglobulin and HLA type in patients with ophthalmic Graves' disease, thyrotoxicosis and Hashimoto's thyroiditis. Acta Endocrinol [Suppl 215] (Copenh) 87:79

Schimpff SC, Diggs CH, Wiswell JG, Salvatore PC Wiernik PH (1980) Radiation related thyroid dysfunction: implications for the treatment of Hodgkin's disease. Ann Intern Med 92:91–98

Schleusener H, Kotulla P, Kruck I, Kruck G, Geissler D, Adlkofer F (1976) Comparison and evaluation of radioligand receptor assay and the mouse bioassay for the protection of human thyroid stimulating immunoglobulins. In: Robbins J, Braverman LE (eds) Thyroid research. Excerpta Medica, Amsterdam, pp 414–416

Schleusener H, Wenzel B, Kotulla P, Wenzel KW (1979) Specific binding of blood lymphocytes and humoral antibodies from patients with Graves' disease to the solubilized TSH receptor. In: Klein E, Horster FA (eds) Autoimmunity in thyroid diseases. Schattauer, Stuttgart, pp 117–124

Schmidt MB (1926) Eine biglandulare Erkrankung (Nebennieren und Schilddrüse) bei morbus Addisonii. Verh Dtsch Ges Pathol 21:212–221

Schultz RO, Van Allen MW, Blodi FC (1960) Endocrine ophthalmoplegia, with an electromyographic study of paretic extraocular muscles. Arch Ophthal mol 63:217–225

Schwartz WL (1973) Hypothyroidism and Addison's disease totally corrected by adrenal replacement. Calif Med 118:57–61

Shearn MA (1971) Sjögren's syndrome. Saunders, Philadelphia (Major problems in internal medicine, vol 2)

Sheets RF (1955) The sequential occurrence of actue thyroiditis and thyrotoxicosis. JAMA 157:139–140

Shenkman L, Bottone EJ (1976) Antibodies to *Yersinia enterocolitica* in thyroid disease. Ann Intern Med 85:735–739

Silverberg J, Trokoudes K, Sugenoya A, Row VV, Volpé R (1978 a) Leukocyte adherence inhibition in thyroid disease. Clin Invest Med 1:93–96

Silverberg J, Row VV, Volpé R (1978 b) Rheumatoid factors in Graves' disease. Ann Intern Med 88:216

Simpson JA (1968) The correlation between myaesthenia gravis and disorders of the thyroid gland. In: Muscular Dystrophy Committee (ed) Research in muscular dystrophy. Proc 4th symposium on current research in muscular dystrophy, National Hospital, Queen's Square, London, January 11–12, 1968. Pitman, London

Skoldstam L, Anderberg B, Norrby K (1978) B and T lymphocytes in toxic diffuse goitre. Clin Exp Immunol 31:524–528

Smith BR (1976) Immunology of the thyrotropin receptor. Immunol Commun 5:345–360

Smith BR, Hall R (1980) The interaction of Graves' immunoglobulin with the TSH receptor. In: Stockigt JR, Nagataki S (eds) Thyroid research VIII. Austral Acad Sci Canberra, pp 715–716

Smith BR, Hall R (1974) Thyroid stimulating immunoglobulins in Graves' disease. Lancet 2:427–431

Smith BR, Pyle GA, Peterson VB, Hall R (1977) Interaction of thyroid stimulating antibodies with the human thyrotropin receptor. J Endocrinol 75:401–407

Solomon DH, Chopra IJ (1972) Graves' disease. Mayo Clin Proc 47:803–813

Solomon DH, Chopra IJ, Chopra U, Smith FJ (1977) Identification of subgroups of euthyroid ophthalmic Graves' ophthalmopathy. N Engl J Med 296:181–185

Sorkin E, Desodovsky H (1976) Hormonal control of immune processes. In: Proc Vth Internat Congr Endocrinol, July 18–24, 1976, Hamburg, West Germany. Excerpta Medica, Amsterdam, Abstract

Staeheli V, Vallotton MB, Burger A (1975) Detection of human anti-thyroxine and anti-triiodothyronine antibodies in different thyroid conditions. J Clin Endocrinol Metab 41:669–675

Strakosch CR, Joyner D, Wall JR (1978) Thyroid stimulating antibodies in patients with subacute thyroiditis. J Clin Endocrinol Metab 46:345–348

Sugenoya A, Trokoudes K, Row VV, Volpé R (1978) The production of thyroid stimulating immunoglobulin (TSI) by lymphocytes from patients with Graves' disease cultured with human thyroid subcellular fractions. J Endocrinol Invest 1:245–251

Sugenoya A, Silverberg J, Trokoudes K, Row VV, Volpé R (1979 a) Macrophage-lymphocyte interaction in Graves' disease and Hashimoto's thyroiditis. Acta Endocrinol (Copenh) 91:99–108

Sugenoya A, Kidd A, Trokoudes K, Row VV, Volpé R (1979 b) Correlation between thyrotropin displacing activity (TDA) and human thyroid stimulating activity (TSA) by immunoglobulins from patients with Graves' disease and other thyroid disorders. J Clin Endocrinol Metab 48:398–402

Sung LC, McDougall IR (1978) Graves' hyperthyroidism: spontaneous occurrence after autoimmune hypothyroidism with persistent infiltrative ophthalmopathy. Arch Intern Med 138:1009–1010

Takahashi H, Bardy MD, Sharma V, Grunt JA (1979) Hyperthyroidism in patients with Down's syndrome. Clin Pediatr 18:273–275

Takeda Y, Kriss JP (1977) Radiometric measurement of thyroglobulin-antithyroglobulin immune complex in human serum. J Clin Endocrinol Metab 44:46–55

Talal N, Roubinian JR (1978) Sex hormones and autoimmunity. In: Rose NR, Bigazzi PE (eds) Genetic control of autoimmune disease. Elsevier/North Holland, New York, pp 163–176

Teng CS, Yeung RTT (1980) Changes in thyroid stimulating antibody activity in Graves' disease treated with antithyroid drug and its relationship to relapse: a prospective study. J Clin Endocrinol Metab 50:144–147

Teng CS, Smith BR, Clayton B, Evered DC, Clark F, Hall R (1977) Thyroid stimulating immunoglobulins in ophthalmic Graves' disease. Clin Endocrinol (Oxf) 6:207–211

Teng CS, Yeung RTT, Khoo RKK, Alagaratnam TT (1980) A prospective study of the changes in thyrotropin binding inhibitory immunoglobulins in Graves' disease treated by subtotal thyroidectomy or radioactive iodine. J Clin Endocrinol Metab 50:1005–1010

Thorsby E, Svejgaard E, Solem JH, Kornstad L (1975) The frequency of major histocompatibility antigens (SD and LD) in thyrotoxicosis. Tissue Antigens 6:54–55

Topliss DJ, White EL, Stockigt JR (1980) Significance of thyrotropin excess in untreated primary adrenal insufficiency. J Clin Endocrinol Metab 50:52–56

Totterman TH (1978) Distribution of T, B and thyroglobulin-binding lymphocytes infiltrating the thyroid gland in Graves' disease, Hashimoto's thyroiditis and DeQuervain's thyroiditis. Clin Immunol Immunopathol 10:270–277

Totterman TH, Gordin A, Hayry P, Andersson LC, Makinen T (1978) Accumulation of thyroid antigen-reactive T lymphocytes in the gland of patients with subacute thyroiditis. Clin Exp Immunol 32:153–158

Totterman TH, Andersson LC, Hayry P (1979) Evidence for thyroid antigen-reactive T lymphocytes infiltrating the thyroid gland in Graves' disease. Clin Endocrinol (Oxf) 11:59–68

Trokoudes KM, Sugenoya A, Hazani E, Row VV, Volpé R (1979) Thyroid stimulating hormone binding to extrathyroidal human tissues. TSH and thyroid stimulating immunoglobulin effects on adenosine 3′, 5′ monophosphate in testicular and adrenal tissue. J Clin Endocrinol Metab 48:919–923

Tunbridge WMG (1979) The epidemiology of hypothyroidism. Clin Endocrinol Metab 8:21–27

Ungar B, Mathews JD, Tait BD, Cowling DC (1977) HLA patterns in pernicious anaemia. Br Med J 1:798–800

Van Boxel JA, Paul WE, Frank MM, Green I (1973) Antibody-dependent lymphoid cell-mediated cytotoxicity: role of lymphocytes bearing a receptor for complement. J Immunol 110:1027–1036

Van der Heide D, Daha MR, Bolk JH, Bussemaker JK, DeBruin TWA, Goslings BM, van Es LA (1980) Circulating immune complexes and thyroid stimulating immunoglobulins before, during and after antithyroid drug therapy in patients with Graves' disease Lancet 1:1376–1379

Van Herle AJ, Uller RP, Matthews NL, Brown J (1973) Radioimmunoassay for measurement of thyroglobulin in human serum. J Clin Invest 52:1320–1327

Van Herle AJ, Vassart G, Dumont JE (1979) Control of thyroglobulin synthesis and secretion. N Engl J Med 301:239–249; 307–314

Van Welsum M, Feltkamp TEW, DeVries MJ, Docter R, Van Zijl J, Henneman G (1974) Hypothyroidism after thyroidectomy for Graves' disease: a search for an explanation. Br Med J 4:755–756

Verhoeven RP, Visser TJ, Docter R, Henneman G, Schalekamp MADH (1974) Plasma thyroxine, 3,3′,5-triiodothyronine and 3,3′,5′-triiodothyronine during beta adrenergic blockade in hyperthyroidism. J Clin Endocrinol Metab 44:1002–1005

Vickery AL, Hamlin E Jr (1961) Struma lymphomatosa (Hashimoto's thyroiditis): observations on repeated biopsies in 16 patients. N Engl J Med 264:226–229

Vladutiu AO, Rose NR (1971) Transfer of experimental autoimmune thyroiditis of the mouse by serum. J Immunol 106:1139–1142

Vladutiu AO, Rose NR (1972) Murine thyroiditis. III. Influence of syngeneic and allogeneic thyroid antigen on induction of the disease. Clin Exp Immunol 2:242–254

Vladutiu AO, Rose NR (1975) Cellular basis of the genetic control of immune responsiveness to murine thyroglobulin in mice. Cell Immunol 17:106–113

Vogel F (1959) Moderne Probleme der Humangenetik. Ergeb Inn Med Kinderheilkd 12:52–125

Volpé R (1976) Acute and subacute thyroiditis. Pharmacol Ther [C] 1:171–181

Volpé R (1977) The role of autoimmunity in hypoendocrine and hyperendocrine function, with special emphasis on autoimmune thyroid disease. Ann Intern Med 87:86–99

Volpé R (1978 a) The pathogenesis of Graves' disease: an overview. Clin Endocrinol Metab 7:3–29

Volpé R (1978 b) The genetics and immunology of Graves' and Hashimoto's diseases. In: Rose NR, Bigazzi PE, Warner NL (eds) Genetic control of autoimmune disease. Elsevier/North Holland, New York, pp 43–56

Volpé R (1978 c) Lymphocytic (Hashimoto's) thyroiditis. In: Werner SC, and Ingbar SH (eds) The thyroid, a fundamental and clinical text, 4th ed. Harper & Row, New York, pp 996–1008

Volpé R (1979 a) Subacute (DeQuervain's) thyroiditis. Clin Endocrinol Metab 8:81–96
Volpé R (1979 b) Autoimmunity in chronic thyroiditis. In: Klein E, Horster FA (eds) Autoimmunity in thyroid diseases. Schattauer, Stuttgart, pp 33–48
Volpé R, Row VV (1975) Proportion of E rosettes normal in Graves' and Hashimoto's diseases: a retraction. N Engl J Med 293:44
Volpé R, Vale J, Johnston MW (1960) The effect of certain physical and emotional tensions and strains on fluctuations in the level of serum protein bound iodine. J Clin Endocrinol Metab 20:415–528
Volpé R, Row VV, Ezrin C (1967) Circulating viral and thyroid antibodies in subacute thyroiditis. J Clin Endocrinol Metab 27:1275–1284
Volpé R, Desbarats-Schonbaum ML, Schonbaum E, Row VV, Ezrin C (1969) The effect of radioablation of the thyroid gland in Graves' disease with high levels of long acting thyroid stimulator (LATS). Am J Med 46:217–226
Volpé R, Edmonds MW, Clarke PV, Row VV (1970) A viewpoint regarding the nature of the emergence of long-acting thyroid stimulator of Graves' disease. Acta Endocrinol Panam 1:155–170
Volpé R, Edmonds MW, Lamki L, Clarke PV, Row VV (1972) The pathogenesis of Graves' disease: a disorder of delayed hypersensitivity? Mayo Clin Proc 47:824–834
Volpé R, Clarke PV, Row VV (1973) The relationship of age-specific incidence rates to immunological aspects of Hashimoto's thyroiditis. Can Med Assoc J 109:898–901
Volpé R, Farid NR, von Westarp C, Row VV (1974) The pathogenesis of Graves' disease and Hashimoto's thyroiditis. Clin Endocrinol (Oxf) 3:239–261
Volpé R, Row VV (1975) Proportion of E rosettes normal in Graves' and Hashimoto's diseases: a retraction. N Engl J Med 293:44
Von Basedow CA (1840) Exophthalmos durch Hypertrophie des Zellgewebes in der Augenhöhle. Wochensch Gesamte Heilkd 13:198–228
von Westarp C, Knox AJS, Row VV, Volpé R (1977) Comparison of thyroid antigens by the experimental production of precipitating antibodies to human thyroid fractions and the identification of an antibody which competes with long acting thyroid stimulator for thyroid binding. Acta Endocrinol (Copenh) 84:759–769
von Westarp C, Garcia A, Wilkins J (1980) Human thyrotropin receptor purification by affinity chromatography. 62nd Meeting, Endocrinol Soc, Washington, DC, June 18–20, 1980, Abstract 307 (to be published)
Walfish PG, Green N (1980) Post-partum recurrence of the transient thyrotoxicosis and painless thyroiditis syndrome. 62nd Meeting, Endocrinol Soc, Washington, DC, June 18–20, 1980, Abstract 513 (to be published)
Wall JR, Ryan EA (1980) Leukocyte migration inhibition factor (LMIF) production in response to bacterial and fungal antigens in patients with Graves' hyperthyroidism: suppression by concanavalin-A induced suppressor cells. In: Pinchera A (ed) Autoimmune aspects of endocrine disorders. Academic Press, New York, pp 235–240
Wall JR, Fang SL, Ingbar SH, Braverman LE (1976 a) Lymphocyte transformation in response to human thyroid extract in patients with subacute thyroiditis. J Clin Endocrinol Metab 43:587–590
Wall JR, Manwar GL, Greenwood DM, Walters BA (1976 b) The in vitro suppression of lectin induced ^{3}H-thymidine incorporation into DNA of peripheral blood lymphocytes after the addition of propylthiouracil. J Clin Endocrinol Metab 43:1406–1409
Wall JR, Gray B, Greenwood DM (1977) Total and "activated" peripheral blood T lymphocytes in patients with thyroid disorders. Acta Endocrinol (Copenh) 85:753–759
Wall JR, Trewin A, Fang SL, Ingbar SH, Braverman LE (1978) Studies of immunoreactivity to human lacrimal gland fractions in patients with ophthalmic Graves' disease. J Endocrinol Invest 1:253–258
Wall JR, Joyner DM, Ryan EA (1979 a) In: Pinchera A (ed) Effect of experimental hyper- and hypothyroidism on B and T lymphocyte reactivity to bacterial, fungal and tissue antigens. In: Autoimmune aspects of endocrine disorders, Pisa, Italy, 19–21 April 1979. Academic Press, New York, 1980, pp 215–220
Wall JR, Strakosch CR, Fang SL, Ingbar SH, Braverman LE (1979 b) Thyroid binding antibodies and other immunological abnormalities in patients with Graves' ophthalmopathy. Effect of treatment with cyclophosphamide. Clin Endocrinol (Oxf) 10:79–91
Wall JR, Henderson J, Strakosch CR, Joyner DM (1981) Graves' ophthalmopathy – a review. Can Med Assoc J 124:855–866
Wartenberg J, Doniach D, Brostoff J, Roitt IM (1973) Leukocyte migration inhibition in human autoimmune thyroid disease. Clin Exp Immunol 14:203–212

Wasnich RD, Grumet FC, Payne RO, Kriss JP (1973) Graves' ophthalmopathy following external neck irradiation for nonthyroidal neoplastic disease. J Clin Endocrinol Metab 37:703–713

Weigle WO, Romball CG (1975) Humoral and cell-mediated immunity in experimental progressive thyroiditis in rabbits. Clin Exp Immunol 21:351–361

Weissel M, Höfer R, Zasmeta H, Mayr WR (1980) HLA-DR and Hashimoto's thyroiditis. Tissue Antigens 16: 256–257

Wekerle H, Begemann M (1978) In vitro induction of experimental autoimmune orchitis. Characterization of a primary T-lymphocyte response against testicular self-antigens. Eur J Immunol 8:294–302

Wenzel KW, Schleusener H, Weise W (1974) Durch externe Schilddrüsenbestrahlung ausgelöste Hyperthyreose und endokrine Ophthalmopathie. Dtsch Med Wochenschr 99:2036–2039

Wenzel B, Kotulla P, Schleusener H (1978) Binding of solubilized human TSH receptor by peripheral blood lymphocytes of patients with Graves' disease (Abstract 37). Ann Endocrinol (Paris) t 39:22 A

Werner SC (1979) Graves' disease following acute (subacute) thyroiditis. Arch Intern Med 139:1313–1315

Werner SC, Fierer JA (1972) Cell-mediated immunity in Graves' disease? N Engl J Med 287:1251

Werner SC, Ingbar SH (1978) The thyroid, a fundamental and clinical text, 4th ed. Harper & Row, New York

Werner SC, Wegelius O, Fierer JA, Hsu (1972) Immunoglobulins (EMG) and complement in the connective tissues of the thyroid in Graves' disease. N Engl J Med 287:421–425

Werner SC, Platman SR (1965) Remission of hyperthyroidism (Graves' disease) and altered pattern of serum thyroxine binding induced by prednisone. Lancet 2:751–756

Whaley K, Webb J, McAvoy BA, Hughes GRV, Lee P, MacSween RNM, Buchanan WW (1973) Sjögren's syndrome. II. Clinical associations and immunological phenomena. Q J Med 42:513–548

Wick G (1975) Experimental animal models in autoimmune thyroid disease. Clin Endocrinol Metab 4:241–266

Wick G, Boyd R (1979) Effector mechanisms in thyroid autoimmune diseases. In: Klein K, Horster FA (eds) Autoimmunity in thyroid diseases. Schattauer, Stuttgart, pp 23–29

Wick G, Graf J (1972) Electron-microscopic studies in chickens of the obese strain with spontaneous hereditary autoimmune thyroiditis. Lab Invest 27:400–411

Wick G, Sundick RS, Albini B (1974) The Obese strain (OS) of chickens: an animal model with spontaneous autoimmune thyroiditis. Clin Immunol Immunopathol 3:272–300

Wick G, Kofler R, Gundolf R, Muller PU, Boyd R (1979) The nature of effector cells in experimental and spontaneous autoimmune thyroiditis. In: Milgrom F, Albini S (eds) Immunopathology. Karger, Basel, pp 101–106

Wigzell H, Binz H, Frischknecht H, Peterson P, Sege K (1978) Possible roles of auto-antiidiotypic immunity in auto-immune disease. In: Rose NR, Bigazzi PE, Warner NL (eds) Genetic control of autoimmune disease. Elsevier/North Holland, New York, pp 327–342

Wilkin TJ, Beck JS, Gunn A, Al Moussah M, Isles TE, Crooks J (1980) Autoantibodies in thyrotoxicosis: a quantitative study of their behaviour in relation to the course and outcome of the disease. J Endocrinol Invest 3:5–14

Witebsky E, Rose NR (1956) Studies on organ specificity. IV. Production of rabbit thyroid antibodies in the rabbit. J Immunol 76:408–416

Wood LC, Maloof F (1975) Thyroid failure after potassium iodide treatment of diffuse toxic goiter. Trans Assoc Am Physicians 88:235–247

Wood LD, Ingbar SH (1979) Hypothyroidism as a late sequela in patients with Graves' disease treated with antithyroid agents. J Clin Invest 64:1429–1436

Wyse EP, McConahey WM, Woolner LB, Scholz DA, Kearns TP (1968) Ophthalmopathy without hyperthyroidism in patients with histologic Hashimoto's thyroiditis. J Clin Endocrinol Metab 28:1623–1629

Yamamoto T, Sakamoto H (1978) Spontaneous remission from primary hypothyroidism. Ann Intern Med 88:808–809

Yamamoto M, Rapaport B, Clark OH (1978) Evidence for increased production of prostaglandin E by the thyroid in Graves' disease. 54th Meeting, Am Thyroid Assoc, Portland, Oregon, 13–16 September 1978, Abstract T2 (to be published)

Yeo PPB, Cheah JS, Sinriah R (1978 a) Pretibial myxoedema. A clinical and pathological study. Aust NZ J Med 8:60–62

Yeo PPB, Chan SH, Lui KF, Wee GB, Lim P, Cheah JS (1978 b) HLA and thyrotoxic periodic paralysis. Br Med J 2:930–932

Yoshida T, Sonozaki H, Cohen S (1973) The production of macrophage migration inhibition factor by B and T cells of the guinea pig. J Exp Med 138:784–797

Yoshida H, Amino N, Yagawa K, Uemura K, Satoh M, Miyai K, Kumahara Y (1978) Association of serum antithyroid antibodies with lymphocytic infiltration of the thyroid gland: study of 70 autopsied cases. J Clin Endocrinol Metab 46:859–862

Zakarija M, McKenzie JM (1978 a) Adsorption of thyroid stimulating antibody (TSAb) of Graves' disease by homologous and heterologous thyroid tissue. J Clin Endocrinol Metab 47:906–908

Zakarija M, McKenzie JM (1978 b) Zoological specificity of human thyroid stimulating antibody. J Clin Endocrinol Metab 47:249–254

Zakarija M, McKenzie JM (1980) Immunochemical characterization of thyroid stimulating antibody (TSAb). In: Stockigt JR, Nagataki S (eds) Thyroid research VIII. Austral Acad Sci Canberra, pp 669–672

Zakarija M (1980) The thyroid stimulating antibody (TSAb) of Graves' disease: evidence for restricted heterogeneity. Horm Res 13:1–15

Ziring PR, Fedun BH, Cooper LA (1975) Thyrotoxicosis in congenital rubella. J Pediatr 87:1002

3 Auto-immunity in Diabetes Mellitus

3.1 Introduction

Diabetes mellitus was a disease known to the ancients (Best 1960). Symptoms of this disorder were first described in the Ebers papyrus of Egypt (1500 B. C.). Aretaeus of Cappadocas termed the disorder diabetes in the second century A. D. The Greek word "diabetes" means "to flow through a siphon". The more recent history of diabetes mellitus constitutes a fascinating story in its own right, culminating in the discovery of insulin by Banting and Best of Toronto in 1921 (Banting and Best 1922) and was summarized by Best in 1960. The current chapter, however, will deal primarily with immune aspects of the disorder, and will not delve further into the metabolic, vascular and other protean aspects of this important malady.

It is a well-known and common clinical observation that spontaneous diabetes mellitus in man can either be insulin-dependent, or insulin-independent. Previous conceptions generally related the insulin-dependent form of diabetes to juvenile-onset diabetes, whereas insulin-independent diabetes was often considered to be a disease of maturity-onset (Table 3.1). However, it is now clear and equally accepted that insulin-dependent diabetes can and does commence in adulthood and indeed even in late adult life, whereas conversely, occasionally insulin-independent diabetes can occur in childhood (Craighead 1978). This has led to a new classification of diabetics which is unrelated to the age of onset, namely type I and type II diabetics (Irvine 1977; Cudworth 1977). Type I includes insulin-dependent diabetics, whether of juvenile or adult-onset, as well as those insulin-dependent diabetics who may be initially controlled by oral hypoglycaemic agents, but who are

Table 3.1. Characteristics of insulin-dependent (type I) and non-insulin-dependent (type II) diabetics (Craighead 1978)

Characteristic	Insulin-dependent	Non-insulin-dependent
Clinical features:		
Weight at onset	Non-obese	Often obese
Age at onset (year)	Usually less than 20	Usually greater than 40
Onset	Rapid-gradual	Insidious
Ketosis	Usual	Uncommon
Epidemiology:		
Peak age of onset (year)	12–14	Greater than 50
Prevalence (percentage)	0.5	2
Pathology:		
Islet beta cell mass (percentage)	Less than 10	Moderate reduction
Insulitis at onset	Often	Probably absent

shown to have islet cell antibodies; this group of patients has a tendency to progress to type I (insulin-dependent) diabetes mellitus. Thus, some prediction of this change is possible in some of the patients who do not (yet) require insulin. Type II diabetes, on the other hand, defines diabetics who are insulin-independent, whether of maturity-onset or juvenile-onset (this would include maturity-onset diabetes of the young (MODY)); in the juvenile-onset type II group, islet cell antibodies are lacking.

Actually, it has been a result of immunological studies that has led to the clear differentiation between type I and type II diabetics (Bottazzo et al. 1974; Bottazzo and Doniach 1978; MacCuish et al. 1974 a, b). Humoral antibodies in diabetes reacting specifically with pancreatic islet cells were first demonstrated only in diabetic patients with insulin-dependent diabetes plus coexisting auto-immune conditions (Bottazzo et al. 1974; MacCuish et al. 1974 b). Later reports, however, have demonstrated islet cell antibodies (ICA) in insulin-dependent diabetics without other coexisting auto-immune conditions (Doniach and Bottazzo 1977). However, these antibodies are found much more commonly in those that are termed by Bottazzo et al. (1978 a) as Ib diabetes, or by Bottazzo and Doniach (1978) as polyendocrine type I diabetes mellitus (i.e. those type I diabetics who have the genetic propensity to have other organ-specific auto-immune diseases), or by Irvine et al. (1978 a, b) as Irl (see below).

It is evident that diabetes mellitus has a familial pattern of transmission, but it is increasingly clear that there is genetic heterogeneity (Fajans et al. 1978). Thus, the disorder may be the result of more than one process (Drash 1979; Notkins 1979). Even amongst juvenile diabetics, there was evidence of genetic heterogeneity recognized before the era of HLA typing by virtue of the incidence of antithyroid and antigastric antibodies in propositi and families of patients with this disorder (Goldstein et al. 1970; Nissley et al. 1973). The sections of this chapter relating to aetiology will deal primarily with type I diabetes, in relation to the immune and genetic factors which may be operative in this particular condition.

3.2 Genetics

Craighead (1978) has stated that fewer than 20% of patients with diabetes have first-degree relatives with a diabetic history, and a definable pattern of transmission has thus not been established in family studies. Thus, autosomal recessive inheritance with variable penetrance has been a widely accepted concept. Rubinstein et al. (1977) have shown evidence that the inheritance is autosomal recessive with 50% penetrance; the predisposing gene is linked with the HLA-D segment.

Pyke and Nelson (1976) have followed over one hundred pairs of identical twins in which one member was affected with diabetes mellitus. It was of great interest that the concordance rate in twins under the age of 40 was only about 50%, rather similar to the concordance rate in twins with Graves' disease (Volpé et al. 1972). Rather surprisingly, studies of twins with diabetes commencing over the age of 40 had a much greater concordance rate (39 out of 42 pairs of twins) (Table 3.2). Similar observations on smaller numbers of patients have been made by Gottlieb and Root (1968) and Then Bergh (1939), and summarized by Fajans et al. (1978).

Table 3.2. Diabetes in identical twins (Pyke 1979)

	No. of pairs		Total
	Concordant	Discordant	
IDD	73	59	132
NIDD	47	6	53
			185

IDD, insulin-dependent diabetes
NIDD, non-insulin-dependent diabetes

Of course, a 50% concordance rate in monozygotic twins in the younger diabetic groups is very much higher than one would anticipate in dizygotic twins or non-twinned siblings. It is thus clear from such studies that there are genetic factors in the genesis of this type of diabetes. The fact that there is *discordance* in 50% of this group suggests that there are also elements other than those which are purely genetic (Tattersall and Pyke 1972; Pyke 1979; Zonana and Rimoin 1976), and such environmental factors as virus diseases have been suggested as a possibility (Craighead 1978; Drash 1979; Fajans et al. 1978; Notkins 1977, 1979). While this will be explored further below, Rosenthal et al. (1976) have argued that diabetes mellitus in man, regardless of age, is primarily genetic in origin, with environmental factors apparently influencing only the time of appearance of the disease. A possibility (favoured by the author) is that in those diabetics suffering from auto-immune isletitis [Irl of Irvine et al. (1978 a) or Ib of Bottazzo et al. (1978 a)], a normally mutating "forbidden" clone of islet-directed helper T-lymphocytes (occuring at random) arises and is not suppressed (because of the genetic defect in immunoregulation). This would thus be analogous to the hypothesis already proposed for auto-immune thyroid disease (Volpé 1978) and reviewed in the preceding chapters. In the author's view, it is possibly *this* random event which may well be the "environmental" factor which precipitates this type of auto-immune diabetes mellitus in the genetically predisposed persons. This possibility will also be discussed further below.

In addition to such twin studies, the association of type I diabetes mellitus with other organ-specific auto-immune diseases certainly has strongly suggested that there must be a common factor in their pathogenesis (Cudworth 1976, 1977; Doniach and Bottazzo 1977; Irvine 1977). Irvine (1977) has pointed out that the association is almost exclusively with ketosis-prone insulin-dependent diabetes, indicating that the common pathogenic factor of auto-immunity is relevant only to insulin-dependent diabetes and not to the insulin-independent group. These associations will be discussed further below.

3.3 HLA Antigens in Type I Diabetes

As with many of the other organ-specific auto-immune diseases, there is consider-able evidence indicating a relationship between certain HLA antigens and type I diabetes. HLA-B8 in linkage disequilibrium with A-1, Dw3, DRw3, on the one hand, and HLA-B15, together with A-2, Cw3, Dw4 and DRw4, on the other, have been demonstrated much more commonly than in control persons, and are thus associated with the development of type I diabetes (Irvine et al. 1978 a, b; Craighead 1978; Galbraith 1979; Doniach and Bottazzo 1981; Irvine 1980). On the other hand, HLA-B7 and A-3, Dw2, DRw2 appear to have a protective role (Irvine et al. 1978 b).

The accurate identification of haplotypes in families with two or more affected siblings has provided evidence for the existence of an HLA-linked gene in insulin-dependent diabetes mellitus, as illustrated by the observed variance from the expected random zygotic assortment of HLA haplotypes in siblings (Craighead 1978). If the insulin-dependent form is due to a single autosomal recessive gene, one would expect more, if not all, pairs of affected siblings to be haplotypes, identical for both HLA chromosome regions. Data accumulated by Cudworth (1978) indicated that this similarity was not demonstrable. Thus, there appears to be at least some genetic heterogeneity in this disease occurring in various families. Moreover, in some population surveys, HLA-B15 has been found with an increasing frequency in diabetic patients lacking HLA-B8 (Solow et al. 1977). Indeed, the risk of developing diabetes is substantially greater in those persons who have both HLA-B8 and HLA-B15 than in those who have either one or the other antigen. It thus seems evident that there may be two genes on the sixth chromosome, each affecting the occurrence of type I diabetes. However, it seems likely that the pathogenesis of the two subtypes of type I diabetes mellitus will be somewhat different with each gene (see below). Only HLA-B8-Dw3 has been shown to be related to the auto-immune endocrinopathies (Friedman and Fialkow 1978) and it would thus appear that HLA-B15-Dw4 might reflect some other mechanism of genetic pathogenesis.

Irvine et al. (1978 a, b) have attempted to investigate the relationship between insulin antibodies, islet cell antibodies and HLA types in insulin-treated type I diabetics. They observed that patients with HLA-B15 and/or Cw3 formed a significantly higher amount of insulin antibodies, while there was an opposite trend in patients with B8 and/or A-1. These workers concluded that there appear to be two main immune response genes in this form of diabetes. One of these, associated with B8 and A-1, seems to be characterized by the tendency of islet-cell antibodies to persist in the serum and by low antibody titres to heterologous insulin, whereas the second, associated with B15 and Cw3, seems to be characterized by high antibody titres to heterologous insulin. The first of these [termed Immune response 1 (Irl) by Irvine et al. (1977 a)] appeared to be concerned with organ-specific auto-immunity, while the second (Ir2) may be concerned with the immune response to certain exogenous antigens. Moreover, those insulin-dependent diabetics who had islet cell antibodies present in their sera for some years after diagnosis had a significantly higher prevalence of HLA-B8 than those insulin-dependent diabetics who did not manifest islet cell antibodies within one month of diagnosis. It is thus likely that Irvine's type Irl may be analogous to auto-immune thyroid disease with respect to its pathogenesis. [A different terminology is employed by Bottazzo et al. (1978 a), as has been mentioned previously; the Ir2 group of Irvine equates with the Ia group of Bottazzo et al., whereas Irvine's Irl group equates with the Ib group of Bottazzo et al. Unfortunately, the problem of having two terminologies will inevitably lead to confusion, and agreement on terminology in this field is urgently required (see Table 3.3).] It may be speculated that in this latter form, there will be no target cell (islet)

Table 3.3. Classification of type I diabetes[a] (Doniach and Bottazzo 1981)

Clinical features:	'Juvenile' type; predominantly in childhood and adolescence, but may occur at all ages; insulin-dependent	
Genetic factors:	Major susceptibility – HLA-linked genes – ? control of immune response to viruses with an affinity for beta cells	
Pathogenesis:	Destruction of beta cells (? immune mediated), failure to regenerate	
	Type Ia	Type Ib
Aetiology	(?) viral	Related to organ-specific auto-immunity
Overall frequency of DM	10%	1%
Insulin-dependent	Yes	Yes
Sex	M=F	F>M
Age	<30	Any age
Associated AI disorders	None	Adrenalitis gastritis, thyroiditis, etc.
Incidence of other auto-antibodies	Low	High
Frequency of ICA	At onset 85% After 1 year 20% Tends to disappear	Not known 38% Remains stable for years
Titre of ICA	1/250 (mean 8)	1/250
First appearance of ICA	(?) at time of viral infection	Years before onset of DM

[a] Type Ia of Doniach and Bottazzo equates to Ir2 of Irvine; type Ib equates to Irl; AI, auto-immune; ICA, islet-cell antibodies; DM, diabetes mellitus

antigenic alteration or stimulation, and that viruses (at least at the target cell level) need not be implicated (see below). Since, by analogy to auto-immune thyroid disease, the likely primary abnormality in this form of the condition is a defect in an antigen-specific clone of suppressor T-lymphocytes, perhaps a more appropriate, albeit speculative designation for this category would be Is (immune suppression) rather than Irl diabetes. At this time, however, it would not seem prudent to add further to the confusion of nomenclature by strongly advocating such a hypothetical designation.

The Irvine Ir2 (Ia of Bottazzo) form of type I diabetes, on the other hand, has no correlation with the other organ-specific auto-immune disorders, and may therefore differ in its aetiology (Doniach and Bottazzo 1981). Irvine (1977) has already pointed out that these patients have abnormalities of immune responsiveness to exogenous antigens. Thus this form is likely to be related to an abnormality of immune *response* to antigens, and possibly could result from islet cell antigenic alteration induced by viral or other agents. This form may prove to be pathogenetically separate and distinct from the Irl (Ib) form of the condition, no matter how close they may seem in terms of hormonal, biochemical, or clinical manifestations (Doniach and Bottazzo 1981; Irvine 1980) (Table 3.3). Clearly, at this time, these proposals are highly speculative and will require considerable further study before they are either proven or discarded. Studies of possible viral involvement in the aetiology of diabetes mellitus will be discussed below. It should additionally be conceded that studies of the relationship between HLA genes and antibodies to viruses have not yet been conclusive (see below).

Schernthaner et al. (1979) have studied the relationship of immune region-associated alloantigens with susceptibility to insulin-dependent diabetes, as well as their possible influence on IgG-insulin antibody production. The incidence of DRw3 and DRw4 was found in significantly increased frequency in the insulin-dependent diabetic patients, when compared to a healthy control group. Subjects positive for DRw3 carry a 4.5 fold increased risk and those positive for DRw4 carry a 2.5 fold increased risk of developing insulin-dependent diabetes. A significant tendency for high insulin-binding capacity by IgG-insulin antibodies was noted in the DRw3-negative patients, yielding a mean insulin-binding capacity of 2.24 units per litre in this group (as opposed to 0.74 in DRw3-positive diabetics). Moreover, a significantly increased insulin dosage was required for adequate metabolic control in those patients with high insulin-binding capacity (greater than 3.0 units per litre). Patients with high insulin-binding capacity and high insulin requirements were predominantly found to be DRw3-negative. This is again consistent with the view that the Dw4 group (Ir2-Ia) is associated with an excessive *immune responsiveness* (and may not be a primary auto-immune disorder in initiation).

Few investigations have been conducted thus far in non-white populations. However, in Japan, where HLA-B8 occurs rarely, and HLA-B15 is common in the general population, a different antigen, HLA-B22J has been found in a statistically significant proportion of patients with insulin-dependent diabetes mellitus (Wakisaka et al. 1976). Still another study in Japan by Nakao et al. (1977) has shown another HLA-B antigen, i. e. HLA-B12, to be increased in type I diabetics. Recently, Sasazuki et al. (1978) have investigated the incidence of the HLA-D specificities associated with Japanese patients with Graves' disease and with juvenile-onset diabetes mellitus. Whereas HLA-Dw3 has been found commonly in Caucasians with Graves' disease and with insulinopenic diabetes mellitus, this gene is virtually absent in the Japanese population, and is also absent in patients with either Graves' disease or diabetes mellitus. It is of interest, however, that HLA-DH0 was found to be significantly increased in Japanese patients with Graves' disease but *not* in those with diabetes mellitus. On the other hand, there was a significant increase in HLA-DYT in the Japanese patients with insulinopenic diabetes mellitus, but there was no such increase in those patients with Graves' disease. These data suggest that there are distinct and separate genetic factors for the development of Graves' disease on the one hand, and diabetes mellitus on the other, each of which is in linkage disequilibrium with either HLA-DH0 or DYT respectively.

The authors pointed out that it might have been reasonable to expect that a chromosome which has HLA-Dw3 and a chromosome which has DH0 or DYT might have a similar biological function responsible for the development of Graves' disease or insulinopenic diabetes mellitus. However, HLA-Dw3, DH0 and DYT seem to be completely different in their antigen specificities so far tested; nevertheless, Sasazuki et al. (1978) pointed out that there still remained the possibility that they might share similar biological functions, although these have yet to be demonstrated. While the point remains to be resolved, it may be proposed that even in Caucasians, the true "disease susceptibility genes" for Graves' disease and Irl diabetes mellitus are separate (however closely they may lie to one another) and the putative defect in antigen-specific clones of suppressor T-lymphocytes responsible for each of these disorders may consequently be separate and distinct. Studies in Black Americans with juvenile-onset diabetes (Rodney et al. 1979) showed a marked increase in HLA-DRw3 and HLA-DRw4 as compared to unaffected persons, similar to Caucasians. Conversely, there was a negative correlation between HLA-DRw2 and juvenile-onset diabetes mellitus. In Mexican-Americans on the other hand, a significant association between HLA-B18 and HLA-DRw3 was found in insulin-dependent diabetics (Zeidler et al. 1980).

3.4 Relationship to Other Organ-specific Auto-immune Diseases

MacCuish and Irvine (1975) have reviewed the clinical associations between diabetes mellitus and other organ-specific auto-immune diseases. These associations certainly provide indirect evidence for a possible immune basis for diabetes mellitus. The first instance of coexisting diabetes mellitus and adrenal insufficiency was reported in 1866 by Ogle. Irvine and Barnes (1972, 1974) reviewed the prevalence of diabetes mellitus in Addison's disease from the literature and from their own studies and found it to be between 7%–23%, with an average of approximately 18%, thus representing a sixfold excess over the estimated prevalence (1%–3%) of diabetes in the overall population of Great Britain or the United States. Conversely, Kozak (1971) and Nerup (1974) have reported that Addison's disease occurs in diabetic populations in the order of 0.023%–0.028%. Mac Cuish and Irvine (1975) estimate that the prevalence of Addison's disease in the general population is between 0.0039% and 0.0060%, thus the excess prevalence of Addison's disease in diabetes mellitus appears to be in the order of fivefold over the general population. Moreover, it is now clear that diabetes mellitus is usually associated with auto-immune adrenalitis, rather than Addison's disease due to other causes, such as tuberculosis (Solomon et al. 1965). It is now clear that the relationship to Addison's disease (and indeed the endocrinopathies to be discussed below) occurs only in type I diabetes of the Irl type (Irvine 1977), or polyendocrine Ib diabetes mellitus (Bottazzo and Doniach 1978). This form of diabetes mellitus is associated with HLA-B8 and HLA-Dw3 in Caucasians (Irvine et al. 1978 a, b), as previously noted.

Parkinson in 1910 was the first to note an association between pernicious anaemia and diabetes mellitus. Ungar et al. (1967) have estimated the prevalence of diabetes mellitus in patients with pernicious anaemia to be about 7%, whereas the prevalence of pernicious anaemia in diabetic populations has been estimated to be between 0.39% and 5% (MacCuish and Irvine 1975).

There is clearly an increased incidence of auto-immune thyroid disease (either Graves' disease or Hashimoto's thyroiditis) in diabetics and an increased incidence of diabetes mellitus in auto-immune thyroid disease (MacCuish and Irvine 1975). The relative incidences of auto-immune thyroid disease in diabetics, and vice versa, are discussed in Chap. 2. Suffice it here to say that the increased incidence of overt thyroid auto-immune disease (Graves' or Hashimoto's disease), or thyroid auto-antibodies, occurs only in type I diabetics (presumably the Irl (Ib) group) and in their families as well (Fialkow et al. 1975; Bottazzo et al. 1978 b).

In addition, auto-antibodies to thyroid and gastric antigens in diabetic patients have been extensively studied. Once again, we are indebted to MacCuish and Irvine for summarizing this material in their excellent monograph in 1975. They point out that thyrogastric antibodies are found most commonly in young female insulin-dependent diabetics. The prevalence of thyrogastric antibodies in older diabetics (above the age of 40) is much closer to that in control populations (Goldstein et al. 1970; MacCuish and Irvine 1975). Again, the excess is mainly associated with female sex and insulin-dependency. The joint occurrence of thyroid and gastric antibodies is almost exclusive to diabetics; however, even among juvenile diabetics and their families, Nissley et al. (1973) found a group in whom both propositi and family members manifested such antibodies, and another group who did not. Such studies were precursors to the present evidence that one group of type I diabetics is of auto-immune origin, and another group is not. A high titre of thyroid cell antibodies in ostensibly euthyroid diabetic children may be associated with chronic (Hashimoto's) thyroiditis.

Moulias et al. (1974) have also investigated cellular thyroid auto-immunity in diabetes mellitus. These authors point out that insulinopenic diabetics have antithyroglobulin antibodies in 17.5% of instances, compared to 4.8% for normal controls, whereas 45% of such diabetics have a positive leukocyte migration inhibition test against one or more thyroid antigenic preparations (as opposed to 9% for normal controls). Thus, there is certainly a very strong association between the presence of cellular immune responses against thyroid antigen and type I diabetics. These associations between type I diabetes and auto-immune thyroid disease are also discussed by Friedman and Fialkow (1978), who again relate the pathogenesis of the various organ-specific auto-immune endocrinopathies (and those non-endocrine organ-specific auto-immune conditions which are frequently associated with them) to factors in some manner related to HLA-Dw3.

Myaesthenia gravis, another organ-specific auto-immune disease associated with HLA-Dw3, is also found in increased incidence in type I diabetes, and vice versa (Osserman 1969). One might expect that those disorders sharing similar linkage disequilibrium with the same HLA gene will share an association, even if not yet appreciated, e. g. chronic active hepatitis.

3.5 Immunologic Disturbances

3.5.1 Morphological Observations

It has long been recognized that mononuclear cell infiltration in the region of the islets of Langerhans is a feature of the pathology of children dying with diabetic ketoacidosis (Von Meyenburg 1940). Indeed, in most patients who have died early in the course of insulin-dependent diabetes mellitus, similar lesions have been observed (Gepts 1965). Furthermore, the suspicion that this lesion might represent an immunological process was further supported by experimental studies of animals immunized with pancreatic extracts and insulin, where similar lesions have been demonstrated, often associated with intolerance to carbohydrate (Craighead 1972). More recently, a strain of animals that suffers from spontaneous diabetes mellitus has been shown to have lesions rather similar to those described above (Nakhooda et al. 1977). This strain will be discussed further below.

3.5.2 Humoral Antibodies

In 1974, Bottazzo and his colleagues were the first to identify islet cell antibodies in patients with type I diabetes mellitus by means of the immunofluorescent technique.

The antibodies so demonstrated appeared to be reactive with cytoplasmic constituents of alpha, beta and delta cells within the islets of Langerhans. In the original observation, Bottazzo et al. (1974) were able to identify these antibodies only in those patients with type I diabetes mellitus who had other auto-immune disorders in association. This observation was soon confirmed by Irvine et al. (1976), as well as Lendrum et al. (1975, 1976 a, b). The antibody was discovered in some patients even prior to the onset of the disease, whereas in other patients, it was demonstrable only after the initiation of the clinical disorder. At the time of diagnosis, approximately 65%–85% of patients were shown to have such circulating islet cell antibodies, although after three years of disease, the proportion of patients manifesting the antibody was reduced to about 20%. Persistence of the antibody was more often associated with the presence of other associated organ-specific auto-antibodies or overt auto immune endocrinopathies (Irvine et al. 1977 a; Bottazzo et al. 1978 b). More recently, Irvine et al. (1978 a, b) have shown that when such antibodies persist for three years or more there is a significantly higher prevalence of HLA-B8 than in those in whom the antibody does not persist. Moreover, those patients with HLA-B15 do not manifest such persistent antibodies, nor do they have evidence of other organ-specific auto-immune disorders. Thus, as mentioned above, there appear to be two forms of insulin-dependent diabetes mellitus, namely, that associated with islet cell antibodies, which may persist for a long time after diagnosis, associated with HLA-B8 and HLA-Dw3, and with a frequent association with other auto-immune conditions, and the second group, as mentioned earlier, associated with HLA-B15 and HLA-Dw4. These conditions may well not have the same aetiology, and will be the subject of speculation below.

Bottazzo and Doniach (1978) have demonstrated that pancreatic islet cell antibodies are important markers for two subtypes of insulin-dependent diabetes mellitus, but conversely also stain the entire islet (not only beta cells) in the standard immunofluorescence test. This could indicate either a mixture of antibodies, each directed against one cell type, or a population of antibodies reacting with a single antigen common to the endocrine pancreas. In the experiments of Bottazzo and Doniach (1978), such a common antigen was observed visually by application of animal antisera raised to each of the four pancreatic hormones, together with islet-cell antibody positive sera in a four-layer double immunofluorescent technique employing green and red anti-IgG conjugates. Double exposure photographs demonstrated that the patients' sera reacted equally with the different endocrine cells. The islet-cell antibodies did not, however, cross-react with gastric glucagon or somatostatin cells. By contrast, human antibodies against glucagon cells or somatostatin cells reacted with discrete antigens specific to each cell type, and in 50% of cases the antibodies also stained with respective endocrine cells in the gastro-intestinal tract. Such antibodies may also be seen in non-diabetics with a family history of diabetes mellitus and may represent another marker for the genetic predisposition to islet cell auto-immunity and for future clinical diabetes in unaffected members of these families.

Ginsberg-Fellner et al. (1980) have studied islet cell antibodies in gestational diabetics. They found that of those patients who were found to have islet cell antibodies during their gestation, at a time when transient diabetes mellitus was present (disappearing after delivery), 73% of such patients had become insulin-dependent within 10 years. Their data suggested that the presence of islet-cell antibodies during pregnancy may enable prediction of which gestational diabetic women will develop true insulin-dependent diabetes in the future.

It is not clear whether the islet cell antibodies in type I diabetes have any role in producing the lesions. Craighead (1978) points out that the immunofluorescent antibody is not cytolytic, and reacts with non-beta cells in the islets. However, in some patients with newly diagnosed disease, Lernmark et al. (1978) have demonstrated an antibody to islet cell membranes which is capable of interfering with the metabolism of beta-cells in tissue culture. This antibody may be separate and distinct from the antibody which is demonstrable by immunofluorescence. Bottazzo et al. (1980) have recently been able to demonstrate complement-fixing islet cell antibodies in type I diabetes, which appear separate from those demonstrated by immunofluorescence. They advanced evidence suggesting that these antibodies might at least monitor beta-cell damage. There has been no demonstrable correlation between the presence of islet cell antibodies and evidence of cell-mediated immunity (Christy et al. 1976).

Currently, therefore, one might speculate that certain islet cell antibodies could be playing a pathogenic role, although this remains to be fully established. While the antibodies may not be destructive when acting alone, it is possible that immune complexes and lymphocyte-dependent antibody-mediated cytolysis may be important cytolytic pathways, and these aspects have only been minimally explored. Irvine et al. (1977 b) have described the presence of immune complexes by means of the Raji cell assay in 7 of 13 newly diagnosed type I diabetics; six of these had islet cell antibodies, but none had antibodies to insulin. The significance of this finding has yet to be determined. One study of lymphocyte-dependent antibody-mediated cytolysis will be discussed in Sect. 3.5.4 (Pozzilli et al. 1979, 1980).

3.5.3 Antibodies to Insulin Receptors

Flier et al. (1979) have studied the curious syndrome of insulin-resistant diabetes associated with the skin condition, acanthosis nigricans. One of these syndromes, known as type B, has been shown to be an auto-immune disease, characterized by immunologically mediated insulin resistance. Ten of 14 patients known to have this disorder were female, and their ages ranged from 12 to 60 years. All but two had clinically important hyperglycaemia, which was initially resistant to insulin therapy – in one patient in doses as high as 25 000 units per day. Plasma insulin levels during fasting and after glucose and other stimuli were 5 to 50 times greater than normal in these patients, exceeding those found in all but the most severely insulin-resistant obese patients. The cause of this condition has been clearly shown to be due to the presence of an antibody directed against the insulin receptor.

Resistance to the glucose-lowering effect of exogenous insulin is very marked in this condition. However, the hypersecretion of insulin is sometimes sufficient to compensate and normoglycaemia may be achieved with extreme hyperinsulinaemia. Most patients with this condition appear to be resistant to the development of ketosis. Moreover, the patients do not show the conditions known to be associated with insulin resistance, such as obesity, lipo-atrophy, Cushing's disease, or acromegaly. Insulin antibodies are absent or present in low titre. Finally, the insulin molecule produced in patients with type B disease appears to be normal in terms of immunoreactivity, fraction of pro-insulin and ability to bind to receptors and activate target cells.

Flier et al. (1979) have also studied the insulin receptors on cells from these patients, utilizing receptors on circulating monocytes. They have clearly demonstrated that the binding of labelled insulin to these receptors is markedly reduced. The most severe binding defect is usually associated with the most severe hormone resistance.

These patients frequently have elevated sedimentation rates, hyperglobulinaemia, leukopenia, hypocomplementaemia, antinuclear antibodies and anti-DNA antibodies. Frequent associated clinical findings include arthralgia, vitiligo, alopecia and parotid enlargements. Some of the patients have had other well-defined syndromes in association, such as systemic lupus erythematosus, Sjögren's syndrome, ataxia telangiectasia and immune complex nephritis.

Roth's group (Flier et al. 1979) has studied these patients in great depth and has shown that the antireceptor antibodies may persist in some patients, whereas in others there have been spontaneous remissions. In some patients there has been increased insulin binding, apparently due to a major increase in receptor molecules on the membrane, i. e. receptor proliferation. Since insulin is a major regulator of the concentration of its receptors, it can well be imagined that interference with the normal hormone-receptor interaction by antireceptor antibodies might change the rate of synthesis or degradation.

In one patient, such proliferation was accompanied by intractable *hypoglycaemia* during fasting. Since the hypoglycaemia occurred in the presence of appropriately low levels of plasma insulin and of an insulin-like peptide, it was apparently caused by an extremely high concentration of receptors, or of receptors bound to (partially agonistic) antireceptor antibodies. Thus, insulin-receptor proliferation in the presence of antireceptor antibodies appears to be a newly identified cause of hypoglycaemia during fasting. (Incidentally, the type A syndrome of insulin resistance and acanthosis nigricans appears to be a specific receptor defect (i. e. a change in the number of receptors), and is not due to antireceptor antibodies.)

3.5.4 Evidence of Cell-mediated Immunity

3.5.4.1 Migration Inhibition Tests

The chief test by which cell-mediated immunity has been studied in diabetes mellitus has been by means of the leucocyte migration inhibition (LIF) test. Nerup et al. (1971, 1973 a, b, 1974) first demonstrated that leucocytes from patients with insulin-dependent diabetes when exposed to human pancreatic antigen would show inhibition of migration. This was not observed when the leucocytes were from non-insulin-dependent diabetic patients. The tests were also positive prior to the initiation of therapy, particularly insulin. Subsequently, Nerup et al. (1973 a, b, 1974), utilizing foetal calf pancreas, confirmed their initial observations, demonstrating cross-reactivity between the two species. These findings have further been confirmed by MacCuish et al. (1974 a) (Fig. 3.1). There have been criticisms of these studies despite the great probability that the results are valid. Firstly, the antigenic preparation contained not only islet tissue, but other pancreatic tissue as well. Secondly, the leucocyte migration inhibition test has been called into question, because of the possible participation of polymorphonuclear leucocytes, immune complexes and B-lymphocytes (see Chap. 2). However, recently, Kowalczyk and Zembala (1978) have confirmed beyond any reasonable doubt that the test is

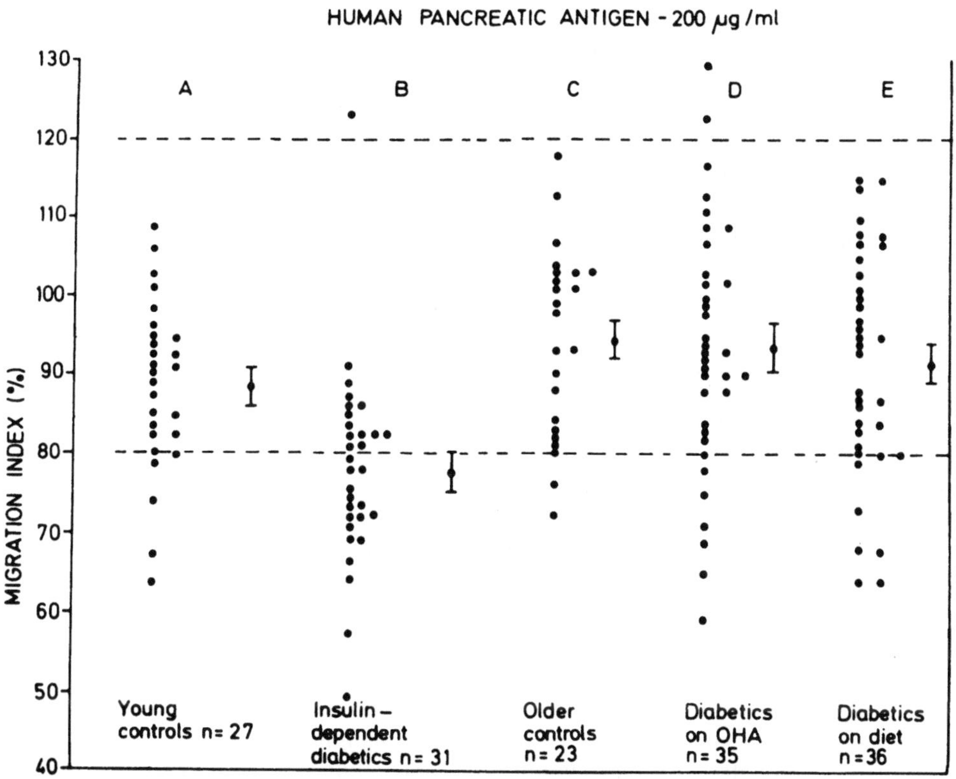

Fig. 3.1. Results of migration inhibition factor test using human pancreatic antigen in various groups of diabetics and control subjects. A positive migration inhibition factor test against human pancreatic antigen was observed in insulin-dependent diabetics, but not in diabetics on oral hypoglycaemia agents or on diet alone. This appears to indicate the presence of T-lymphocytes sensitized against pancreatic antigen in the insulin-dependent diabetic group. (Mac Cuish et al. 1974 a)

dependent upon sensitized T-lymphocytes, and thus is, after all, a true test of T-lymphocyte sensitization, i.e. cell-mediated immunity. This has again been confirmed by Totterman et al. (1979), who likewise showed that the procedure is T-lymphocyte dependent. However, from experience gained with preparations of T-lymphocytes alone in auto-immune thyroid disease, it would seem preferable to use such isolated T-lymphocytes preparations in further studies (see Chap. 2). Moreover, an antigenic preparation prepared from a human beta cell adenoma would be more appropriate as antigen than the antigens prepared from the entire pancreas.

In any event, MacCuish and Irvine (1975) point out that by means of this procedure a state of cell-mediated immunity can be demonstrated in insulin-dependent diabetics in response to an antigen which is present in the pancreas, is species non-specific (demonstrable with porcine, bovine, human and rat pancreas), and is probably different from insulin. The phenomenon may be found in both juvenile-onset and maturity-onset diabetics, and may occur in both insulin-independent, as well as insulin-dependent, patients. However, it is much more commonly found in patients who are insulin-dependent, than in those who are not.

Unfortunately, in the same patients, the leucocyte migration inhibition test may also be positive when antigens from other organs are employed. Liver mitochondrial antigen is particularly capable of inhibiting leucocyte migration in diabetics, as has also been demonstrated in Hashimoto's thyroiditis, primary biliary cirrhosis and pernicious anaemia (MacCuish and Irvine 1975).

In addition to studies of cell-mediated immunity employing the leucocyte migration test, MacCuish and Irvine (1975) have demonstrated the effects of adding purified insulins and insulin chains to cultured lymphocytes from newly diagnosed diabetics and insulin-taking patients without evidence of allergy. The extent of blastogenesis in these cultures was assessed both by morphological examination and tritiated thymidine uptake. They observed that lymphocytes from about 25% of insulin-taking diabetics, who have no clinical signs of insulin allergy, undergo significant blastogenesis when cultured in the presence of insulin. Of interest, however, the lymphocytes from five of ten newly diagnosed diabetics also underwent significant transformation when exposed to bovine or porcine insulin. Of these five patients, two had been treated with insulin for less than 3 weeks, while three had never received insulin prior to the procedure.

The LIF assay has not been widely used to investigate cell-mediated immunity in response to insulin (in contrast to pancreatic cell antigenic preparations). Moulias and Goust (1974) found that of 40 patients with insulin-dependent diabetes, 8 (20%) demonstrated migration inhibition, and 10 (25%) stimulation of migration (normal range 0.8–1.11) in response to bovine insulin at a concentration of 0.1 μU/ml. However, utilizing human insulin at the same concentration, only three patients gave abnormal results, and of these the two showing migration inhibition both had lipoatrophic diabetes. It seems evident, therefore, that LIF in response to bovine insulin may represent immunization by the heterologous insulin (see below). Lymphocyte transformation assays have shown similar results.

3.5.4.2 Cytotoxic Assays

Huang and MacLaren (1976) and MacLaren et al. (1975) have devised a cytotoxicity assay using target cells derived from an insulinoma cell line. Peripheral blood mononuclear cells from 23 patients with insulin-dependent diabetes, one of whom had not been treated prior to the study, and from 12 healthy patients were studied. Effector and target cells were mixed at a ratio of 50:1, and incubated at 37°C at 5% CO_2 in air for 18, 40 and 60 h. Following incubation, cytotoxic effects in the insulinoma cells were assessed by eosin exclusion. Cytotoxic indices of 21% or greater were observed in 15 (65%) of the 23 diabetic patients, but in none of the healthy controls. In parallel experiments, target cells were incubated with patients' mononuclear cells plus serum at 1:5 dilution, and in patient serum at 1:5 together with complement. These studies showed that the majority of patients in whom mononuclear cells demonstrated elevated cytotoxic indices demonstrated similar results when serum was also added, whereas serum with complement without mononuclear cells had no effect. Further experiments in which mononuclear cells were fractionated into T-lymphocyte enriched and T-lymphocyte depleted populations by means of E-rosetting indicated that both populations were capable of causing cytotoxic effects, in the majority of cases. These experiments have provided important additional evidence of the potential importance or organ-specific reactions in diabetes mellitus. One caveat might be that the insulinoma cells might

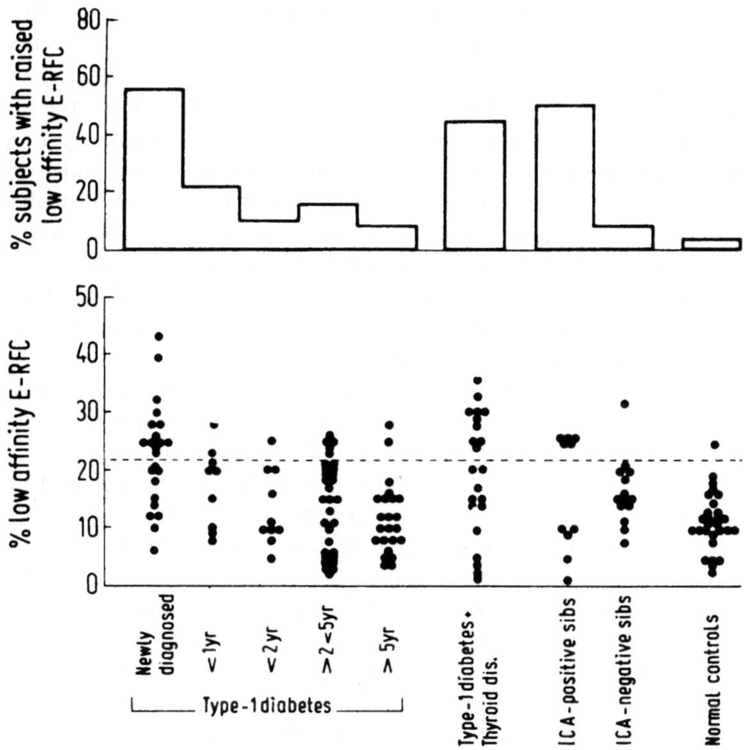

Fig. 3.2. Distribution of blood mononuclear cells forming low affinity rosettes with sheep erythrocytes ("killer" cells) in type I diabetics, unaffected siblings, patients with type I diabetes as well as coexistent auto-immune thyroid disease, and healthy subjects. (Pozzilli et al. 1979)

not bear the same antigenic configuration on their cell membranes as do normal islet cells.

Moreover, Pozzilli et al. (1979, 1980) have demonstrated that there is an increased number of K cells in auto-immune diabetes mellitus when associated with other organ-specific auto-immune disorder (Fig. 3.2). In addition, there appeared to be a relationship between the increase in K cells and the appearance of the last endocrinopathy. In addition, antibody-dependent cytotoxicity was demonstrable and felt to be a useful marker of active tissue damage in patients affected with polyendocrine auto-immune disease. However, Ludwig et al. (1980) have reported a *decreased* K cell activity in a group of insulin-dependent diabetics. Thus, the question of K cell involvement in insulin-dependent diabetes remains to be resolved.

A number of laboratories are currently attempting to test human lymphocytes in cytotoxicity assays, using normal islet cell suspensions of non-human origin. Such experiments may provide misleading results, as it is clearly important to avoid immunological heterogeneity in such studies (Galbraith 1979).

3.5.4.3 Evidence for a Defect in Immunosuppression

Fairchild et al. (1980) have studied non-specific suppressor cell function and specific suppressor cell function in insulin-dependent diabetic patients. Non-specific suppressor cell function was evaluated by measuring pokeweed mitogen stimulated B-lymphocyte IgG biosynthesis in concanavalin-A suppressor cell-activated (experimental) and non-activated (control) cultures. Antigen-specific suppressor cell function was evaluated by suppressor cell activation with 100 μg of guinea pig islet cell homogenate (experimental culture) or splenic cell homogenate (control culture) for 24 h. Experimental and control cultures were washed and co-cultured with fresh cells stimulated with islet cell homogenate. Co-culture cell proliferation rates were measured by tritiated thymidine incorporation. Suppressor cell activity was scored by dividing the values obtained for experimental cultures by those for control cultures. They demonstrated that in insulin-dependent diabetes, non-specific suppressor cell function was less efficient than for controls. Moreover, they also demonstrated that specific suppressor cell activity was also lower than for the control population. However, there appeared to be a decline with time, and the authors concluded that these effects may be an early transient event, although possibly playing a key role in the induction of the disease.

Buschard et al. (1980) studied non-specific suppressor cell function by a similar technique to that described by Fairchild et al. (1980). They demonstrated that there was non-specific suppressor cell depression in newly diagnosed insulin-dependent diabetic patients, which soon returned to normal within 1 month. They suggested that this effect might be important in initiating insulin-dependent diabetes, but could not distinguish whether this was a primary or secondary event.

Clearly, further investigation is needed so as to determine the role of defective immunoregulation in the pathogenesis of type I diabetes. Studies such as have been reported in Chap. 2 for auto-immune thyroid disease would be worth doing in the context of diabetes, and might prove to be quite revealing.

3.5.5 Animal Experiments

Attempts have been made to induce experimental diabetes by immunological means. Nerup et al. (1973 a, b) injected extracts of bovine pancreas with Freund's adjuvant into female Wistar rats. Evidence of cell-mediated immunity was demonstrated using a modified leucocyte migration inhibition assay. A second group of animals, immunized by an equivalent amount of bovine purified insulin (also with complete Freund's adjuvant), failed to induce evidence of cell-mediated immunity; moreover, control groups of animals that were not injected, or which were injected with adjuvant alone, also failed to show positive results for cell-mediated immunity. Additionally, these investigators showed that this effect was organ-specific since injections of adrenal and liver extracts failed to result in cell-mediated immunity directed against the islet-cell tissue. They were able to demonstrate the presence of mononuclear cell infiltration within the pancreas of the affected rats, most marked between day 8 and day 15 following the injections. Electron-microscopic studies also showed some abnormalities of the beta cells of the islets. Nevertheless, there was no evidence of glycosuria or impairment of glucose tolerance.

Subsequently, Andersen et al. (1974) immunized inbred mice with a preparation of islets derived from OB/OB mice in complete Freund's adjuvant. Electron-microscopic studies showed degranulation of alpha-2 and beta cells, reaching a maximum on day 15 following the injection. At the time, plasma glucose levels were abnormally elevated. By the day 21, glucose tolerance had reverted to normal.

It would thus seem possible to be able to induce a diabetic syndrome in animals by means of injection of pancreatic antigens. However, it may be added that it has also been possible to induce lymphocytic infiltration of islets with destruction of beta cells and fibrosis in heifers by means of injection of emulsions of both homologous and heterologous insulins, along with Freund's adjuvant (LeCompte et al. 1966). Similar studies in rabbits have also resulted in diabetes following immunization with insulin (Grodsky et al. 1966).

Of considerable interest is the study of Buschard et al. (1978), who transferred lymphocytes from human subjects into athymic "nude" mice. When lymphocytes from diabetic patients were injected, there was a marked rise in the blood glucose levels, whereas when normal lymphocytes were similarly utilized there was only a minimal rise in blood sugar values. The Buschard experiment with the "nude" mice would be consistent with the view that there is no necessity for initial islet-cell damage, but merely a defect in immunoregulation. This would militate against the notion that islet-cell damage (i.e. antigenic stimulation) is a *sine qua non* in the initiation of insulinopenic diabetes. Unfortunately, two groups have been unable to confirm these results (Lipsick et al. 1979; Thurneyssen et al. 1979).

It is of considerable interest that diabetes in animals experimentally induced by Streptozotocin has been shown to be due, at least in part, to T-lymphocyte functions. Buschard and Rygaard (1977) were able to show that diabetes induced by Streptozotocin in mice could be transferred to athymic "nude" mice after transplantation of spleen cells from the original diabetic animals. Moreover, the same authors in 1978 (Buschard and Rygaard 1978) produced Strepozotocin-induced diabetes in a group of normal mice and "nude" mice, and found that the "nude" mice had significantly lower blood glucose values. This result supported the original suggestion by Buschard and Rygaard that a thymus-dependent immune reaction is, in part, responsible for the diabetogenic effect of Streptozotocin. These results were further confirmed by Paik et al. (1980), who demonstrated that the development of diabetes in mice treated with repeated low doses of Streptozotocin required host T-lymphocyte functions (presumably involving T-lymphocytes sensitized against beta cell associated self-antigens). Moreover, Arquilla et al. (1980) were able to show impairment of cell-mediated immunity in chronic alloxan-treated diabetic mice, which is related to the persistent insulinopenia. It would thus appear that the original drug-induced beta cell damage is further enhanced and aggravated by immune factors.

A spontaneous form of diabetes mellitus has been observed in approximately 30% of non-obese, outbred colony of Bio Breeding/Worcester (BB/W) rats. Without insulin replacement therapy most animals succumb within 1 to 2 weeks of the detection of glycosuria. A unique feature of this model is the presence of profound insulitis before and shortly after the syndrome develops with lymphocytes, macrophages and occasionally eosinophils infiltrating into the pancreatic islets. Late in the disease the islets are small with no insulin-synthesizing beta cells. The physiological and morphological characteristics of these animals closely resemble those of insulin-dependent humans with juvenile-onset diabetes. Both the demonstration that selective inbreeding of diabetic animals increases the frequency of diabetes and the lymphocyte and macrophage nature of the insular infiltrate suggest a cell-mediated auto-immune pathogenesis for this syndrome (Nakhooda et al. 1977). Recently, Like et al. (1979) have shown that injections of rabbit antiserum to rat lymphocytes reversed the hyperglycaemia in 36% of the spontaneous diabetic rats, and prevented diabetes in susceptible non-diabetic controls. These findings strengthen the hypothesis that cell-mediated auto-immunity plays a role in the pathogenesis of diabetes in this animal model which mimics many morphological and physiological characteristics of human insulin-dependent diabetes mellitus.

3.5.6 Insulin as an Antigen

There have been several studies indicating the presence of sensitized T-lymphocytes and of humoral antibodies against insulin in patients with insulin-dependent diabetes mellitus. As mentioned above, Moulias and Goust (1974) have studied the leucocyte migration inhibition factor (LIF) assay and have shown migration inhibition in response to bovine insulin in at least a minority of patients with insulinopenic diabetes mellitus. However studies by Nerup et al. (1971, 1973a, b, 1974) and MacCuish et al. (1974a) have also examined the LIF test in relation to sensitization of T-lymphocytes against bovine and porcine insulin, but their studies have been consistently negative.

Antibodies which bind insulin were demonstrated by Berson's group as early as 1956 (Berson et al. 1956; Yalow and Berson 1957; Berson and Yalow 1959 a, b). The basic method as described by these workers involved radio-iodination of insulin and reaction with human serum suspected to contain insulin antibodies. The presence of insulin-binding antibodies was demonstrated by a shift in the radioactive insulin peak towards the gammaglobulin region on paper chromatography or electrophoresis. Berson and his colleagues were able to demonstrate insulin-binding antibodies in the serum of all of a group of diabetics who had been treated with insulin for 3 months or longer, although not in those patients who had never received insulin therapy. Subsequently, a significant correlation was demonstrated between insulin antibody levels and daily insulin requirements, the insulin-binding capacity being less than 10 units per litre of serum in well-controlled insulin-treated patients, but 60 to 500 units per litre or more in insulin-resistant patients.

As a result of these studies, Yalow and Berson (1960, 1961) developed a radioimmunoassay for insulin, the first of the now ubiquitous radioimmunoassays. They also carried out a series of studies of plasma insulin levels in normal persons and diabetic patients, as well as of species specificity of antigen-antibody interactions.

Insulin-binding antibodies have subsequently been detected by a variety of separate techniques. These have included haemagglutination, complement-consumption, precipitin reaction, and immunofluorescence (Galbraith 1979).

However the antibodies are measured, they generally represent antibodies to heterologous insulins. Since there are some differences in amino acid sequences between the various mammalian insulins, it has been possible to determine the degree of cross-reactivity based on structural similarities. For example, it was anticipated by Berson and Yalow (1959 a, b, 1961) that porcine insulin would be less immunogenic than bovine insulin, which differs from human insulin at two positions of the 8-10 residues segment of the a-chain. This group of investigators demonstrated that insulin antibodies from patients treated with bovine and porcine insulins bound bovine and ovine insulins, which possess identical amino acids at positions 8 and 10 of the a-chain, much more strongly than porcine, equine and human insulins, in which the amino acids at positions 8 and 10, while shared, are different from those of bovine and ovine insulin. Moreover, significantly higher titres of antibodies are produced in diabetics receiving bovine insulin than in patients treated with insulin of porcine origin. Feldman et al. (1963) have reported that some patients who are clinically resistant to bovine insulin will respond to porcine insulin. Despite these species differences in amino acid sequence, Galbraith (1979) has stressed that differences in secondary or tertiary structure of insulin may also contribute to their immunogenicity; despite identical primary structures, sperm whale and pig insulins have been found to possess distinct immunochemical properties. Galbraith (1979) also points out that impurities present in commercial preparations of insulin may also be immunogenic. The possibility that such contaminants contribute to the immunogenicity of insulins has led to attempts to obtain pure monospecies (MS), single peak (SP) and monocomponent (MC) insulins. The introduction of these modifications has led to variable results, although Galbraith (1979) states that there has been a general decrease in the titres of insulin-binding antibodies with such insulins and a corresponding fall in insulin requirements. Further studies will clearly be necessary to study the clinical consequence of treatment with MC insulin, although it may be mentioned that severe hypoglycaemic reactions have been reported after change-over.

Until recently, it was generally felt that insulin antibodies do not normally occur in patients who have not been treated with insulin, but conversely are found in the majority of patients who receive such therapy. This would certainly strongly suggest that insulin antibodies are probably a result of treatment rather than related to the cause of the disorder. However, this may not be universally so. Folling and Norman (1972) have reported the case of an untreated diabetic patient with IgG insulin antibodies as detected by ultracentrifugation, electrophoretic and immunoelectrophoretic studies. Several similar patients have been described by Ohneda et al. (1974), Anderson et al. (1978) and Kawazu et al. (1975).

3.6 The Possible Role of Viruses in the Induction of Insulinopenic Diabetes

3.6.1 Clinical and Pathological Evidence

As has been mentioned above, pathological studies of the islets of Langerhans in type I diabetes have shown mononuclear cell infiltration in at least a proportion of such patients. Moreover, these cells are primarily lymphocytes, and polymorphonuclear leucocytes have been observed only rarely, even in children dying within a week of clinical presentation. Nevertheless, the hypothesis that viruses are one cause of insulinopenic diabetes has been suggested by the abrupt onset in such cases, a possible seasonal incidence in type I diabetes, the presence of inflammatory cells in the islets and the destruction of beta cells (Craighead 1978; Notkins 1977, 1979; Galbraith 1979). While the circumstantial evidence will be presented below, the only direct evidence that human diabetes mellitus can be virus-induced in some instances has come from the study of one 10-year-old boy dying with diabetic ketoacidosis (Yoon et al. 1979). This child had been admitted to hospital in diabetic ketoacidosis within three days of onset of symptoms of a "flu-like" illness. He died 7 days later, and post-mortem examination showed lymphocytic infiltration of the islets of Langerhans and necrosis of beta cells. Inoculation of mouse, monkey and human cell cultures with homogenates from the patient's pancreas led to isolation of a virus. Serological studies revealed a rise in the titre of neutralizing antibody to this virus from less than 4 on the second hospital day to 32 on the day of death. Neutralization data showed that the virus was related to a diabetogenic variant derived from Coxsackie virus B4. Inoculation of mice with the human isolate produced hyperglycaemia, inflammatory cells in the islets of Langerhans and beta cell necrosis. Staining of mouse pancreatic sections with fluorescein-labelled antiviral antibody revealed viral antigens in beta cells. Both the clinical picture and animal studies suggested that in this child diabetes was indeed virus-induced.

The possibility that viruses might induce diabetes mellitus was first suggested at the turn of the century when a patient was described who developed diabetes mellitus shortly after having had mumps (Notkins 1979). The mumps virus was further proposed as a possible cause of diabetes mellitus by Gunderson (1927), Kremer (1947) and Melin and Ursing (1958). However, to date, there is still not firm evidence that the relationship between mumps and diabetes is anything more than a chance association. As Notkins (1979) points out, if the mumps virus does infect beta cells and cause diabetes mellitus in human beings, it must do so under some very special circumstances. In such cases, a rare strain of mumps virus may be involved, or an individual who develops diabetes may have an unusual and possibly genetically determined susceptibility to the virus.

3.6.2 Experimental Evidence

Experimental studies in laboratory animals have shown that viruses possess the capacity to multiply in pancreatic tissue and cause lesions of the islets of Langerhans. This has been clearly shown to cause a disorder in these animals which clinically and pathologically resembles human abrupt onset diabetes mellitus (Craighead and McLane 1968; Craighead and Steinke 1971; Wellmann et al. 1972; Muntefering 1974; Hayashi et al. 1974). Moreover, there are some epidemiological observations that at least are in keeping with the view that viruses could cause diabetes mellitus in humans (Gamble et al. 1969; Gamble et al. 1973; Craighead 1974). Craighead (1974) has reviewed the published reports on human pathologic material in relation to this suggestion. It was his feeling that the prominent accumulations of lymphocytes within the islets, the severe focal necrosis, the presence of macrophages and the localized accumulation of immunoglobulins which are seen in human patients dying of spontaneous diabetes mellitus, were similar to those observed in experimental viral-induced diabetes mellitus. Craighead thus reasoned that these findings provided additional evidence to support the hypothesis that group B Coxsackie viruses or other common viruses possess the capability to damage the islets of Langerhans during the course of an infection and cause abrupt onset diabetes mellitus. However, he also conceded that such lesions could be immunologically induced rather than induced by viruses alone.

Specific viruses were studied by Craighead and McLane (1968), as well as From et al. (1968). These workers were able to show that the M variant of the encephalomyocarditis (EMC) virus produces exclusively lesions of the islet cells

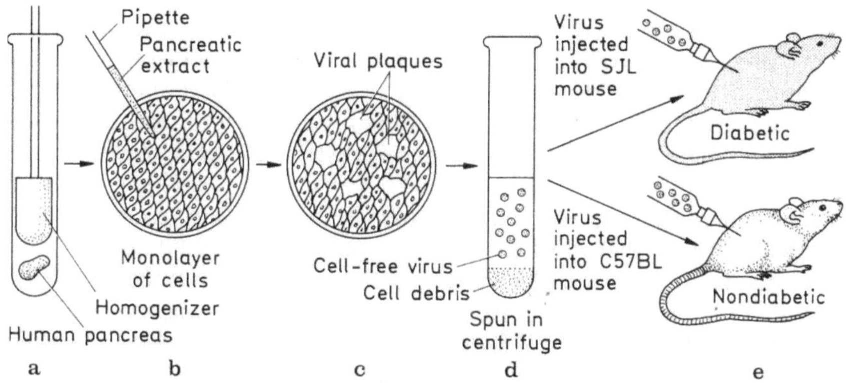

Fig. 3.3. Passaging a virus repeatedly through cultures of beta cells increases its ability to induce diabetes, although, of course, it may do so at the time of the first experimental infection. It is thought that passaging selects for those variants of the virus that reproduce most successfully in beta cells. For example, Coxsackie B4 virus does not normally cause diabetes in mice, although encephalomyocarditis virus may do so. If the Coxsackie B4 virus is passaged several times, however, its capacity to kill beta cells and cause diabetes is increased. (Notkins 1979)

accompanied by a diabetes-like syndrome in animals. Only those animals respond who are genetically susceptible, and this susceptibility has been demonstrated to be under polygenic control (Ross et al. 1976). Specific viral infection of islets has also been studied by Muntefering (1974), who studied the consequent sequential infiltration of the islets of Langerhans by inflammatory cells, followed by necrosis of the islets. Taylor (1974) similarly studied experimental diabetes using Coxsackie B4 virus. This virus, too, was capable of inducing islet cell infiltration and of inducing diabetes mellitus. Coxsackie B virus is not generally capable of inducing experimental diabetes in mice; however, after passaging the virus through beta cell cultures repeatedly, the virus can become diabetogenic in the mice (Notkins 1979) (see Fig. 3.3). Susceptibility to Coxsackie B4 experimental diabetes has been associated with a genetic predisposition in the animals (Webb et al. 1976). The picorna virus group (which includes the Coxsackie group) has also been demonstrated to be diabetogenic in animals by Rayfield and Seto (1978); the severity of the islet cell inflammation has, once again, been genetically related to the H2 tissue type of the animals (Onodera et al. 1978).

3.6.3 Seasonal Variation in Incidence of Diabetes Mellitus

Adams (1926) was the first to note that the incidence of acute onset diabetes seemed to reach a peak between September and January, and suggested that this could have been related to the respiratory infections that occur frequently at that time of year. This seasonal variation was confirmed by Gamble and Taylor (1969) in Great Britain, particularly in those insulin-dependent patients younger than 19 years of age; this prevalence seemed to correlate with the annual patterns of the incidence of Coxsackie B4 infections. While in a second study Gamble et al. (1973) found the same peak period for new cases of diabetes, this differed somewhat from the results of Bloom et al. (1975); they surveyed over 2000 new cases of diabetes mellitus and found the peak incidence to be between October and March, with the seasonal variation largely confined to the 11 to 15 year age group. The interval between October and March was also the peak months for the onset of new cases of diabetes mellitus in the study of Rolles et al. (1975). In the latter study, the authors felt that the patients positive for HLA-B8 far more commonly had their onset of disease between October and February, whereas patients negative for this gene did not have such a peak incidence.

A somewhat different peak incidence was observed by Barbosa et al.(1977); these workers studied families in which two or more siblings were diabetics, and found that the disease developed in the winter months between November and April more frequently in the HLA identical siblings than in the haplo-identical siblings. In the twin studies of Nelson et al. (1975) the diabetes presented clinically in the months of January to March more frequently in cases where both monozygotic twins had diabetes (concordant) in comparison to the situation when one of the twin pair was not diabetic (discordant).

Since there are some discrepancies between the various studies noted above, it is still difficult to be certain whether there is a true seasonal variation in the onset of diabetes mellitus, or whether such a seasonal variation occurs in some groups of diabetics but not in others, and indeed what the peak season truly is. Nevertheless, the suggestion that a seasonal variation does exist in precipitating diabetes mellitus has been one of the elements leading investigators to study the possible role of viruses in the aetiology of at least some patients with diabetes mellitus.

3.6.4 Immune Responses to Viruses in Diabetes

Gamble et al. (1969) have studied antibodies to a number of viruses in 123 patients with diabetes of recent onset, 155 patients who had suffered diabetes for over two years, and 250 normal persons. With the exception of antibodies to Coxsackie B viruses, antibodies to a large variety of other viruses were present no more often than in the normal subjects. However, antibodies to Coxsackie B viruses were present more often in the diabetic population (particulary those of recent onset) than in the control population, and this difference was most pronounced in the case of Coxsackie B4. Subsequently, Gamble et al. (1973) confirmed their own findings in a larger group of insulin-dependent diabetics, with the elevated titres against the Coxsackie viruses most common in the 10–19 year age group of diabetics. However, Richens et al. (1976) studied the leucocyte migration inhibition test in response to Coxsackie B4 (as a measure of cellular immunity) and found this test to be positive no more commonly in insulin-dependent diabetics than in the age and sex matched control persons.

There have been several studies of concordant and discordant twins with respect to viral antibodies against Coxsackie B4 and other viruses. Nelson et al. (1975) could find no significant difference between concordant and discordant twins with respect to Coxsackie B antibodies. On the other hand, Nerup et al. (1975) and Cudworth et al. (1977) have shown somewhat higher titres of antibodies to Coxsackie B4 in those diabetics with HLA-B8 and in concordant twins with the disease. Of course, it is clear that antibody response may be influenced by a number of factors and may not represent causation.

Riley et al. (1980) have studied the role of inherited auto-immunity versus Coxsackie B virus antibodies in insulin-dependent diabetics. While their data indicated a strong familial predisposition for organ-specific auto-immunity, they also found that islet cell antibodies were absent in patients convalescing from proven Coxsackie illnesses, that antibodies to Coxsackie were similar in the household contacts and the probands at the time of diagnosis, and that transient islet-cell antibodies were not seen amongst relatives of probands at the time of diagnosis. Thus, these workers concluded that an acute viral illness with Coxsackie B4 is not a frequent aetiological factor in the pathogenesis of insulin-dependent diabetes mellitus. Indeed, Notkins (1979) also points out that diabetes does not seem to be a common consequence of Coxsackie B4 infection, if in fact Coxsackie B4 is the truly appropriate virus. Moreover, many juvenile-onset diabetics do not have antibodies to Coxsackie B4 (Galbraith 1979).

As mentioned above, experimental viral-induced diabetes mellitus in animals has been associated with genetic susceptibilities. One would thus anticipate that there might be some markers of genetic susceptibilities in those humans suspected of having viral-induced diabetes mellitus. However, it is not yet clear whether there is a relationship between the presence of antibodies to various viruses, such as Coxsackie B4 virus, and particular HLA antigens. Nerup et al. (1975) have reported that antibodies to Coxsackie B4 were found more commonly in sera which were positive for islet-cell antibodies, and in the presence of HLA-B8 or Bw15. Similarly, Cudworth et al. (1977) have also found higher titres of antibodies to Coxsackie B1, B2, B3 and B4 in patients with HLA-B8 or Bw15, and most commonly in patients who had both antigens. The differences however were significant only in the case of Coxsackie B4, and antibodies to other viruses showed no differences from control groups.

Further studies are clearly necessary in this area. One should look closely for correlations between the two D loci which are found commonly in diabetes mellitus, i. e. Dw3 and Dw4, and the occurrence of viral antibodies at the time of onset of the diabetic state. It certainly would be of considerable interest if there were an increased incidence of viral antibody titres in one or other of these groups, and one might even anticipate that such antibodies would be more common with Dw4. However, there are no such available data at present, and thus a final position for the precise role of viruses and a possible genetic predisposition towards viral induction of diabetes mellitus awaits further clarification.

Certainly, many investigators are interested in the relationship of viral infection to diabetes mellitus, and the search is on for other viruses that might cause diabetes in man. Notkins (1979) adds that it is quite possible that viruses may be only one of many causes of diabetes (and perhaps a minor one), and that perhaps other insults from the environment, such as drugs and toxic chemicals, might similarly damage beta cells and given rise to diabetes. Freytag (1974) has suggested a number of mechanisms by which viruses might possibly induce diabetes mellitus. Firstly, the viruses might damage the host cell and cause the lesions directly. Moreover, they may result in chemical alteration of certain proteins, resulting in structures sufficiently different from "self", so that antibodies are produced which may cross-react with the original proteins. In some instances, the mechanism may induce an underlying disease by self-perpetuation. Secondly, antibodies to viruses may be induced resulting in immune complexes, which could localize on the basement membranes in certain organs. A more differentiated pathogenic mechanism that may lead to a pathological immune response is suggested for some RNA viruses which may carry on their surface host-specific antigens in addition to virus-specific antigens. They may thus incorporate into their own structures parts of the membranes of the cells in which they propagate. Viruses may also induce an immunological disease, depending upon the close relationship between lipid-containing RNA viruses and the lipids in the cell membranes, as mentioned above. Alternatively, the infected cell membrane may become altered because of virus infection, and incorporation may result in the uncovering of pre-existing masked antigens. A further alternative may be that the viral DNA or a part of it becomes integrated in the chromosomal DNA of the host cell, leading to essential changes in cell metabolism. This could involve insulin synthesis in the beta cells, perhaps leading to formation of an insulin with altered antigenic sites.

Finally, the virus may involve the immunologically competent cells. A loss of immunological memory may be the result of incorporation of virus-DNA into the nucleus of leucocytes. This might lead to auto-immunity in two possible ways: the first would be to allow a mutation of an organ-directed "forbidden" clone of helper T-lymphocytes to arise because of the virus-lymphocyte interaction, in a person who lacks normal immunoregulation (e.g. lacks a specific clone of suppressor T-lymphocytes, or a specific anti-idiotypic antibody). Secondly, virus-lymphocyte interactions may lead to a defect in a suppressor T-lymphocyte clone, thus leading to a defect in immunoregulation. In summary, Freytag noted that there are many different pathogenic pathways by which viral infections might give rise to diabetes, including: (1) ne antigenic sites in the proteins of cells, (2) the production of cell-specific antibodies, (3) virus-lymphocyte interaction changing immune processes.

It has been common, both in the world of immunology and in the field of investigation of diabetes mellitus, for workers to consider that there should be some alteration in the antigen, i.e. the beta cells, to account for the precipitation of diabetes mellitus in the genetically predisposed hosts. While such antigenic alteration, whether induced by viruses or other means, certainly may account for some cases of diabetes mellitus, it is by no means clear that antigenic alteration is necessary for the many type I patients, particularly those with HLA-B8-Dw3, who manifest other organspecific auto-immune diseases, such as auto-immune thyroid disease (Irl of Irvine, Ib of Doniach and Bottazzo). Indeed, both Irvine (1980) and Doniach and Bottazzo (1981) have reasoned that this group of type I diabetics have their disease as a result of primary immunological processes. On the other hand, the Ir2-Ia form could be due to other causes, such as viral isletitis, based on a different form of genetic predisposition. Hence, considerable attention should be given to the possibility that in the Irl-Ib group of patients the immune system is solely at fault; there would thus be no need for any antigenic alteration, only the availability of the antigen. In still others, of course, there may be a combination of factors which may include abnormalities of the immune system, and in addition, some abnormality or alteration of the host antigen, possibly viral-induced (see Table 3.3).

Jansen et al. (1978) have examined the hypothesis that the diabetic symptoms provoked by encephalomyocarditis (EMC) virus in DBA_2 mice might be due to immune reactions initiated by the virus. Studies were carried out in DBA_2 male mice aged 8–12 weeks infected subcutaneously with EMC virus. It was found that glucose levels remained normal after 500 rads of x-ray radiation plus virus infection, although virus-infected mice had significantly higher mean glucose levels.Immune suppression by a cyclophosphamide derivative led to a significantly increased mean glucose level and increased insulitis, compared with the effects in controls that were only infected. These findings indicated an important role for the cellular immune reaction, insulitis, in islet cell destruction. At the other extreme, viral infection alone without any abnormality of the immune system might suffice. Clearly, a great deal of further investigation is needed to clarify the possible role of viruses in the aetiology of diabetes mellitus. Such a role, if confirmed, would result almost certainly in attempts to immunize against certain viral strains in genetically susceptible small children, but at present this is not justifiable.

3.7 The Role of Immunity in the Pathogenesis of Complications of Diabetes Mellitus

It does not appear likely that any of the complications of diabetes mellitus are due to the same aetiological factors (immune or otherwise) which induce the diabetes in the first place. However, it is probable that secondary immune factors (either secondary to the disease itself, or secondary to the use of insulin as treatment) may well be involved in inducing some of the complications attributed to the disease. Acute reactions of the immediate hypersensitivity type may well occur (urticaria, or even acute systemic allergic reactions) and these have clearly been a result of the antigenicity of the insulin preparations employed (most probably related to contamination of insulin with pro-insulin, glucagon, VIP, PPP, and other pancreatic hormones). Moreover, increasing resistance to insulin, resulting in insulin-resistant diabetes mellitus has been clearly shown to be due to antibodies against insulin (Berson and Yalow 1961). Indeed, insulin antibodies are present in virtually all diabetic patients who receive insulin for long-term therapy for their disorder. Insulin requirements may well be related to titres of these insulin-binding antibodies in virtually all instances.

The most serious late complication of long-standing diabetes mellitus is microangiopathy, whether it manifests itself as diabetic retinopathy, neuropathy, nephropathy, or lesions elsewhere. In this condition, there is deposition of certain plasma proteins within the basement membrane of small blood vessels, with basement membrane thickening and hyalinization. Berson et al. (1956) noted that microangiopathy had not been observed prior to the insulin era, and suggested that the vascular lesion in diabetes mellitus could be the result of insulin therapy possibly by deposition of insulin-antibody complexes on the basement membrane of small vessels throughout the body. Indeed, subsequently, Anderson (1976) observed that insulin requirements were higher in patients with retinopathy or intercapillary glomerulosclerosis than in those patients without such complications. The titres of insulin antibodies were somewhat higher in those patients with microangiopathy than in those without. While it is true that immune complexes of insulin-antibody can be demonstrated in renal lesions associated with diabetes (Freedman et al. 1960; Burkholder 1965; Coleman et al. 1962; Werner and Larsen 1969), nevertheless, immunohistopathological studies have shown that the basement membrane in diabetic glomerulosclerosis contains not only insulin, IgG, IgM and BlC fraction of complement, but also contains non-immunological plasma proteins (such as albumin and others), deposited in a linear fashion (Westberg and Michael 1972; Larsson 1967; MacCuish and Irvine 1975; Galbraith 1979). Indeed, Churg and Dolger (1971) have provided evidence that this might be a metabolic disorder rather than an immunological one. Moreover, microangiopathic complications have been observed in diabetics who have not taken insulin. Galbraith (1979) states that "it would be premature and imprudent on the basis of existing information to ascribe a definite role to immune complexes of insulin-antibody in the causation of tissue damage, particulary since the characteristic appearances of glomerulosclerosis may develop in patients who have never been treated with insulin". While immune complexes may even be demonstrable prior to and unrelated to insulin administration, the biological relevance of immune complexes remains to be determined. Finally, there is no evidence that HLA-related genetic factors play a role in producing these lesions (Deckert et al. 1979; Jervell and Solheim 1979).

Aside from the development of insulin antibodies, secondary to the prolonged administration of this material, there is some evidence that the metabolic disorder of diabetes mellitus may also have secondary immune consequences. It is a common observation that diabetic patients are particularly prone to certain infections such as tuberculosis, furunculosis and fungal and viral infections (Handwerger et al. 1980). There is certainly considerable evidence that the chemotactic function of phagocytes is significantly impaired by the metabolic abnormalities of poorly controlled diabetes mellitus (Galbraith 1979). There also appears to be impaired opsonizing properties (a property of non-immune IgG and complement components and other unidentified serum factors to react with other micro-organisms and render them increasingly susceptible to phagocytosis). The nature of this impairment is not yet clear. The ability of diabetics to produce antibodies to bacteria has been reported to be impaired (particularly in children with persistent hyperglycaemia, glycosuria and ketonuria) (Bates and Weiss 1941). However, in well-controlled diabetics, or in animals with experimental diabetes mellitus, several workers have been unable to show that the antibody production of diabetics and non-diabetics clearly differs (Galbraith 1979).

The blastogenic response of lymphocytes to mitogenic stimulation has been reported to be diminished in poorly controlled diabetics, and normal in well-controlled diabetics (Handwerger et al. 1980). Similar results have been observed in experimental diabetes in mice and rats (Handwerger et al. 1980). These authors have also summarized the poor response to allogeneic stimulation and delayed hypersensitivity observed in experimental diabetes.

The ability of phagocytes to ingest micro-organisms or latex particles has also been studied. Once again, diabetics have shown deficiencies in the ability to ingest either organisms or particles. Bagdade et al. (1974) have shown a close relationship between the degree of hyperglycaemia and the impairment of ingestion. It is not clear whether this abnormality is due to hyperglycaemia per se. Since it has been shown (Esmann 1964) that glucose utilization is impaired in leucocytes from diabetic patients, it may not be surprising that there is a disorder in leucocyte function, including phagocytic ingestion. Dumm (1957) showed that glucose utilization becomes increasingly impaired in relationship to the severity of the disorder, and that addition of insulin in vitro improved glucose utilization towards normal. Thus, the defect in ingestion of particles or micro-organisms by leucocytes may be directly related to this metabolic abnormality.

Ingestion of micro-organisms is followed by intracellular degranulation and subsequent killing. Bagdade et al. (1974) have demonstrated a definite defect in intracellular killing in poorly controlled diabetic patients utilizing S. pneumoniae as the organism. Tan et al.(1975) showed similar results, while noting that the impairment in bactericidal activity involved defective ingestion in some patients, whereas there was decreased intracellular killing in others. Once again, these abnormalities are associated with poor metabolic control.

It would thus appear that several aspects of phagocytic cell function are impaired in poorly controlled diabetics. This may be related to impaired glucose utilization that occurs under these circumstances. While more data are required to fully understand the consequences of the metabolic process, the evidence is emerging that there is a relationship between the severity of the disease process (in terms of hyperglycaemia, ketonaemia and other metabolic disturbances) and the degree of impairment of phagocytic function.

3.8 Immunological Aspects of Islet and Pancreas Transplantation in Diabetes

Matas et al. (1976) have summarized the current status of islet and pancreas transplantation in diabetes mellitus. Moreover, a recent symposium has also dealt with this problem (Brown 1980). They have summarized the experimental evidence indicating that islet and whole pancreas transplants can ameliorate the metabolic abnormalities of experimental diabetes. Islet cell transplantation in diabetic patients has continued to be exceedingly difficult. No patient so far has been cured of diabetes by this means, and the only successful transplants have been in patients who have been markedly immunosuppressed (generally because they have received renal allografts for end-stage diabetic nephropathy). Some of these patients did obtain reduction in insulin requirements, which was occasionally quite marked in degree. However, the experimental evidence that a critical mass of islet cell tissue evokes a particularly vigorous immunological rejection response would indicate that larger quantities of islet cell tissue will be necessary in the future and that donor-recipient pairs must be well matched in terms of their HLA typing. Moreover, it is evident that "passenger" leucocytes present in allografts might play a significant role in initiating immune rejection of the transplanted organ by the recipient (Lacy et al. 1981). There is some evidence that cultured human foetal islet cell tissue may be less antigenic than adult tissue (Brown 1980; Lacy et al. 1981).

Aside from the question of the number of potential pancreatic donors, and the technical difficulties in obtaining islet cell tissue from whole pancreatic tissue, major problems remain in allograft rejection, even with foetal pancreatic tissue (Brown 1980). However, Lacy et al. (1981) have reported a series of new findings which indicate that it is possible to prevent rejection of islet allografts and islet xenografts in animals without the continued use of immunosuppressive agents. The survival of allografts of rat islets has been prolonged for more than 3 months by in vitro culture of the islets at low temperatures 1 week prior to transplantation in conjunction with a single injection of rat anti-lymphocyte serum at the time of transplantation. Similar techniques have allowed xenograft survival of rat islets transplanted in diabetic mice for more than 3 months by the use of culture of rat islets at low temperatures with a single injection of anti-serums to mouse and rat lymphocytes at the time of transplantation. These pretreatment regimens employed for prolonging islet allograft and xenograft survival would appear to destroy or alter passenger leucocytes in the grafts since the latter cells may be necessary for the induction of immune recognition by the recipient.

These advances bring the possibility of human islet cell transplantation for the treatment of diabetes mellitus closer. However, it is clear that at least in many patients with type I diabetes mellitus, auto-immune processes were important in producing the lesions in the first place. Thus it may readily be conjectured that this may prove to be a continuing problem for the new, transplanted islets even when every other obstacle is overcome.

3.9 Summary

There is much evidence to indicate that the clinical disorder of diabetes mellitus is genetically heterogeneous and that the pathogenesis is likewise heterogeneous. The possible involvement of immune mechanisms in the initiation of diabetes mellitus has been extensively studied over the past several years, and it is now increasingly evident that immune mechanisms do play a role in at least many of the patients who suffer from the insulinopenic (type I) form of diabetes mellitus. However, even this group of diabetics appears to have genetic heterogeneity, since subgroups of type I have HLA-B8 and HLA-Dw3 and/or HLA-B15 and Dw4. The combination of Dw3 and Dw4 increases the risk of diabetes mellitus beyond that seen with either gene alone. Those diabetics with HLA-Dw3 often have antibodies to organs other than the islets of Langerhans, such as the thyroid and stomach. Moreover, other organ-specific auto-immune diseases are much more common in this group, termed Irl by Irvine. The finding of islet cell antibodies and evidence of cell-mediated immunity directed against islet-cell antigens in these patients provide further evidence implicating auto-immune reactions in type I diabetes mellitus. In addition to the immune phenomena observed in this condition, the possibility of viral infection has been extensively studied. However, despite some circumstantial evidence implicating viruses in the aetiology of diabetes mellitus (and one case now reported which clearly resulted from viral infection), it is still unclear whether viral disease does cause the disorder, or whether it may cause the disorder in one subgroup and not in the other.

One form of diabetes mellitus, namely, that associated with acanthosis nigricans, has been extensively studied, primarily by one group of investigators. It is quite clear that in one category of patients with this condition, the cause of the diabetes is directly due to the presence of antibodies directed against insulin receptors. This remarkable disorder has led to extensive studies of the role of insulin receptors in glucose metabolism. This antibody is capable of inducing such receptors in some instances, and thus occasionally resulting in hypoglycaemia (the antibody in this instance acting as an agonist, rather than antagonist).

While anti-insulin antibodies are primarily a result of chronic treatment with insulin preparations, occasionally antibodies to insulin may precede such treatment, and thus may be spontaneous. However, in the vast majority of patients in which insulin antibodies are demonstrated, they are the result of treatment and are not causative. Such antibodies may result in certain complications of the treatment, such as allergic reactions, or insulin resistance, but there is not clear evidence relating such antibodies to the long-term micro-angiopathic complications of diabetes mellitus.

It should also be noted that the metabolic disorder itself has immunological consequences. These seem to relate most directly to leucocyte and phagocytic functions and may be a result of impaired glucose utilization in these cells during periods of poor diabetic control. It may be that these impaired functions are involved in the increased susceptibility to bacterial and fungal infection as observed in diabetes mellitus.

The role of immunology in the future management of diabetes mellitus is of further interest. The continued search for a less immunogenic form of insulin may result in improved management, since insulin dosage as currently utilized depends greatly upon the level of insulin-binding antibodies which develop in the course of treatment. Another very interesting possibility for the future is that of pancreatic islet cell transplants. This has now become feasible, although major problems relating to rejection still exist. Moreover, there does not appear to have been careful consideration given to the question of the continuing auto-immune processes which may be present in at least one large subgroup of the diabetic population. Thus, even if the question of immediate rejection of the islet cells was solved, it is possible that the auto-immune process will reassert itself, and that the transplant will thus be susceptible to immunological destruction once more.

Whether improved genetic identification of risk may be helpful in future remains to be seen. If it becomes possible to identify a "disease susceptibility" gene by relatively simple means in infants, then the matter of disease prevention becomes at least a possibility. There are at least a number of avenues where immunological research might point the way towards possible means of prevention. Since such possibilities are at present highly conjectural, it does not seem appropriate to discuss them at this point. It is nevertheless clear that much remains to be learned about the basis of this disorder, and the next decade should provide exciting new perspectives on aetiology, management, and possibly even prevention.

3.10 References

Adams SF (1926) The seasonal variation in the onset of acute diabetes; the age and sex factor in 1000 diabetic patients. Arch Intern Med 37:861–864

Andersen OO (1976) Anti-insulin antibodies and late diabetic complications. Acta Endocrinol (Copenh) 83:329–340

Andersen OO, Nerup J, Bendixen G, Egeberg J, Gunnarsson R, Kromann H, Poulsen JE (1974) Experimental induction of anti-pancreatic cell-mediated immunity associated with B-cell degeneration and glucose intolerance in rodents. In: Bastenie PA, Gepts W (eds) Immunity and autoimmunity in diabetes mellitus. Excerpta Medica, Amsterdam, pp 211–217

Anderson JH, Blackard WG, Goldman J, Rubinstein AH (1978) Diabetes and hypoglycaemia due to insulin antibodies. Am J Med 64:868–873

Arquilla ER, Michalski RE, Roth MD (1980) Involvement of cell-mediated immunity in chronic alloxan diabetic mice (Abstract 206). Diabetes [Suppl 2]29:52A

Bagdade JD, Root RK, Bulger RJ (1974) Impaired leucocyte function in patients with poorly controlled diabetes. Diabetes 23:9–15

Banting FG, Best CH (1922) Pancreatic extracts. J Lab Clin Med 7:464–472

Barbosa J, King R, Noreen H, Yunis EJ (1977) The histocompatibility system in juvenile, insulin-dependent diabetic multiple kindreds. J Clin Invest 60:989–998

Bates G, Weiss C (1941) Delayed development of antibody to *Staphylococcus* toxin in diabetic children. Am J Dis Child 62:346–351

Berson SA, Yalow RS (1959 a) Recent studies on insulin-binding antibodies. Ann NY Acad Sci 82:338–344

Berson SA, Yalow RS (1959 b) Quantitative aspects of the reaction between insulin and insulinbinding antibody. J Clin Invest 38:1996–2016

Berson SA, Yalow RS (1961) Preparation and purification of human insulin-I^{131}; binding to human insulin-binding antibodies. J Clin Invest 40:1803–1808

Berson SA, Yalow RS, Bauman A, Rothschild MA, Newerly K (1956) Insulin I_{131} metabolism in human subjects: demonstration of insulin binding globulin in the circulation of insulin treated subjects. J Clin Invest 35:170–190

Best CH (1960) Epochs in the history of diabetes. In: Williams RH (ed) Diabetes. Hoeber, New York, pp 1–13

Bloom A, Hayes TM, Gamble DR (1975) Register of newly diagnosed diabetic children. Br Med J 3:580–583

Bottazzo GF, Doniach D (1978) Islet cell antibodies (ICA) in diabetes mellitus. Evidence of an autoantigen common to all cells in the islets of Langerhans. Ric Clin Lab 8:29–38

Bottazzo GF, Florin-Christensen A, Doniach D (1974) Islet cell antibodies in diabetes mellitus with autoimmune polyendocrine deficiencies. Lancet 2:1279–1283

Bottazzo, GF, Cudworth AG, Moul DJ, Doniach D, Festenstein H (1978 a) Evidence for a primary autoimmune type of diabetes mellitus (type Ib). Br Med J 2:1253–1255

Bottazzo GF, Mann JI, Thorogood M, Baum JD, Doniach D (1978 b) Autoimmunity in juvenile diabetics and their families. Br Med J 2:165–168

Bottazzo GF, Dean BM, Gorsuch AN, Cudworth AG, Doniach D (1980) Complement fixing islet-cell antibodies in type I diabetes: possible monitors of active beta cell damage. Lancet 1:668–672

Brown J (ed) (1980) Proceedings of a conference on pancreas transplantation, June 8–9 1979 Diabetes 29 (Suppl 1) 1–128

Burkholder PM (1965) Immunohistopathologic study of localized plasma proteins and fixation of guinea pig complement in renal lesions of diabetic glomerulosclerosis. Diabetes 14:755–770

Buschard K, Rygaard J (1977) Passive transfer of streptozotocin induced diabetes mellitus with spleen cells. Acta Pathol Microbiol Scand [C] 85:469–472

Buschard K, Rygaard J (1978) Is the diabetogenic effect of streptozotocin in part thymus dependent? Acta Path Microbiol Scand [C] 86:23–27

Buschard K, Madsbad S, Rygaard J (1978) Passive transfer of diabetes mellitus from man to mouse. Lancet 1:908–910

Buschard K, Madsbad S, Rygaard J (1980) Depressed suppressor cell activity in patients with newly diagnosed insulin-dependent diabetes mellitus. Clin Exp Immunol 41:25–32

Christy M, Nerup J, Bottazzo GF, Doniach D, Platz P, Svejgaard A, Ryder LP, Thomsen M (1976) Association between HLA-B8 and autoimmunity in juvenile diabetes mellitus. Lancet 2:142–143

Churg J, Dolger H (1971) Diabetic renal disease. In: Strauss MB, Welt LG (eds) Diseases of the kidney 2nd ed. Little Brown, Boston, pp 873–889

Coleman SL, Becker B, Canaan S, Rosenbaum L (1962) Fluorescent insulin staining of the diabetic eye. Diabetes 11:375–377

Craighead JE (1972) Inflammatory lesions of the islets of Langerhans. In: Greep RO, Astwood EB, Steiner DR, Frienkel N, Geiger SE (eds) Handbook of physiology, vol 1/7. American Physiological Society, Washington DC, pp 315–321

Craighead JE (1974) Insulitis associated with viral infection. In: Bastenie PA, Gepts W (eds) Immunity and autoimmunity in diabetes mellitus. Excerpta Medica, Amsterdam, pp 227–233

Craighead JE (1978) Current views on the etiology of insulin-dependent diabetes mellitus. N Engl J Med 299:1439–1445

Craighead JE, McLane MF (1968) Diabetes mellitus: induction in mice by encephalomyocarditis virus. Science 162:913–914

Craighead JE, Steinke J (1971) Diabetes mellitus-like syndrome in mice infected with encephalomyocarditis virus. Am J Pathol 63:119–134

Cudworth AG (1976) The aetiology of diabetes mellitus. Br J Hosp Med 16:207–216

Cudworth AG (1977) The aetiology of diabetes. In: Besser M (ed) Advanced medicine, vol 13. Pitman, London, pp 163–172

Cudworth AG (1978) Type I diabetes mellitus. Diabetologia 14:281–291

Cudworth AG, Gamble DR, White GSB, Lendrum R, Woodrow JC, Bloom A (1977) Aetiology of juvenile onset diabetes: a prospective study. Lancet 1:385–388

Deckert T, Egeberg J, Frimoldt-Moller C, Sander E, Svejgaard A (1979) Basement membrane thickness, insulin antibodies and HLA antigens in long standing insulin-dependent diabetics with and without severe retinopathy. Diabetologia 17:91–96

Doniach D, Bottazzo GF (1977) Autoimmunity in the endocrine pancreas. In: Joachim HL (ed) Pathobiology annual. Appleton-Century Crofts, New York, pp 327–346

Doniach D, Bottazzo GF (1981) Viruses, autoimmunity, genes and receptors in diabetes. In: Bajaj JS (ed) Insulin and metabolism. Elsevier/North Holland, New York

Drash AL (1979) The etiology of diabetes mellitus. N Engl J Med 300:1211–1313

Dumm ME (1957) Glucose utilization and lactate production by leukocytes of patients with diabetes mellitus. Proc Soc Exp Biol Med 95:571–574

Esmann V (1964) Effect of cell concentration on the metabolism of normal and diabetic leukocytes in vitro. Metabolism 13:354–360

Fairchild RS, Kyner JL, Abdou NI (1980) Suppressor cell dysfunction in insulin dependent diabetes (Abstract 208). Diabetes [Supple. 2] 29:52 A

Fajans SS, Cloutier MC, Crowther RL (1978) Clinical and etiologic heterogeneity of idiopathic diabetes mellitus. Diabetes 27:1112–1125

Feldman R, Grodsky GM, Kohout FW, McWilliams NB (1963) Immunologic studies in a diabetic subject resistant to bovine insulin but sensitive to porcine insulin. Am J Med 35:411–417

Fialkow PJ, Zavala C, Nielsen R (1975) Thyroid autoimmunity: increased frequency in relatives of insulin-dependent diabetes patients. Ann Intern Med 83:170–176

Flier JS, Kahn CR, Roth J (1979) Receptors, antireceptor antibodies and mechanism of insulin resistance. N Engl J Med 300:413–419

Folling I, Norman N (1972) Hyperglycemia, hypoglycemic attacks and production of anti-insulin antibodies without previous known immunization; immunological and functional studies in a patient. Diabetes 21:814–826

Freedman P, Peters JH, Kark RM (1960) Localization of gamma-globulin in the diseased kidney. Arch Intern Med 105:524–535

Freytag G (1974) Do viruses serve as mediators of immunological reactions? In: Bastenie PA, Gepts W (eds) Immunity and autoimmunity in diabetes mellitus. Excerpta Medica, Amsterdam pp 247–251

Friedman JM, Fialkow PJ (1978) The genetics of Graves' disease. Clin Endocrinol Metab 7:47–65

From GLA, Craighead JE, McLane MF, Steinke J (1968) Virus-induced diabetes in mice. Metabolism 17:1154–1158

Galbraith RM (1979) Immunological aspects of diabetes mellitus. CRC, Boca Raton

Gamble DR, Taylor KW (1969) Seasonal incidence of diabetes mellitus. Br Med J 3:627–630

Gamble DR, Kinsley ML, Fitzgerald MG, Bolton R, Taylor KW (1969) Viral antibodies in diabetes mellitus. Br Med J 3:627–630

Gamble DR, Taylor KW, Cumming H (1973) Coxsackie viruses and diabetes mellitus. Br Med J 4:260–262

Gepts W (1965) Pathologic anatomy of the pancreas in juvenile diabetes mellitus. Diabetes 14:619–633

Ginsberg-Fellner F, Dobersen M, Mark EM, Nechemias C, Hausknecht RU, Rubinstein P, Notkins AL (1980) Islet cell antibodies in gestational diabetes mellitus: prognostic value (Abstract 211). Diabetes [Suppl 2]29:53 A

Goldstein D, Drash A, Gibbs J, Blizzard RM (1970) Diabetes mellitus. The incidence of circulating antibodies against thyroid, gastric and adrenal tissue. J Pediatr 77:304–306

Gottlieb MS, Root HF (1968) Diabetes mellitus in twins. Diabetes 17:693–704

Grodsky GM, Feldman R, Toreson WE, Lee JC (1966) Diabetes mellitus in rabbits immunized with insulin. Diabetes 15:579–585

Gunderson E (1927) Is diabetes of infectious origin? J Infect Dis 41:197–202

Handwerger BS, Fernandes G, Brown DM (1980) Immune and autoimmune aspects of diabetes mellitus. Human Pathology 11:338–352

Hayashi K, Boucher DW, Notkins AL (1974) Virus-induced diabetes mellitus. II. Relationships between beta cell damage and hyperglycemia in mice infected with encephalomyocarditis virus. Am J Pathol 75:91–102

Huang SW, McLaren NK (1976) Insulin-dependent diabetes: a disease of auto-aggression. Science 192:64–66

Irvine WJ (1977) Classification of idiopathic diabetes. Lancet 1: 638–642

Irvine WJ (1980) Polyglandular autoimmune diseases. In: Cumming IA, Funder JW, Mendelsohn FAO, Endocrinology 1980. Austral Acad Sci Canberra, pp 100–105

Irvine WJ, Barnes EW (1972) Adrenocortical insufficiency. Clin Endocrinol Metab 1:549–594

Irvine WJ, Barnes EW (1974) Addison's disease and associated conditions with particular reference to premature ovarian failure, diabetes mellitus and hypoparathyroidism. In: Gell PH, Coombs RRA, Lachman PJ (eds) Clinical aspects of immunology,3rd ed. Blackwell Scientific, Oxford, pp 1301–1354

Irvine WJ, Gray RS, McCallum CJ (1976) Pancreatic islet cell antibody is a marker for asymptomatic and latent diabetes and prediabetes. Lancet 2:1097–1102

Irvine WJ, McCallum CJ, Gray RS, Duncan LJP, Farquhar JW, Vaughan H, Morris PJ (1977 a) Pancreatic islet cell antibodies in diabetes mellitus correlated with the duration and type of diabetes, coexistent autoimmune diseases and HLA type. Diabetes 26:138–147

Irvine WJ, Al Khateeb SF, Di Mario U, Feek CM, Gray RS, Edmond B, Duncan LJP (1977 b) Soluble immune complexes in the sera of newly diagnosed insulin-dependent diabetics and in treated diabetics. Clin Exp Immunol 30:16–21

Irvine WJ, DiMario U, Feek CM, Gray RS, Ting A, Morris PJ, Duncan LJP (1978 a) Autoimmunity and HLA antigens in type I diabetes. J Clin Lab Immunol 1:111–114

Irvine WJ, DiMario U, Feek CM, Ting A, Morris PJ, Gray RS, Duncan LJP (1978 b) Insulin antibodies in relation to islet cell antibodies and HLA antigens in type I diabetes. J Clin Lab Immunol 1:107–110

Jansen FK, Muntefering H, Schmidt WAK (1978) Virus induced diabetes and the immune system. I. Suggestion that the appearance of diabetes depends on immune reactions. Diabetologia 13:545–549

Jervell J, Solheim B (1979) HLA antigens in longstanding insulin dependent diabetics with terminal nephropathy and retinopathy with and without loss of vision. Diabetologia 17:391

Kawazu S, Kanazawa Y, Kajinuma H, Miki E, Kuzuya T, Kosaka K (1975) Demonstration of anti-"a-component" antibody: a possible means to differentiate patients with auto-antibodies to endogenous insulin from insulin-treated patients. Diabetologia 11:169–173

Kowalczyk D, Zembala M (1978) Migration inhibition of T lymphocytes from human peripheral blood by specific antigen and lymphokines. Clin Exp Immunol 32: 333–338

Kozak GP (1971) Diabetes and other endocrinological disorders. In: Marble A, White P, Bradley RF, Krall LP (eds) Joslin's diabetes mellitus, 11th ed. Lea & Febiger, Philadelphia, pp 666–694

Kremer HU (1947) Juvenile diabetes as a sequel to mumps. Am J Med 3:257–258

Lacy PE, Davie JM, Finke EH (1981) Transplantation of insulin producing tissue. Am J med 70:589–594

Larsson O (1967) Studies of small vessels in patients with diabetes. Acta Med Scand [Suppl] 480:1–66

LeCompte PM, Steinke J, Soeldner JS, Renold AE (1966) Changes in the islets of Langerhans in cows injected with heterologous and homologous insulin. Diabetes 15:586–596

Lendrum R, Walker G, Gamble DR (1975) Islet cell antibodies in juvenile diabetes mellitus of recent origin. Lancet 1:880–883

Lendrum R, Walker G, Cudworth AG, Woodrow JC, Gamble DR (1976 a) HLA-linked genes and islet cell antibodies in diabetes mellitus. Br Med J 1:1565–1567

Lendrum R, Walker G, Cudworth AG, Theophanides C, Pyke DA, Bloom A, Gamble DR (1976 b) Islet cell antibodies in diabetes mellitus. Lancet 2:1273–1276

Lernmark A, Freedman ZR, Hofmann C, Rubinstein AH, Steiner DF, Jackson RL, Winter RJ, Traisman HS (1978) Islet-cell-surface antibodies in juvenile diabetes mellitus. N Engl J Med 299:375–380

Like AA, Rossini AA, Guberski DL, Appel MC, Williams RM (1979) Spontaneous diabetes mellitus: reversal and prevention in the BB/W rat with antiserum to rat lymphocytes. Science 206:1421–1423

Lipsick J, Beattie G, Osler AG, Kaplan NO (1979) Passive transfer of lymphocytes from diabetic man to athymic mouse. Lancet 1:1290–1291

Ludwig H, Schernthaner G, Kraft D, Scheiner O, Mayr WR (1980) Antibody-dependent killer cell function in insulin-dependent diabetes mellitus. J Endocrinol Invest 3:39–44

MacCuish AC, Irvine WJ (1975) Autoimmunological aspects of diabetes mellitus. Clin Endocrinol Metab 4:435–471

MacCuish AC, Jordan J, Campbell CJ, Duncan LJP, Irvine WJ (1974 a) Cell-mediated immunity to human pancreas in diabetes mellitus. Diabetes 23:693–697

MacCuish AC, Barnes EW, Irvine WJ, Duncan LJP (1974 b) Antibodies to pancreatic islet cells in insulin-dependent diabetes with coexistent autoimmune disease. Lancet 2:1529–1531

MacLaren, NK, Huang SW, Fogh J (1975) Antibody to cultured human insulinoma cells in insulin-dependent diabetes. Lancet 1:997–1000

Matas AJ, Sutherland DER, Najarian JS (1976) Current status of islet and pancreatic transplantation in diabetes. Diabetes 25:785–795

Melin K, Ursing B (1958) Diabetes mellitus som komplikation till parotitis epidemica. Nord Med 60:1715–1717

Moulias R, Goust JM (1974) Cell-mediated immune responses against insulin in low insulin output diabetes and in diabetes with lipo-atrophy. In: Bastenie PA, Gepts W (eds) Immunity and autoimmunity in diabetes mellitus. Excerpta Medica, Amsterdam, pp 121–123

Moulias R, Goust JM, Bernard S, Croisier B, Attali A, Berthaux P (1974) Humoral and cellular thyroid auto-immunity and diabetes mellitus. In: Bastenie PA, Gepts W (eds) Immunity and autoimmunity in diabetes mellitus. Excerpta Medica, Amsterdam, pp 140–148

Muntefering H (1974) Experimental virus-induced diabetes mellitus accompanied by insulitis. In: Bastenie PA, Gepts W (eds) Immunity and autoimmunity in diabetes mellitus. Excerpta Medica, Amsterdam, pp 234–241

Nakao Y, Fukunishi T, Koide M, Akasawa K, Ikeda M, Mikio Y, Imura H (1977) HLA antigens in Japanese patients with diabetes mellitus. Diabetes 26:736–739

Nakhooda AF, Like AA, Chappel CI, Murray FR, Marliss EB (1977) The spontaneously diabetic Wistar rat; metabolic and morphologic studies. Diabetes 26:100–112

Nelson PG, Pyke DA, Gamble DR (1975) Viruses and the aetiology of diabetes: a study in identical twins. Br Med J 4:249–251

Nerup J (1974) The clinical and immunological association of diabetes mellitus and Addison's disease. In: Bastenie PA, Gepts W (eds) Immunity and autoimmunity in diabetes mellitus. Excerpta Medica, Amsterdam, pp 149–152

Nerup J, Andersen OO, Bendixen G, Egeberg J, Poulsen JE (1971) Anti-pancreatic cellular hypersensitivity in diabetes mellitus. Diabetes 20:424–427

Nerup J, Andersen OO, Bendixen G, Egeberg J, Poulsen JE, Vilien M, Westrup M (1973 a) Anti-pancreatic cellular hypersensitivity in diabetes mellitus: experimental induction of anti-pancreatic cellular hypersensitivity and associated morphological B-cell changes in the rat. Acta Allergol 28:231–249

Nerup J, Andersen OO, Bendixen G, Egeberg J, Poulsen JE (1973 b) Anti-pancreatic cellular hypersensitivity in diabetes mellitus. Antigen activity of fetal calf pancreas and correlation with clinical type of diabetes. Acta Allergol 28:223–230

Nerup J, Andersen OO, Bendixen G, Egeberg J, Poulsen JE (1974) Cellular hypersensitivity to islet cell antigen(s) different from insulin in diabetes mellitus. In: Bastenie PA, Gepts W (eds) Immunity and autoimmunity in diabetes mellitus. Excerpta Medica, Amsterdam, pp 107–111

Nerup J, Andersen OO, Christy M, Platz P, Thomsen M, Svejgaard A, Bottazzo GH, Pouplard A, Doniach D (1975) HLA factor, autoimmunity, virus and juvenile diabetes mellitus. Diabetologia 11:365–366

Nissley SP, Drash AL, Blizzard RM, Sperling M, Childs, B (1973) Comparison of juvenile diabetics with positive and negative organ-specific antibody titers. Evidence for genetic heterogeneity. Diabetes 22:63–65

Notkins AL (1977) Virus-induced diabetes mellitus: a brief review. Arch Virol 54: 1–17

Notkins AL (1979) The causes of diabetes. Sci Am 241:62–73

Ogle JW (1866) On disease of the brain as a result of diabetes mellitus. St. George's Hosp Rep 1:157–188

Ohneda A, Matsuda K, Sato M, Yamagata S, Sato T (1974) Hypoglycaemia due to apparent autoantibodies to insulin: characterization of insulin-binding protein. Diabetes 23:41–50

Onodera T, Jenseon AB, Yoon JW, Notkins AL (1978) Virus-induced diabetes mellitus: reovirus infection of pancreatic beta cells in mice. Science 201:529–531

Osserman KG (1969) Muscles (myasthenia gravis). In: Miescher PA, Muller-Eberhard HJ (eds) Textbook of immunopathology, vol 2. Grune & Stratton, New York, pp 607–623

Paik SG, Fleischer N, Shin SI (1980) Induction of diabetes by streptozotocin is mediated by T-cell functions (Abstract 205). Diabetes [Suppl 2]29:52 A

Parkinson J (1910) A case of pernicious anaemia terminating in acute diabetes. Lancet 2: 543–546

Pozzilli P, Sensi M, Gorsuch A, Bottazzo GH, Cudworth AG (1979) Evidence for raised K cell levels in type I diabetes. Lancet 2:173–175

Pozzilli P, Andreani D, Sensi M, Wolf E, Taylor M, Bottazzo GF, Cudworth AG (1980) K cells and

antibody dependent cytotoxicity in autoimmune polyendocrine disease. 6th Internat Endocrinol Cong, Melbourne, Australia, 10–14 February 1980, Abstract 639, p 529 (to be published)
Pyke DA (1979) Diabetes: the genetic connections. Diabetologia 17:333–344
Pyke DA, Nelson PG (1976) Diabetes mellitus in identical twins. In: Creutzfeldt W, Kobberling J, Neel JV (eds) The genetics of diabetes mellitus. Springer, Berlin Heidelberg New York, pp 194–202
Rayfield EJ, Seto Y (1978) Viruses and the pathogenesis of diabetes mellitus. Diabetes 27:1126–1140
Richens ER, Ancil RJ, Hartog M (1976) Autoimmunity and viral infection in diabetes mellitus. Clin Exp Immunol 23:40–46
Riley W, MacLaren N, Rand K, Bejar R (1980) Inherited autoimmunity versus Coxsackie B4 in insulin dependent diabetes (Abstract 211). Diabetes [Suppl 2]29:53 A
Rodney G, White N, Frazer TE, Duquesnay RJ, Santiago JV (1979) HLA DR specificities among black Americans with juvenile-onset diabetes. N Engl J Med 301:810–812
Rolles CJ, Rayner PHW, MacKintosh P (1975) Aetiology of juvenile diabetes. Lancet 2:230
Rosenthal MB, Goldfine ID, Siperstein MD (1976) Genetic origin of diabetes: re-evaluation of twin data. Lancet 2:250–251
Ross ME, Onodera T, Brown KS, Notkins AL (1976) Virus-induced diabetes mellitus. IV. Genetic and environmental factors influencing the development of diabetes after infection with the M variant of encephalomyocarditis virus. Diabetes 25:190–197
Rubinstein P, Suciu-Foca N, Nicholson JF (1977) Genetics of juvenile diabetes mellitus. A recessive gene clearly linked to HLA D and with 50% penetrance. N Engl J Med 297:1036–1040
Sasazuki T, Kohno Y, Iwamoto I, Kosaka K, Okimoto K, Maruyama H, Ishiba S, Konishi J, Takeda Y, Naito S (1978) HLA and Graves' disease or diabetes mellitus in Japan. N Engl J Med 298:630–631
Schernthaner G, Ludwig H, Mayr WR (1979) Immunoglobulin G-insulin antibodies and immune-region associated alloantigens in insulin-dependent diabetes mellitus. J Clin Endocrinol Metab 48:403–407
Solomon N, Carpenter CJC, Bennett IL, Harvey AM (1965) Schmidt's syndrome (thyroid and adrenal insufficiency) and coexistent diabetes mellitus. Diabetes 14:300–304
Solow H, Hidalgo R, Blajchman M, Singal DP (1977) HLA, B, C and B lymphocyte alloantigens in insulin-dependent diabetes. Transplant Proc 9:1859–1861
Tan JS, Anderson JL, Watanakunakorn C, Phair JP (1975) Neutrophil dysfunction in diabetes mellitus. Diabetes 14:300–304
Tattersall RB, Pyke DA (1972) Diabetes in identical twins. Lancet 2:1120–1125
Taylor KW (1974) The diabetogenic effect of Coxsackie B viruses. In: Bastenie PA, Gepts W (eds) Immunity and autoimmunity in diabetes mellitus. Excerpta Medica, Amsterdam, pp 242–244
Then Bergh H (1939) Zur Frage der psychischen und neurologischen Erscheinungen bei Diabeteskranken und deren Verwandten. Z Gesamte Neurol Psychiatr 165:278–283
Thurneyssen O, Jansen FK, Vialettes B, Vague Ph, Selam JL, Mirouze J (1979) Passive transfer of lymphocytes from diabetic man to athymic mouse. Lancet 1:1291–1292
Totterman TH, Andersson LC, Hayry P (1979) Evidence for thyroid antigen-reactive T lymphocytes infiltrating the thyroid gland in Graves' disease. Clin Endocrinol (Oxf) 11:59–68
Ungar B, Whittingham S, Francis CM (1967) Pernicious anaemia; incidence and significance of circulating antibodies to intrinsic factor and to parietal cells. Aust Ann Med 16:226–229
Volpé R (1978) The pathogenesis of Graves' disease: an overview. Clin Endocrinol Metab 7:3–29
Volpé R, Edmonds M, Lamki L, Clarke PV, Row VV (1972) The pathogenesis of Graves' disease: a disorder of delayed hypersensitivity? Mayo Clin Proc 47:824–834
Von Meyenburg H (1940) Über "insulitis" bei Diabetes. Schweiz Med Wochenschr 70:554–557
Wakisaka A, Aizawa M, Matsurra N, Nakazawa S, Nakayama E, Ilakura K, Okuno A, Wagatsuma Y (1976) HLA and juvenile diabetes mellitus in the Japanese. Lancet 2:970
Webb SR, Loria RM, Madge GE, Kilbrick S (1976) Susceptibility of mice to Group B Coxsackie virus is influenced by the diabetic gene. J Exp Med 143:1239–1248
Wellmann KF, Amsterdam D, Brancato P, Volk BW (1972) Fine structure of the pancreatic islets of mice infected with the M variant of the encephalomyocarditis virus. Diabetologia 8:349–357
Werner AU, Larsen HW (1969) Immunohistological studies on human diabetic and non-diabetic eyes. I. Fluorescent labelling of insulin and insulin antibodies. Acta Ophthalmol 47:937–955
Westberg NG, Michael AF (1972) Immunohistopathology of diabetic glomerulosclerosis. Diabetes 21:163–174
Yalow RS, Berson SA (1957) Apparent inhibition of liver insulinase activity by serum and serum fractions containing insulin binding antibody. J Clin Invest 36:648–655

Yalow RS, Berson SA (1960) Immunoassay of endogenous plasma insulin in man. J Clin Invest 39:1157–1175

Yalow RS, Berson SA (1961) Immunological specificity of human insulin: application to immunoassay of insulin. J Clin Invest 40:2190–2198

Yoon JW, Austin M, Onodera T, Notkins AL (1979) Virus-induced diabetes mellitus: isolation of a virus from the pancreas of a child with diabetic ketoacidosis. N Engl J Med 300:1173–1179

Zeidler A, Loon J, Fraser SD, Kunar D, Perry R, Terasaki P (1980) HLA DRw antigens in Mexican-American and black American diabetic patients. Diabetes 29:247–256

Zonana J, Rimoin DL (1976) Inheritance of diabetes mellitus. N Engl J Med 295:603–605

4 Auto-immunity of the Anterior Pituitary

Since the endocrine organs seem unduly susceptible to auto-immune disorders, one might have expected that the anterior pituitary would not be excluded from such lesions. This has indeed been the case, although auto-immune hypophysitis has (so far) appeared to be a rare disorder. Lymphoid involvement of the pituitary was observed as early as 1953, but auto-immune processes were not suspected (Rapp and Pashkis 1953). The first patient in whom there was a suspicion of this condition was reported by Goudie and Pinkerton (1962); they described a young woman, aged 22, who died of a peripheral vascular collapse following removal of a gangrenous appendix. She had felt fatigued following the birth of a second child 14 months previously, and had had only two scanty menstrual periods between that time and her subsequent death. She also had been found to have an enlarging goitre, and had been treated with thyroid therapy. At autopsy, her very large goitre was proven to result from Hashimoto's thyroiditis. A shrunken anterior pituitary gland was discovered; histology of the latter showed extensive lymphocytic infiltration of the anterior pituitary surrounding atrophic pituitary cells. Goudie and Pinkerton proposed that the coexistence of the lymphocytic hypophysitis and Hashimoto's thyroiditis might well be explained by an auto-immune mechanism. Goudie (1968) again discussed this proposal.

Hume and Roberts (1967) have described a similar case with lymphocytic thyroiditis and chronic atrophic gastritis, associated with pernicious anaemia. Kiaer and Rytter Norgaard (1969) studied a patient at autopsy with granulomatous hypophysitis, lymphocytic thyroiditis and diffuse lymphocytic adrenalitis. Two further patients suffering from lymphocytic hypophysitis have been described by Egloff et al. (1969) and Lack (1975). Doniach (1977) reviewed these cases. In addition, Gleason et al. (1978) have described a 59-year-old woman with attacks of hypoglycaemia and unexplained arthralgias who at post-mortem showed an enlarged pituitary gland, with lymphoid follicles, interstitial round cell infiltrates, fibrosis and focal collections of pituitary cells. The condition was not diagnosed during life. In a recent report, antibodies to adrenal, thyroid, stomach and pituitary were detected in the serum of a patient with an 8-year history of Addison's disease. At necropsy, focal lymphoid hypophysitis was observed, although pituitary function studies had been virtually normal throughout life (Ludwig and Schernthaner 1978).

Laboratory studies have been reported in only a few publications. Goust et al. (1972) have reported the results of leucocyte migration inhibition tests in four patients with non-tumorous hypopituitarism, utilizing anterior pituitary antigen, and have shown positive values in all of these patients. Bottazzo and Doniach (1978) have recently studied antibodies to anterior pituitary cells under various conditions. Since systematic examination by immunofluorescence on all endocrine glands of sera from Addisonian and hypoparathyroid cases actually had led to the first description of islet cell antibodies (Bottazzo et al. 1974), the same group of investigators decided to examine the same series of stored polyendocrine sera for antibodies to normal human pituitary glands (obtained at hypophysectomy for alleviation of carcinoma of the breast). They were able to show, by immunofluorescent techniques, that 19 of 278 cases had antibodies reacting specifically with the prolactin-secreting cells of the anterior pituitary (Bottazzo et al. 1975). In their study, Bottazzo and Doniach were unable to find pituitary antibodies in cases of panhypopituitarism. However, in their 1978 case review, they note that prolactin cell antibodies were detected in two cases showing mild or partial pituitary deficiency (Bottazzo and Doniach 1978). They suggested that these antibodies are weak and may well disappear from the blood in advanced stages of pituitary atrophy.

Mori et al. (1978) have reported the presence of antibodies to TSH in a patient with Sheehan's syndrome and chronic thyroiditis. Bottazzo et al. (1980) additionally have found antibodies against the growth hormone-secreting cells. These antibodies were found in a young girl who showed retarded growth from age 6 years, and whose mother suffered from Addison's disease and thyroiditis. This group (Bottazzo and Doniach 1978) also have some sera under study where the antibodies react neither with lactotrophs nor with somatotrophs, and may possibly be against LH- or FSH-secreting cells. They speculate that it is possible that antibodies to each of the anterior pituitary cells will finally be identified.

Experimental auto-immune hypophysitis was first induced by Levine (1967) in rats by means of the injection of pituitary tissue and adjuvant. No spontaneous animal model has yet been discovered.

While, therefore, the literature still remains scant with respect to overt anterior pituitary deficiency of auto-immune origin, the studies of Bottazzo and Doniach at least suggest that occult auto-immune hypophysitis in the human may not be quite so rare, at least as judged by the presence of antibodies directed against anterior pituitary cells. Indeed, with increased awareness of the possibility of such entities, the rate of detection of both occult and clinically evident auto-immune pituitary disorders will almost surely rise.

4.1 References

Bottazzo GF, Florin-Christensen A, Doniach D (1974) Islet cell antibodies in diabetes mellitus with autoimmune polyendocrine deficiencies. Lancet 2:1279–1283

Bottazzo GF, Pouplard A, Florin-Christensen A, Doniach D (1975) Autoantibodies to prolactin-secreting cells of the human pituitary. Lancet 2:97–101

Bottazzo GF, Doniach D (1978) Pituitary autoimmunity: a review. Proc R Soc Med 71:433–436

Bottazzo GF, McIntosh C, Stanford W, Preece M (1980) Growth hormone cell antibodies and partial growth hormone deficiency in a girl with Turner's syndrome. Clin Endocrinol (Oxf) 12:1–9

Doniach I (1977) Histopathology of the anterior pituitary. Clin Endocrinol Metab 6:21–52

Egloff B, Fischbacher W, Von Goumoens E (1969) Lymphomatose Hypophysitis mit Hypophyseninsuffizienz. Schweiz Med Wochenschr 42:1499–1502

Gleason TH, Stebbins PL, Shanahan MF (1978) Lymphoid hypophysitis in a patient with hypoglycemic episodes. Arch Pathol Lab Med 192:46–48

Goudie RB (1968) Anterior hypophysitis associated with autoimmune disease. Proc R Soc Med 61:275

Goudie RM, Pinkerton RH (1962) Anterior hypophysitis and Hashimoto's thyroiditis in a young woman. J Pathol Bacteriol 83:584–585

Goust JM, Moulias R, Reinert P, Deville-Chabrolle A, Buffet C, Muller-Berat CN (1972) Cellular immunity to antigens of the organs in endocrine disease. Studies of the leukocyte migration test. Rev F Endocrinol Clin 13:410-411

Hume R, Roberts GH (1967) Hypophysitis and hypopituitarism; report of a case. Br Med J 2:548–550

Kiaer W, Rytter Norgaard JO (1969) Granulomatous hypophysitis and thyroiditis with lymphocytic adrenalitis. Acta Pathol Microbiol Scand 76:229–238

Lack EE (1975) Lymphoid "hypophysitis" with end organ insufficiency. Arch Pathol 99:215–219

Levine S (1967) Allergic adrenohypophysitis: new experimental disease of the pituitary gland. Science 158:1190–1191

Ludwig H, Schernthaner G (1978) Multiorganspezifische Autoimmunität bei idiopathischer Nebennierenrindeninsuffizienz. Wien Klin Wochenschr 90:736–741

Mori T, Kato H, Tatsumi S, Igarashi T, Takayama H (1978) Anti-TSH autoantibody in a patient with Sheehan's syndrome and chronic thyroiditis. 6th Asia and Oceania Congr Endocrinol, Singapore, January 22–27, 1978, Abstract 125 (to be published)

Rapp JJ, Pashkis KE (1953) Panhypopituitarism with idiopathic hypoparathyroidism. Ann Intern Med 39:1103–1107

5 Auto-immune Diseases of the Adrenals, Gonads and Paraythyroids: Auto-immune Polyendocrine Disease

5.1 Addison's Disease

The term "Addison's disease" refers to a clinical state due to primary adrenal failure, characterized by hypotension or shock, weight loss, hyponatraemia, hyperkalaemia, hypoglycaemia and increased pigmentation – all due to deficient adrenocortical hormone production and consequent increased secretion of anterior pituitary adrenocorticotrophic hormone (ACTH) (Liddle 1974). The original description by Addison in 1855 of 11 examples of this disorder includes cases now recognizable as idiopathic adrenal atrophy, as well as tuberculosis of the adrenal gland and metastatic carcinoma (Addison 1868). Subsequently, many other rare causes of primary adrenal failure have been observed, including fungal or viral infections, amyloidosis, haemachromatosis, Hodgkin's disease, periarteritis nodosa, systemic lupus erythematosus, haemorrhages, infarction, trauma (including surgical removal) and overwhelming bacterial infection (Irvine and Barnes 1975 a). Even enzymatic intra-adrenal defects of hormone biosynthesis may produce an Addison-like picture (Liddle 1974). However, the most important causes of spontaneous Addison's disease in the world are idiopathic atrophy of the adrenals and tuberculosis. While tuberculosis once accounted for the majority of cases of this condition, in recent decades tuberculosis has declined as a cause (at least in many countries).

It is currently estimated that about one-third of patients with Addison's disease in Europe and North America suffer from tuberculosis of the adrenal gland, the remainder being non-tuberculous (Stuart-Mason et al. 1968). The overall prevalence of Addison's disease may be in the order of 60 per million (Nerup 1974 a). The vast majority of patients with non-tuberculous Addison's disease are found to have "idiopathic adrenal failure". Nevertheless, Irvine and Barnes (1975 a) point out that a diagnosis of idiopathic Addison's disease, as opposed to Addison's disease due to some established cause, is reached by excluding, as far as possible, known causes of adrenal destruction. Since, however, it is sometimes extremely difficult to be certain that such known causes have been excluded, some cases thought to be idiopathic have turned out at autopsy to be actually due to some other specific cause, such as tuberculosis, metastatic carcinoma and others. They point out that cases of Addison's disease thought to be immunological in nature have sometimes turned out to be not of that origin, thus creating some difficulties in interpreting immunological findings in large groups of patients.

There is now ample evidence that idiopathic Addison's disease is an auto-immune disorder. This evidence as so superbly summarized by Irvine and Barnes (1975 a, b) rests upon many lines of investigation, including the histology of the disorder, the finding of auto-antibodies against the adrenal cortex in many patients with this condition, the association with other organ-specific auto-immune diseases, studies of HLA antigens and the genetics of Addison's disease, and experimental observations. These elements will be amplified below.

5.2 Experimental Auto-immune Adrenalitis

Attempts to detect organ-specific antigens in the adrenal were reported as early as 1908 by Ritchie, who used duck antisera to guinea-pig adrenals (Ritchie 1908). It is difficult, however, to interpret the results of Ritchie's experiment precisely, since the techniques employed at that time seem somewhat primitive. Nevertheless, it seems that Ritchie did succeed in demonstrating adrenal specificity. Witebsky and Klinke (1933) studied adrenal specificity by means of antisera from rabbits immunized with bovine adrenal. They demonstrated a thermostable ethanol-soluble antigen characteristic for adrenal medulla and structurally related to the brain antigen.

Experimental auto-immune adrenalitis has now been produced in guinea-pigs, rabbits, rats and monkeys, using the classic injection protocol with autologous, homologous or heterologous adrenal homogenate and adjuvants (Werdelin 1972). The first report of experimental auto-immune adrenalitis was that of Colover and Glynn (1958) who immunized guinea-pigs with homologous adrenal antigen in Freund's complete adjuvant; they reported adrenal necrosis and round cell invasion of the adrenal cortex. Milcou et al. (1959) were the first to immunize animals with adrenal antigen from the same species or autologous adrenal antigen. Steiner et al. (1960) and Barnett et al. (1963) reported similar observations. Moreover, in studies on experimental auto-immune adrenalitis, anti-adrenal antibodies could be induced which did not cross-react with ovary or testis (Witebsky and Milgrom 1962). Similar antibody production was reported by Barnett et al. in 1963; these antibodies, however, also cross-reacted with interstitial cells of the ovary and testis. These workers also noted that the adrenal lesions were more severe, and the antibody titres higher, if heterologous rather than homologous adrenals were employed as antigen (Barnett et al. 1963). Andrada et al. (1968) injected inbred Lewis rats with rat adrenal extract in complete Freund's adjuvant and observed the formation of antibodies to adrenals in rats receiving multiple injections. These antibodies reacted only to the adrenal cortex and not to the medulla. The titre of the antibodies was low, but no antibodies to the adrenals were detected in the sera of rats immunized with rat tissue other than adrenal. This was confirmed by Irino and Grollman in 1968. However, the pathological importance of these adrenal antibodies has not yet been elucidated in the experimental disorder, and it seems evident that antibodies alone are not pathogenic (Wick 1975). Thus, Witebsky and Milgrom (1962) found no correlation between the presence of adrenal antibodies and the development of histopathological changes.

Autoradiographic studies have suggested that the arrival in the adrenal of a few specifically sensitized lymphocytes migrating from the bloodstream is the initiating event of auto-immune adrenalitis in the rat (Werdelin 1972). The histological lesions which follow in the experimental animal consist initially of foci of lymphocytes and histiocytes with a small number of plasma cells and eosinophilic leucocytes, with degenerative changes of the adrenocortical cells in these foci. Usually the lesions are most numerous and most extensive in the deeper layers of the cortex, but similar infiltrates have been described in the medulla, and may be related to isolated adrenocortical cells which may occur there (Steiner et al. 1960).

Kracht et al. (1962) and Barnett et al. (1963) have also observed adrenal lesions in their experimental animals. Extensive infiltrates composed of round cells were located in peripheral portions of the adrenal cortex. Infiltrating cells were found in all layers of the cortex and on the margins of the medulla. The cortical cells frequently appeared abnormal in the vicinity of the infiltrates. Andrada et al. (1968) observed adrenalitis in 70% of female rats and 27% of male rats injected with homologous adrenal extract in complete Freund's adjuvant. The adrenal lesions consisted of mononuclear cell infiltration, localized in the zona fasciculata and zona reticularis of the adrenal cortex. The infiltrating mononuclear cells, mainly lymphocytes and plasma cells, were grouped in foci of various sizes. In these areas the cortical cells were frequently abnormal, exhibiting eosinophilia and vacuolization of the cytoplasm, as well as loss of nuclear definition. Infiltrates were not found in the zona glomerulosa or in the medulla, although occasionally they were prominent at the corticomedullary junction. The initial lesions were observed 9 days after the injection of adrenal extract, but most pronounced lesions were seen 11 to 19 days after injection.

Hoenig et al. (1970) studied the early phase of the inflammatory lesions of experimental auto-immune adrenalitis by both light and electron-microscopic observations. Lymphocytes appeared in the adrenal sinusoids intruding into the adrenal parenchyma through defects of the sinusoidal endothelium. Oedema and adrenal parenchymal cell damage were observed in the vicinity of the lymphocytes, and in areas of ischaemia produced by the obstruction of sinusoids with inflammatory cells and fibrin.

Irino and Grollman (1968) studied animals immunized with adrenocortical tissue in complete Freund's adjuvant. They detected reduced plasma corticosterone levels, fasting hypoglycaemia and increased excretion of salt and water during a salt-free diet. This was correlated with degenerative changes throughout the adrenal cortex, similar to those described above.

While it has not been possible to produce passive transfer adrenalitis by means of the passive transfer of serum as yet, Levine and Wenk (1968) have transferred lymph node cells from Lewis rats with auto-immune adrenalitis to normal recipients, thereby producing adrenalitis in the passively transferred recipients. This was confirmed by Werdelin et al. (1971).

Similar to the experience with other auto-immune diseases, the genetic background of the immunized animals is important for the successful production of experimental allergic adrenalitis (Wick 1975). Thus, BSVS mice which readily develop auto-immune encephalomyelitis and orchitis are also very susceptible to adrenalitis (Werdelin and Boehme 1969).

It can thus be concluded that experimental adrenalitis has some characteristics of other established experimental auto-immune models. The histological lesions consist of mononuclear cell infiltrations and can be induced by active immunization, as well as passive transfer of lymph node cells in histocompatible animals. The lesions are organ-specific, but there is no correlation between the presence of the lesions and circulating auto-antibodies to adrenal antigen, and adrenalitis has not yet been transferred passively by injection of serum. As with other experimental auto-immune models, some strains of animals are more susceptible than others to the induction of experimental auto-immune adrenalitis. However, these experimental models are not truly analogous to human Addison's disease, since atrophy of the adrenal gland, which is typical of the human disorder, is not seen under these conditions. Moreover, no spontaneous animal model has yet been described.

5.3 Pathology of Idiopathic Addison's Disease

Even in the first report of Addison's disease by Addison in 1855, at a time when tuberculosis of the adrenal gland was by far the most common cause of Addison's disease, one case was found to be extremely contracted, small and atrophied. Irvine and Barnes (1975 a) list the various descriptive names that have been employed to describe this condition, perhaps the most well-known of which is "idiopathic atrophy". (It is expected that "auto-immune adrenal failure", or "auto-immune adrenalitis", will be the terms employed in the future for this condition.) In any event, in this disease, both adrenal glands are found to be exceedingly small, and difficult to locate at autopsy. The capsule is generally thickened, and the cortex is usually completely destroyed. The remaining adrenocortical cells may be in small clusters or present as single cells. These cells are often enlarged, with pleomorphism and eosinophilia. A mononuclear cell infiltration is invariable, with lymphocytes, plasma cells, macrophages and occasionally germinal centres. Generally, the few remaining parenchymal cells are surrounded by the heaviest infiltration of lymphocytes. There is a variable amount of fibrosis in these glands.

Diffuse mononuclear cell infiltration is the rule, and focal adrenalitis is rare. The adrenal medulla is generally well preserved, but may have considerable infiltration with lymphoid cells (Petri and Nerup 1971). It seems evident that a diffuse chronic mononuclear inflammation associated with progressive destruction of the adrenal cortex is specific to idiopathic Addison's disease (Symington 1969). The subtypes of infiltrating lymphocytes in this lesion have not yet been identified.

5.4 Humoral Immunity in Human Addison's Disease

Anderson et al. (1957) reported that anti-adrenal antibodies could be detected in two of ten patients with Addison's disease using a complement fixation test and saline extracts of human adrenal and human thyroid tissue. Subsequent to this original observation, several workers have demonstrated antiadrenal antibodies in Addison's disease, using either the complement fixation test, or the immunofluorescent technique, and these series have been summarized by Irvine and Barnes (1975 a, b). The overall presence of anti-human adrenocortical antibodies has been detected in about 70% of cases of idiopathic (auto-immune) Addison's disease, whereas these antibodies are absent in patients with tuberculous destruction of the adrenal. Wuepper et al. (1969) and Nerup (1974 b) have indicated that adrenal antibodies are more common in those patients with a short duration of disease, and in those who develop the disorder at an early age. The titres of antiadrenal antibodies tend to be lower than those for thyroid and gastric antibodies in auto-immune thyroid disease or pernicious anaemia respectively, but may persist for many years following adequate medical therapy (Irvine 1978). Adrenal auto-antibodies are found very rarely in the control population (Nerup 1974 b). They are also quite rare in first-degree relatives of patients with Addison's disease, provided that these relatives do not have idiopathic hypoparathyroidism (Wuepper et al. 1969; Irvine and Barnes 1972).

Curiously, antiadrenal antibodies have been detected in occasional sera from patients with Cushing's syndrome (Wuepper et al. 1969; Irvine and Barnes 1972) and Andrada et al. (1979) have recently suggested that some cases of Cushing's syndrome might be a result of an auto-immune process (analogous to the situation in Graves' disease), although their data do not prove the relationship in their case report. As mentioned above, such antibodies are not found in tuberculous Addison's disease, nor in adrenal insufficiency secondary to pituitary failure, but may occasionally be seen in sera from patients with auto-immune thyroid disease and insulin-dependent diabetes mellitus. Only in idiopathic hypoparathyroidism do adrenal antibodies occur more frequently, and they are found in 25%–30% of such patients (Spinner et al. 1969).

The majority of these auto-antibodies react only with the adrenal cortex, but others may react with ovary, testis and placenta (steroid-producing cells). Often this cross-reacting antibody is associated with evidence of primary ovarian failure (see below). These antibodies, which are all IgGs, tend to persist in the serum for many years, or even many decades, after the onset of adrenocortical and/or gonadal failure (Irvine 1978). Being IgG, they are transported across the placenta into the foetal circulation, but there is no evidence that they are able to cause damage to the foetal adrenal (Gamlen et al. 1977).

It is of very considerable interest that in patients with idiopathic Addison's disease, there is a very high incidence of antibodies to other organ antigens, including ovary, testis, parathyroids, thyroid, islet cell antigens, or gastric antigens, although there may be no overt functional deficiencies in any of those organs to which antibodies are detectable. (Of course, there is an increased incidence of the other overt organ-specific auto-immune diseases in association with Addison's disease, as will be presented below.) Irvine and Barnes (1975 a) have reported the incidence of various auto-antibodies in patients with Addison's disease, as is depicted on Table 5.1. It is curious that patients with auto-immune Addison's disease or auto-immune hypoparathyroidism have a much higher incidence of auto-antibodies to other organ-specific antigens (e. g. thyrogastric antibodies) than is the converse, i. e. patients with auto-immune thyroid disease or type I diabetes mellitus

Table 5.1. Number of patients with antibodies found in Addison's disease (Irvine and Barnes 1975 a)

Addison's disease	Sera	Steroid-producing cells		Stomach		Thyroid	
		Adrenal	Ovary, testis	Parietal cells	IF[a]	Cytoplasm	Thyro-globulin
Idiopathic	174	109	30	50	16	66	38
Tuberculous	46	0	0	3	0	6	5
Others	4	0	0	0	0	0	0
Control subjects	224	1	0	23	0	27	15

[a] IF, intrinsic factor

only occasionally have antibodies to the adrenal or to steroid-secreting cells (Irvine and Barnes 1975 a; Doniach and Bottazzo 1981).

Doniach and Bottazzo (1981) have tested 600 sera from patients with auto-immune endocrine diseases in the *absence* of clinical Addison's disease. They found a total of 44 (7%) positive reactions for antibodies against the adrenal cortex. They studied clinical correlations in 31 of these patients; they found that there was a high incidence of auto-immune thyroid disease in diabetes mellitus, but in addition 19% had steroid-secreting cell antibodies (although it was not clear whether they had any clinical gonadal abnormality).

5.5 Cell-mediated Immunity in Addison's Disease

The first study of cell-mediated immunity in relation to adrenal antigen in Addison's disease was that of Nerup and Bendixen (1969 a), who used the leucocyte migration inhibition factor test employing pooled foetal adrenal extracts as antigen. (This procedure has been used to demonstrate the sensitization of T-lymphocytes against the antigen being tested: see Chap. 2 for a discussion of the procedure, as well as below.) They showed positive results in 8 of 11 males and 6 of 19 females with idiopathic Addison's disease, and this proved to be organ-specific. However, it was not species-specific, as Nerup and Bendixen themselves later showed that the cells from those patients were positive in the leucocyte migration test in response to monkey adrenal antigen (Nerup and Bendixen 1969 b), and this was confirmed by Moulias and Goust (1971) and Moulias et al. (1970, 1971). Porcine adrenal tissue also produced positive results with the human lymphocytes from patients with Addison's disease (Nerup and Bendixen 1969 b).

Our own group has shown similar findings using the leucocyte migration inhibition test in response to a human adult adrenal extract (Volpé 1977) (see Fig. 5.1). Between 40% and 80% of patients with idiopathic Addison's disease will be found to be positive with this procedure in various series in the literature (Irvine and Barnes 1975 a). There is no correlation between these results and the appearance of adrenal antibodies in the serum, the patient's age, or the duration of the disorder (Nerup and Bendixen 1969 b).

Nerup and Bendixen (1969 a) demonstrated the occurrence of positive leucocyte migration inhibition tests in response to adrenal antigen in some patients with insulin-dependent diabetes mellitus (without any clinical evidence of Addison's disease). However, there has been no systematic study in Addison's disease of the incidence of cell-mediated immunity against other organ antigens, or conversely the incidence of positive responses against adrenal antigens in patients with other organ-specific auto-immune diseases.

In Chap. 2 of this monograph, there is considerable discussion about the place of the leucocyte migration inhibition test, including the criticism that has been levelled at this procedure because of the possible participation of B-lymphocytes and immune complexes in producing positive results (see Chap. 2). While it now seems evident that the leucocyte migration inhibition test does indeed measure sensitization of T-lymphocytes against the antigen employed, it would be useful to repeat this work using preparations of isolated T-lymphocytes as has now been performed in auto-immune thyroid disease (see Chap. 2). This would lay to rest any remaining

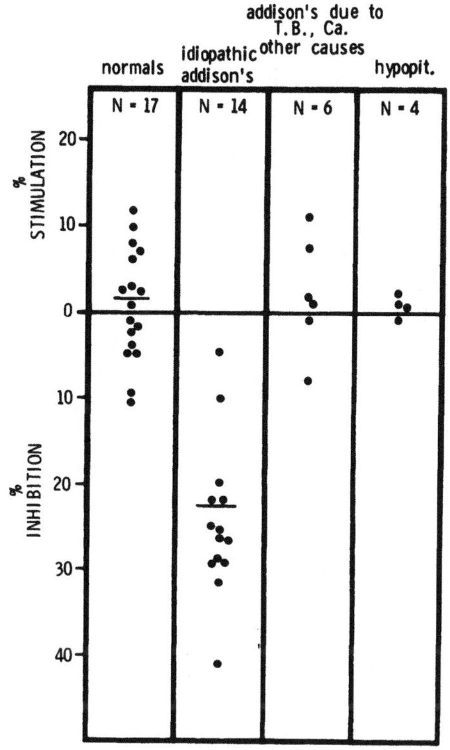

Fig. 5.1. Results of migration inhibition factor test in Addison's disease using crude adrenal homogenate as antigen. In "idiopathic" Addison's disease, there was a highly significant migration inhibition factor test result, using the adrenal antigen, whereas in Addison's disease due to other causes (four due to tuberculosis, two due to secondary carcinoma), the test was negative. Once again this indicates the presence of T-lymphocytes sensitized against the adrenal antigen in "idiopathic" Addison's disease. Other organ antigens employed were kidney and muscle antigens which were non-reactive in these patients. However there is a considerable overlap with other organ-specific auto-immune endocrine diseases, as is discussed in the text. (Volpé 1977)

concern about the participation of antigen-sensitized T-lymphocytes in the immune process in idiopathic Addison's disease (although it seems almost certain that similar results to those already published with the leucocyte migration inhibition test would again be observed using the isolated T-lymphocyte preparations).

Delayed-type hypersensitivity reactions have also been demonstrated in a small series of patients by Nerup et al. (1970). These workers showed that hypersensitivity skin reactions correlate well with the results obtained with the leucocyte migration inhibition test, again consistent with the notion that cell-mediated immunity is indeed involved in this disorder. Attempts to show increased blast transformation by leucocytes in response to adrenal antigen in idiopathic Addison's disease have not been successful, but this has been a notably difficult technique to demonstrate such abnormalities in organ-specific auto-immune disorders (Nerup et al. 1970).

Studies of suppressor T-lymphocyte function have not been carried out extensively. One such study by Verghese et al. (1980), studying general suppressor cell function in patients with Addison's disease combined with other auto-immune disorders (and suggesting a generalized defect in suppressor T-lymphocytes), will be discussed further below in relation to auto-immune polyglandular disease. However, what is required here is the type of study that has been performed in auto-immune thyroid disease by Okita et al. (1981) which will help to determine whether or not there is an antigen-specific defect in suppressor T-lymphocytes responsible for idiopathic Addison's disease. (The author is prejudiced to the view that such a defect will indeed be found.)

5.6 Genetic Aspects of Auto-immune Addison's Disease

5.6.1 HLA Antigens Associated with Addison's Disease

There has been shown to be an increased incidence of HLA-B8 and HLA-Dw3 in Caucasians with auto-immune Addison's disease (Ludwig et al. 1975; Thomsen et al. 1975; Irvine 1978). The relative risk of developing Addison's disease if one has HLA-B8 is 3.7 times the risk within the general population, whereas for HLA-Dw3 the relative risk is 10.5. There has been some controversy as to whether there is any correlation between adrenocortical antibodies in the serum and the presence of HLA-B8. Thomsen et al. (1975) showed a positive correlation, while Irvine (1978) has shown no such correlation. Since the presence of HLA-Dw3 appears to be closer to the putative "disease susceptibility" gene for Addison's disease, studies of HLA-Dw3, in relationship to the presence of adrenal antibodies, the association with other auto-antibodies and auto-immune diseases, and the severity of the disease, will be awaited with anticipation.

5.6.2 Family Studies

It is evident that auto-immune Addison's disease aggregates in families and tends to be familial (Rimoin and Schimke 1971). Auto-immune Addison's disease is seen much more commonly in females than in males, thus differentiating it from tuberculosis of the adrenal glands. Irvine and Barnes (1975 a) have shown that the sex ratio of new patients with auto-immune Addison's disease when occurring alone is equal in the first three decades, and predominantly female thereafter; on the other hand, the sex ratio in patients with auto-immune Addison's disease associated with other organ-specific auto-immune disorders is predominantly female in all decades. Spinner et al. (1968) and Nothiger (1967) have suggested that the inheritance is by an autosomal recessive gene. No familial cases showing an unequivocal X-linked inheritance pattern have been described, and indeed one family with both father and son has been described (Toccafondi and Borghi 1962). In addition, the disorder has also been reported transmitted through an unaffected male (DeCock et al. 1957). Moreover, both two and three generation transmission of Addison's disease has been observed (Bamatter et al. 1966; Nothiger 1967; DeCock et al. 1957; Toccafondi and Borghi 1962; Gambaro 1962). On the basis of these families, an autosomal dominant form of adrenal failure with decreased penetrance was postulated (Bamatter et al. 1966). Rimoin and Schimke (1971) point out that it seems likely that idiopathic adrenal insufficiency can be inherited in at least two (autosomal dominant and recessive) and possibly three (X-linked recessive) ways (Rimoin and Schimke 1971). Indeed, four pairs of identical twins with idiopathic Addison's disease have now been reported. In two of these pairs adrenal antibodies were not looked for, but a diagnosis of auto-immune aetiology was made by exclusion of other causes and by post-mortem evidence of adrenocortical atrophy in one of the patients (Smith et al. 1963; Heggarty 1968). In the other pair, adrenal antibodies were demonstrated in one twin only, but both twins had idiopathic hypoparathyroidism as well (Irvine and Barnes 1975 b). In the final pair of twins, published in 1978 by Simmonds and Lister, identical male twins were described, one of whom presented with clinical symptoms of Addison's disease, while the other was shown to have a deficient adrenocortical response to stimulation tests. Both of these twins were positive for antibodies to adrenocortical antigen (Simmonds and Lister 1978).

Familial idiopathic Addison's disease and hypothyroidism (Schmidt's syndrome) has been reported and thought to be an autosomal recessive character (Frey et al. 1973; Beaven et al. 1959; Carpenter et al. 1964). The incidence of auto-immune disease in first- and second-degree relatives of patients with Addison's disease has been described by Irvine and Barnes (1975 a); about 45% of patients with idiopathic Addison's disease have a history of auto-immune disease in other relatives within the family. These are more than twice as common in first-degree relatives when compared to second-degree relatives. Moreover, of 42 first-degree relatives of patients with idiopathic Addison's disease, three were positive for adrenal antibodies.

The auto-immune diseases discovered in first-degree relatives of patients with Addison's disease have been listed by Irvine and Barnes (1975 a) to include hypothyroidism, thyrotoxicosis, diabetes mellitus, pernicious anaemia, asthma, rheumatoid arthritis, Addison's disease and hypoparathyroidism. Spinner et al. (1968) found that when hypoparathyroidism occurs in association with Addison's disease, a number of disorders, including pernicious anaemia, moniliasis, thyroid disease and diabetes, tend to occur in the family of these patients, in contrast to the situation when hypoparathyroidism occurs without Addison's disease.

A further discussion of the frequent association of idiopathic Addison's disease and other organ-specific auto-immune diseases follows below, and indeed will be discussed again in polyendocrine auto-immune disease at the end of this chapter.

5.7 Other Organ-specific Auto-immune Diseases Associated with Idiopathic Addison's Disease

Irvine and Barnes (1975 a) have summarized the literature and added considerable material of their own emphasizing that patients with idiopathic Addison's disease are remarkably prone to develop a variety of other auto-immune disorders of the organ-specific type. They have compared the incidence of such disorders in patients with idiopathic Addison's disease with those suffering from tuberculous adrenal failure. This comparison makes it clear that the other organ-specific auto-immune diseases occur in association with auto-immune adrenal disease, and not in relation to tuberculous adrenal destruction. These disorders include premature ovarian failure, auto-immune thyroid disease, pernicious anaemia, diabetes mellitus, hypoparathyroidism, alopecia totalis or areata, vitiligo, myaesthenia gravis and others. Similar observations have been made by Doniach and Bottazzo (1981) (see Table 5.2). A discussion of associated disorders follows below.

5.7.1 Thyroid Disease

Carpenter et al. (1964) have reviewed the coexistence of adrenal and thyroid insufficiency, first described by Schmidt (1926) (and termed Schmidt's syndrome). Thyroid auto-antibodies, even in the absence of overt thyroid disease, are very common in patients with idiopathic Addison's disease, occurring in about one-quarter of patients (Irvine and Barnes 1975 a). Moreover, there is a high incidence of

Table 5.2. Associated organ-specific auto-immune diseases in patients with auto-immune adrenalitis (Addison's disease) (Doniach and Bottazzo 1981; Irvine 1977)

Associated disorders	Middlesex Hospital series		Edinburgh series	
	No.	%	No.	%
Primary ovarian failure	25	8	51	18
Thyroid disease	(56)	(19)	(46)	(16)
Primary thyrotoxicosis	20	7	21	7
Primary myxoedema	33	11	20	7
Goitrous AI thyroiditis	3	1	5	2
Insulin-dependent diabetes (type Ib, AI variant)	45	15	27	9
Idiopathic parathyroid deficiency (CE syndrome)	12	4	16	5.5
Pernicious anaemia	7	2	12	4
Positive prolactin-cell antibodies (? subclinical hypophysitis)	(12)	(4)	–[b]	–[b]
Number of patients affected	118[a]	40	106	37
Total number of patients	294		289	

[a] Discrepancy in numbers due to polyendocrine cases
[b] Not tested

subclinical hypothyroidism in Addison's disease (McHardy-Young et al. 1972; Faber et al. 1979; Topliss et al. 1980). McHardy-Young et al. (1972) found increased levels of serum thyrotropin (TSH) in 10 of 13 patients with idiopathic Addison's disease who had thyroid auto-antibodies in their serum and in three of 14 others whose serum was negative for thyroid auto-antibodies. Faber et al. (1979) studied 14 patients with idiopathic Addison's disease in order to detect possible subclinical hypothyroidism. All 14 were clinically euthyroid and serum thyroxine and serum total tri-iodothyronine values were within normal limits. However, 11 of the 14 had circulating thyroid antimicrosomal antibody in their blood. Moreover, the mean basal serum TSH was significantly higher than in a control group, although only three patients had values above the upper limit of the normal range. The prevalence of thyroid microsomal antibodies found in sera from patients with idiopathic Addison's disease and without overt thyroid disease has been found to be between 20% and 79% (Faber et al. 1979).

Topliss et al. (1980) have studied the significance of thyrotropin excess in untreated primary adrenal insufficiency. They measured the level of circulating thyroid hormones and TSH before and after steroid replacement in 10 consecutive patients with non-tuberculous primary adrenal insufficiency in order to study the numerous interactions between corticosteroids and thyroid function tests. Although none had clinical features of thyroid disease, six showed increased levels of plasma TSH before treatment in association with a wide range of circulating thyroid hormone levels. In one patient with positive thyroid auto-antibodies, biochemical features of primary hypothyroidism resolved after steroid replacement, although TSH excess persisted. In five patients, two of whom had adrenal insufficiency due to metastatic carcinoma, TSH decreased to normal after steroid replacement; in one of these the TSH decrease occurred without a change in normal circulating thyroid hormone levels, consistent with a direct influence of glucocorticoids on TSH release.

It thus may be seen that glucocorticoid deficiency may unmask occult thyroid auto-immune disease, which reverts to the occult stage even with physiological doses of replacement corticosteroid therapy. Thus thyroid function can return towards normal after such replacement. Alternatively, TSH may be released (and thus increased) as a direct result of steroid deficiency, without thyroid malfunction. Hence, when TSH is assessed in adrenal insuficiency, a distinction must be made between values obtained before and after adrenocortical replacement. Gharib et al. (1972) and Schwartz (1973) have also described similar patients in whom reduced thyroid function returned to normal following physiological replacement doses of corticosteroids.

The current prevalence of thyrotoxicosis (Graves' disease) in idiopathic Addison's disease is about 9%, whereas for tuberculous Addison's disease it has been reported to be 2% (Irvine and Barnes 1975 a). The former incidence is much greater than in the general population, where the incidence of thyrotoxicosis has been reported to be approximately 1% (Tunbridge 1979). In addition, Irvine and Barnes (1975 a) have estimated the prevalence of auto-immune thyroiditis (either Hashimoto's disease or myxoedema) in idiopathic Addison's disease to be about 9%, as opposed to about 1%—3% in the population (Tunbridge 1979).

5.7.2 Ovarian Failure

Approximately 25% of women with idiopathic Addison's disease will be found to have premature menopause or amenorrhoea (Turkington and Lebovitz 1967; Irvine and Barnes 1975 a). Anderson et al. (1968) detected antibodies against components of ovaries and testis, as well as placental trophoblasts and adrenal cortex, in two male patients with idiopathic Addison's disease, but no overt evidence of gonadal insufficiency. Irvine and Barnes (1975 a) have noted that steroid-secreting cell antibodies are commonly found in the serum of patients with idiopathic Addison's disease, once again even without any overt evidence of gonadal failure (see Table 5.1). On the other hand, as mentioned above, amenorrhoea or oligomenorrhoea does occur in as many as 30% of patients with idiopathic Addison's disease, and the majority of these have circulating antibodies against steroid-secreting cells in their serum (Irvine and Barnes 1975 a). In fact, if patients have *primary* amenorrhoea associated with idiopathic Addison's disease, then virtually all such patients will be found to have circulating steroid-secreting cell antibodies. However, it should be emphasized that such antibodies are *not* detectable in patients with amenorrhoea *not* associated with Addison's disease. Irvine and Barnes (1975 a) have also grappled with the significance of antibodies to the gonads in Addison's disease under these circumstances, and more importantly, how destruction of the gonads is brought about. The question arises as to whether auto-immune ovarian or testicular failure is a closely associated, but separate, organ-specific auto-immune disease, or whether it represents and is a result of cross-reactivity by antibodies primarily reacting against adrenal constituents. The evidence would suggest that steroid cell antibodies are not organ-specific but cross-reactive, with specific antigens shared between the adrenal cortex and some of the steroid-producing cells in the gonads and the placenta. This would then explain the finding of antibodies against ovarian constituents in some male patients with auto-immune adrenal failure. Thus, most patients with idiopathic Addison's disease make antibodies directed against the adrenal cortex, while a few patients develop similar antibodies that also cross-react with other steroid-producing cells in such organs as the gonads and placenta.

The finding of auto-antibodies against the ovaries in the absence of overt ovarian disease might be explained on the basis of at least two different antibody populations (McNatty et al. 1975). These workers have shown that some sera containing anti-ovarian antibodies produce complement-dependent cytotoxic changes in cultured granulosa cells, together with a fall in progesterone production. On the other hand, some patients with Addison's disease and ovarian antibodies are known to have normal menstrual function (Murthy et al. 1976). These discrepancies may be the result of different antibody populations, since sera positive in the cytotoxicity assay produce a clumped staining pattern on immunofluorescence, whereas sera causing a confluent staining immunofluorescent pattern produce no cytotoxic changes (McNatty et al. 1975).

In any event, it would appear that the cross-reactivity between ovarian and adrenal antigens is not confined only to the humoral arm of the immune response. Our own group (Edmonds et al. 1973) have described a young woman of 18 years with auto-immune adrenalitis, oophoritis and thyroiditis, with premature menopause. Her menses had ceased at about age 16. In this patient, antithyroid and anti-adrenal antibodies were detectable, but antibodies to the testis and ovary were not demonstrable. On the other hand, however, the leucocyte migration inhibition test was positive in response to thyroid, adrenal, testicular and ovarian antigens, but not to other organ-specific antigens (Fig. 5.2).

This may well not be surprising, since it might be expected that cross-reactivity depends on the presence of cross-reactive sensitized T-lymphocytes, just as much as on auto-antibodies which are likewise cross-reactive. Tissue damage might well be antibody-mediated, by means of the formation of immune complexes and "killer" cells (Pozzilli et al. 1979, 1980), but T-lymphocytes may also exert a cytotoxic role (see Chap. 1).

Histological features of the ovaries of patients with amenorrhoea (either primary or secondary) associated with auto-immune Addison's disease show only fibrous tissue, or lymphocytic infiltration, similar to that seen in thyroid auto-immune disease (Irvine and Barnes 1975 a).

In the *absence* of idiopathic Addison's disease, it would appear that premature menopause is only rarely due to auto-immune processes. On the other hand, when present with auto-immune Addison's disease, it may well be due to cross-reactivity of sensitized T-lymphocytes and auto-antibodies which are primarily reactive against the adrenal cortex. Thus, it is not yet clear whether premature ovarian failure as a result of auto-immune processes ever occurs alone, or if it does so, it may well be quite rare (Gottesman et al. 1980).

Of interest, Doniach and Bottazzo (1981) have found that steroid cell antibodies are present in almost all cases where idiopathic hypoparathyroidism is associated with Addison's disease, as well as in all patients with gonadal atrophy complicating auto-immune adrenalitis. However, Doniach and Bottazzo point out that these antibodies may be present several years before the onset of clinical symptoms, and may vary *independently* of adrenal antibodies. This statement thus suggests that

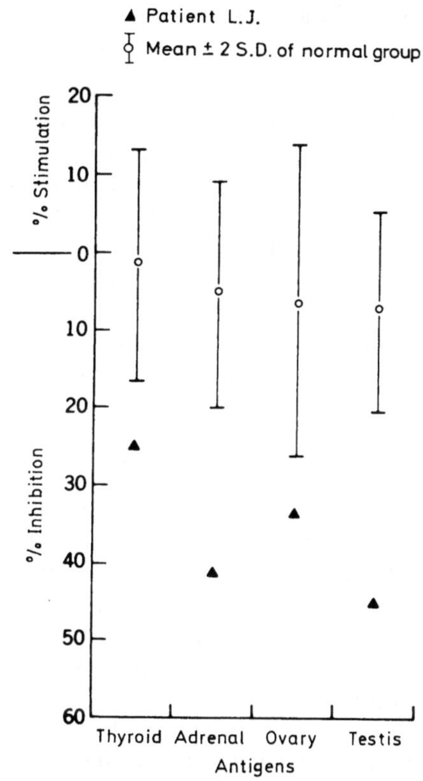

Fig. 5.2. Migration inhibition factor test against thyroid, adrenal, ovarian and testicular antigen in a patient who suffered auto-immune thyroiditis, adrenalitis (with Addison's disease), and oophoritis (with premature menopause), all occurring before the age of 20. The patient's results are depicted by triangles, with the normal ranges vertically above these. The patient's leucocytes produced migration inhibition factor in response to thyroid, adrenal, ovarian, and testicular antigen, but not against other organ antigens tested. There was a very poor correlation between the presence of migration inhibition factor and humoral antibodies in this patient. (Edmonds et al. 1973)

cross-reactivity may not be the sole reason for auto-immune gonadal failure, and that at least occasional cases of the latter condition may occur independently of auto-immune adrenal failure. Ruehsen et al. (1972) have additionally pointed out that women with menstrual irregularities or amenorrhoea together with auto-immune disorders *other* than Addison's disease or hypoparathyroidism occasionally show immunofluorescent anti-ovarian antibodies, although (as stated above) this is much less common than the incidence observed when Addison's disease is present.

5.7.3 Auto-immune Testicular Failure

Auto-immune testicular failure associated with Addison's disease is quite uncommon. In the series of Irvine and Barnes (1975 a), only 3 of 79 male patients with idiopathic Addison's disease had antibodies in the serum reactive with interstitial (Leydig) cells within the testis. Only one of these three males actually showed clinical hypogonadism. In our own experience, we have observed only two males with auto-immune orchitis and hypogonadism; these patients both had not only Addison's disease, but also manifested hypoparathyroidism, alopecia and candidiasis (polyendocrine auto-immune failure). This will be discussed further below.

5.7.4 Pernicious Anaemia

There is a marked increased incidence of antibodies to gastric parietal cells and intrinsic factor in the sera of patients with idiopathic Addison's disease. In the series of Irvine and Barnes (1975 a), of 246 patients with idiopathic Addison's disease, 21 were positive for anti-intrinsic factor antibodies. Moreover, approximately 15 cases of pernicious anaemia have now been reported occurring in close association with idiopathic Addison's disease (Whittingham 1974; Irvine and Barnes 1975 a, b; Doniach and Bottazzo 1981). Either disorder occurred before the other with equal frequency. It is therefore clear that there is a markedly increased incidence of overt pernicious anaemia and/or of antibodies to gastric antigens in patients with auto-immune Addison's disease (Doniach and Bottazzo 1981), when compared to the general population (see Table 5.1).

5.7.5 Diabetes Mellitus Associated with Addison's Disease

Ogle (1886) was the first to describe coexisting adrenal insufficiency and diabetes mellitus. It is now very clear that these two disorders have a true association (Nerup 1974 a, b; Irvine and Barnes 1975 a, b; Doniach and Bottazzo 1981). The incidence of diabetes mellitus in Addison's disease is reported as high as between 8% and 23%, with an approximate average of 18% (Irvine and Barnes 1975 a). This may be compared with the prevalence of diabetes in the general population which is approximately 1%–1.3% (Knowles 1960). It is evident that the type of diabetes found in association with idiopathic Addison's disease is the insulin-dependent variety and it has been determined that it is the HLA-Dw3 group of diabetics which is associated with Addison's disease and the other organ-specific auto-immune diseases (see Chap. 3).

5.7.6 Hypoparathyroidism

Hypoparathyroidism occurs mostly in children and adolescents, is equally prevalent in the two sexes, and is often associated with mucocutaneous candidiasis (Doniach and Bottazzo 1981). When present, it is frequently associated with auto-immune Addison's disease. Thus, in children with hypoparathyroidism it is very common to have associated auto-immune Addison's disease, occurring at an age which is otherwise unusually early. Irvine and Barnes (1975 a) point out that the mean age at the time of diagnosis of Addison's disease in patients who have subsequently developed hypoparathyroidism is 12 years, in contrast to 32 years for patients with diabetes mellitus, 41 years for patients with thyroid disease, and 41 years for patients with pernicious anaemia. Moreover, in many instances, there is associated hypogonadism, which becomes manifest after puberty. Diabetes mellitus, alopecia and vitiligo, chronic active liver disease and episodes of intestinal malabsorption or coeliac syndrome are occasional accompaniments (Doniach and Bottazzo 1981). These authors point out that this combination is frequently familial.

The histology of idiopathic hypoparathyroidism is characterized by lymphocytic infiltration and atrophy, indicative of an auto-immune process (Irvine and Barnes 1975 a, b). Moreover, Blizzard et al. (1966) and Irvine and Scarth (1969) have demonstrated the presence of antiparathyroid antibodies in such patients. Indeed,

Blizzard et al. (1966) have found such antibodies by the immunofluorescent technique in about 40% of patients with idiopathic hypoparathyroidism, 26% of patients with idiopathic Addison's disease, and in 12% of patients with Hashimoto's thyroiditis. However, this group also found positive antiparathyroid antibodies in 6% of normal control persons. Cell-mediated immunity has been demonstrated by Moulias et al. (1971) by the leucocyte migration inhibition test in seven of ten cases of idiopathic hypoparathyroidism.

Experimental auto-immune parathyroiditis has been induced in rats and dogs (Lupulescu et al. 1965, 1968). In these studies, the disorder was manifested by histological, serological and metabolic abnormalities. Complement-fixing antibodies to homologous parathyroid antigens were demonstrable in low titres in the dog but not in the rat sera. Experimental parathyroiditis has also been demonstrated by the passive transfer of antiparathyroid antibody in rats (Altenahr and Jenke 1974).

Hypoparathyroidism in the human, when associated with other organ-specific auto-immune diseases, will be discussed further below (see Sect. 5.8).

5.8 Polyendocrine Auto-immune Disease

From the preceding chapters, as well as the material described above with respect to auto-immune adrenal disease and its relationship to other organ-specific auto-immune diseases, it is evident that several of the endocrine glands can become affected during the course of a patient's life, often accompanied by typical lymphoid infiltration and subsequent replacement by fibrous tissue (Doniach and Bottazzo 1981). The thyroid gland is by far the most common endocrine organ involved in auto-immunity and the four syndromes, i.e. Graves' disease with its variants; endocrine exophthalmos (which is considered as a separate, overlapping, organ-specific auto-immune process) (see Chap. 2); primary myxoedema; and goitrous thyroiditis, may all be implicated in polyendocrine auto-immune disorders. While it is true that the above conditions occur more often as single disorders in a given patient, the same patient may alternate between the above four conditions during the course of a lifetime. Moreover, in a minority of patients with auto-immune thyroid disease, there will occur other organ-specific auto-immune disorders, as have been listed in Chap. 2. Another interesting aspect relates to the distinction between those patients that have overt auto-immune organ-specific disease and those in whom the expression is occult (i.e. the presence of auto-antibodies alone). The possible subtle genetic, immunological and environmental variations which lie behind these distinctions remain to be determined. The antibody markers for these disorders are listed on Table 5.3.

5.8.1 Relative Incidence of Auto-immune Disease

Another interesting question relates to the relative incidence of certain auto-immune diseases, either within the general population as single disorders, or in combination with one another. It is clear that auto-immune thyroid disease and type Irl (Ib) diabetes are common, and certainly thyroid disease and auto-antibodies are very common amongst the older population (see Chaps. 2, 3). On the other hand,

Table 5.3. Circulating auto-antibody markers in polyendocrine syndromes (Doniach and Bottazzo 1981)

Disease	Antibody markers to	Frequency in normal populations
Primary thyrotoxicosis	TSH receptors	nyd[a]
Primary myxoedema	Thyroid microsome	F > M; 0%–20% according to sex and age[b]
Hashimoto goitre	Thyroglobulin	F > M; 0%–20% according to sex and age
Endocrine exophthalmos	Extraocular muscle (immune complexes)	nyd
	Retro-orbital tissue (ophthalmic Ig, OIg)	
Pernicious anaemia	Intrinsic factor	0.1%
	Gastric parietal cell	F > M; 0%–16% according to sex and age
Fundal (type A) gastritis	Gastric parietal cell	F > M; 0%–16% according to sex and age
Antral (type B) gastritis	Gastrin cell	< 0.1%
Addison's disease	Adrenal cortex	< 0.1%
Premature menopause	Adrenal cortex	< 0.1%
with adrenalitis	Steroid cells, gonadal and placental	< 0.01%
Primary gonadal deficiency	Sperm and ovum	7%
Diabetes mellitus	Pancreatic islet-cells	0.5%
(type I a and b)	Pancreatic glucagon-cell	0.2%
	Pancreatic somatostatin cell	0.5%
Partial pituitary deficiency	Prolactin cell	< 0.1%
	Growth hormone cell	< 0.01%
Idiopathic hypoparathyroiditis	Parathyroid chief cell	nyd
Vitiligo	Melanocyte	nyd
Myaesthenia gravis	Acetylcholine receptors	< 1%
Auto-immune liver disorders		
Chronic active liver disease		< 1%
Lupoid variant	Nuclei (mostly diffuse)	F > M; 0%–20% according to sex and age
	Smooth muscle (mostly actin)	12%
Liver and kidney microsome variant	Liver and kidney microsome	0.3%
Cholestatic variant	Mitochondria	0.4%–0.7%
Primary biliary cirrhosis	Mitochondrial inner membrane	0.4%–0.7%

[a] nyd, not yet determined
[b] F, females; M, males

auto-immune Addison's disease and auto-immune idiopathic hypoparathyroidism are rare. Indeed, when one finds an increased incidence of other antibodies and auto-immune diseases amongst those afflicted with auto-immune thyroid disease or auto-immune diabetes mellitus, the incidence of Addison's disease and hypoparathyroidism remains very *uncommon* even in such patients (Irvine and Barnes 1975 a, b; Doniach and Bottazzo 1981). Conversely, however, in patients with either overt idiopathic Addison's disease or in patients who make auto-antibodies to the adrenal cortex without manifesting clinical Addison's disease, there is a *very high* chance of such patients also making antibodies to the thyroid, gastric parietal cells, intrinsic factor, parathyroid, as well as other steroid-producing cells (Irvine and Barnes 1975 a, b; Doniach and Bottazzo 1981). Similarly, in patients with idiopathic hypoparathyroidism, there is a very high incidence of anti-adrenal antibodies, as well as the other organ-specific antibodies noted above; moreover, in both idiopathic Addison's disease and hypoparathyroidism there is a high incidence of other overt auto-immune disorders, much greater than that seen in auto-immune thyroid disease or diabetes mellitus.

5.8.2 Mechanism of Cellular Destruction

The mechanism of cellular destruction has not been thoroughly studied in patients with polyglandular auto-immune disease. However, Pozzilli et al. (1979) did study the proportion of blood mononuclear cells forming low affinity rosettes with sheep's erythrocytes ("killer" or K cells) in patients with type I diabetes and coexistent auto-immune thyroid disease, a form of polyendocrine auto-immune failure. In 10 (45%) of 22 patients of this type there was a raised proportion of K cells, which was not related to the duration of the diabetes or the presence of islet cell antibodies. Thus it may be that the means of cellular destruction in these disorders could relate to "killer" cell activity and thus this circumstantial evidence supports the involvement of cell-mediated cytotoxicity in organ-specific auto-immune endocrinopathies. In a further study of 44 patients affected by polyendocrine auto-immune endocrinopathies (Pozzilli et al. 1980), once again, there was a high proportion of "killer" cells, as well as a positive correlation between antibody-dependent cytotoxicity and the level of "killer" cells. In addition, there appeared to be a relationship between the increase of "killer" cells and the appearance of the last endocrinopathy. These data suggested that abnormal "killer" cell function is pathogenetically involved in auto-immune endocrinopathies. It was also concluded that the measurement of "killer" cells and antibody-dependent cytotoxicity might be useful markers of active tissue damage in patients affected by polyendocrine auto-immune disease (Pozzilli et al. 1980).

5.8.3 Association with Various Non-Endocrine Auto-immune Disorders

It should also be emphasized that while there seems to be a propensity for the endocrine glands to be involved with these auto-immune processes, a number of non-endocrine organ-specific auto-immune diseases are also similarly associated.

Vitiligo, for example, is found in 0.7% of the population; these patient have a higher prevalence of organ-specific auto-antibodies than would be anticipated in the general population (Brostoff et al. 1969). Conversely, the frequency of vitiligo is 10–20 times greater in patients with polyendocrine syndromes that in the general population; this vitiligo may precede or postdate the onset of the endocrine disorder.

Pernicious anaemia, another organ-specific auto-immune disease, is also found commonly in association with auto-immune endocrinopathies. Ten per cent of patients with pernicious anaemia give a history of thyroid diseases, and conversely pernicious anaemia is five-eight times more common in thyroid patients than would be expected by chance (Doniach and Roitt 1964; Doniach et al. 1965 a). It is also more common than expected in diabetes (see Chap. 3) and in Addison's disease (see above).

Myaesthenia gravis, still another organ-specific auto-immune disease is found much more frequently in association with auto-immune endocrinopathies (Doniach et al. 1972; Bundey et al. 1972; Bosch et al. 1977). Other non-endocrine auto-immune diseases commonly associated with the auto-immune endocrinopathies include Sjögren's syndrome and chronic active hepatitis (Doniach and Bottazzo 1981). Even less well characterized disorders such as alopecia totalis and alopecia areata are commonly associated with those patients who have severe multiple endocrine auto-immune disorders, usually in association with auto-immune gonadal failure, hypoparathyroidism, Addison's disease and candidiasis (Arulanantham et al. 1979).

Doniach and Bottazzo (1981) have noted that there is an overlap between the polyendocrine auto-immune diseases and the "collagen disorders", which is quite striking in some families and has been reported many times especially in children. Rheumatoid arthritis is seen quite often in patients with Graves' and Hashimoto's diseases, and also in the relatives of polyendocrine patients. In classical systemic lupus erythematosus, there is no increased incidence of organ-specific antibodies, but conversely patients with endocrine or polyendocrine auto-immune disorders have antinuclear antibodies with some frequency. In children with auto-immune thyroiditis, 30% were positive for antinuclear antibodies, and two of 64 patients actually developed a lupus-like syndrome (Doniach et al. 1965 b). Moreover, drug sensitivities, food allergies, gluten hypersensitivity and coeliac syndrome have already been mentioned in relation to severe polyendocrine auto-immune disease (Cooper et al. 1978; Walsh et al. 1978). Chronic active hepatitis has also been found not infrequently in association with polyendocrine auto-immune disease (Kunin et al. 1963). Nearly half of the sera from such patients contains thyroid or gastric antibodies, and there is an increased incidence of auto-immune thyroid disease and diabetes mellitus associated with this condition (Galbraith and Fudenberg 1977).

5.8.4 Defect in Immunoregulation

It is clear that the occurrence of auto-immunity in idiopathic Addison's disease is not related to adrenal insufficiency *per se*, as it has not been noticed in tuberculous Addison's disease (Irvine and Barnes 1975 a). Moreover, candidiasis is commonly associated with those patients who have polyendocrine auto-immune failure, including parathyroid and adrenal failure, whereas it is not seen with auto-immune thyroid disease alone, or in those without Addison's disease or hypoparathyroidism.

Thus it would appear that the immune abnormality responsible for causing idiopathic Addison's disease and idiopathic hypoparathyroidism must be much more profound, albeit much more rare, than that which brings about auto-immune thyroid disease or diabetes mellitus. For some reason, at present unknown, if one has the propensity for developing auto-immune parathyroid or adrenal disease, then it is likely that one has a much more severe defect in immune control or regulation than that seen with the more common auto-immune disorders, such as thyroid disease or diabetes. The precise mechanism by which these differences occur is unknown. However, Verghese et al. (1980) have shown that in polyglandular auto-immune failure there is evidence of depressed skin test reactivity and depressed anti-Coxsackie viral titres. They have also evaluated the concanavalin A induced suppressor cell function of lymphocytes from eight unrelated patients with polyglandular auto-immune disease, and screened their sera for antibodies to human lymphocyte cell lines. Characteristic abnormalities of suppressor cell function were found in two patients. Lymphocytes from one patient on repeated testing with multiple stimulator and suppressor cell combinations failed to suppress either autologous or heterologous lymphocytes (mixed lymphocyte culture assay). Lymphocytes from another patient on repeated testing were capable of suppressing cells from unrelated donors but were unable to suppress her own lymphocytes. In contrast, lymphocytes from the remaining six patients and all controls exhibited significant suppressor cell function. However, quantitatively, polyglandular failure patients had decreased suppressor activity; 67% of normal for autologous suppression ($p < 0.05$), and 35 % of normal for heterologous suppression ($p < 0.01$). Serum from these patients bound more antibody to a human lymphocyte line than serum from control patients. The abnormalities of the suppressor cell function did not, however, correlate with antilymphocyte antibodies. The authors proposed the hypothesis that the phenotypic expression of several immunological lesions can result in polyglandular auto-immune failure.

However, it is not clear from this study that there was indeed generalized suppressor T cell deficiency. It seems equally possible that there are inherited multiple defects (each one antigen-specific) in suppressor T-lymphocytes, but this does not necessarily denote a generalized suppressor T cell deficiency state. Thus it would be more appropriate to study antigen-specific T-lymphocyte suppressor abnormalities which is now possible to do (see Chap. 2). Such studies should soon be forthcoming. It is quite possible, however, that those patients with polyendocrine auto-immune failure *associated with mucocutaneous candidiasis* may have a more profound and even generalized defect in immunoregulation (Arulanantham et al. 1979; Vladimarsson et al. 1973). However, there is preliminary evidence suggesting that this particular category of patients is *not* related to HLA-B8-DW3, and thus may represent a different genetic and pathogenetic mechanism than may be operative in those without candidiasis (Arulanantham et al. 1979; Neufeld et al. 1980). Similarly, those multi-system immunologically mediated diseases, such as systemic lupus erythematosus, polymyositis and sarcoidosis, in which a generalized T-lymphocyte deficiency has been demonstrated, may be associated with auto-immune endocrine disease (Wall et al. 1978). However, such cases do not constitute a model for auto-immune endocrine disease generally.

Farid et al. (1980) studied several categories of patients with polyendocrine auto-immune disease (without candidiasis) and found that most were positive for HLA-DRw3. However, they found that the disease susceptibilities for polyendocrine glandular auto-immune disease occurred in the same haploptype in the same families, but in different haplotypes between families. They concluded that separate HLA associated genes code for different auto-immune endocrine diseases, and that these genes may be carried on the same haplotype, which may not necessarily be B8 or DRw3 positive. These observations were similar to those of Eisenbarth et al. (1978, 1979) who found the overt disorders occurred in members of the families who shared more haplotypes with the propositus, when compared to those who manifested antibodies only.

Since there appear to be many different antigens involved in the various organ-specific auto-immune diseases, only some of which are related to the endocrine system, it may be suggested that the basic immunological disorder does not depend on close antigenic relationships. Rather one could speculate that the defects are in closely related immunoregulatory mechanisms, probably suppressor T-lymphocytes, controlled by specific genes. Thus there appears to be a close genetic relationship of different clones of suppressor T-lymphocytes, each of which would react with particular self-directed helper T-lymphocyte surface antigens; when there is an abnormality in two or more of these closely related clones of suppressor T-lymphocytes, then this family of associated organ-specific auto-immune disorders results, rather than because of any particular antigenic similarity. The interrelationships between the various disorders may be schematically represented as on Fig. 5.3 (Moulias et al. 1974). Of course, other immunoregulatory mechanisms could also be playing a role, e. g. anti-idiotypic antibodies (Wigzell et al. 1978). It thus may further be suggested that the gene responsible for each of the specific disorders is actually separate in some of the patients with polyendocrine auto-immune failure, however closely such genes may lie to one another in linkage disequilibrium with HLA-DRw3. In others, not necessarily related to the same HLA antigen, the immunoregulatory defect may be a diffuse one, as seems possible in those cases associated with candidiasis. It remains to be explained, however, why thyroid auto-immune disease is common, whereas idiopathic Addison's disease is rare; conversely when one has thyroid auto-immune disease, it is much less common to have multiple endocrine deficiencies, when compared once again to the reverse situation in idiopathic Addison's disease where such multiple associated immune disorders are common.

There is indeed some evidence that for each organ-specific disorder there is one specific genetic abnormality. It has been possible to show evidence to support the view that the genetic tendency to insulin-dependent diabetes is separate from that which leads to auto-immune thyroid disease (Gorsuch et al. 1980). Moreover, pernicious anaemia appears to have different genetic implications when it occurs on

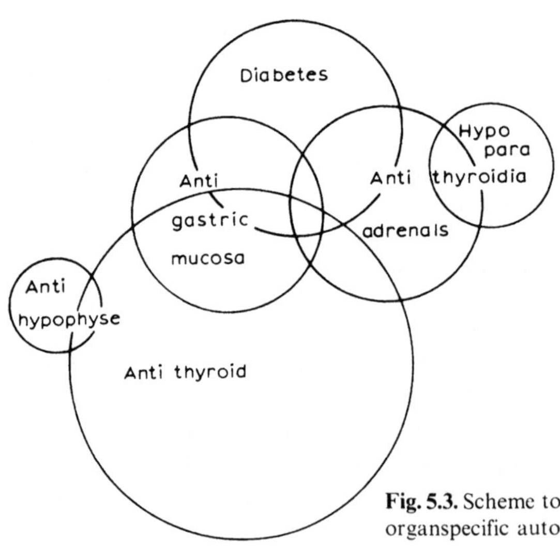

Fig. 5.3. Scheme to show interrelationships between the various organspecific auto-immune disorders. (Moulias et al. 1974)

Table 5.4. Classification of polyglandular auto-immune disease (Neufeld and Blizzard 1980)

I.	Candidiasis, hypoparathyroidism, Addison's disease (two or three present)
II.	Addison's disease and thyroid auto-immune disease and/or insulin-dependent diabetes mellitus
III. A.	Thyroid auto-immune disease and insulin-dependent diabetes mellitus
B.	Thyroid auto-immune disease and pernicious anaemia
C.	Thyroid auto-immune disease and vitiligo and/or alopecia and/or other organ-specific auto-immune diseases not falling into above categories

its own than when it is associated with type I diabetes, or with adrenal insufficiency (Ungar et al. 1977). Indeed, it seems evident that relatives of patients with Hashimoto's thyroiditis will tend to have thyroid disorders most commonly, whereas the relatives of patients suffering from pernicious anaemia are more likely to have auto-antibodies against gastric antigens or overt pernicious anaemia itself.

Moreover, Doniach and Bottazzo (1981) have pointed out that preliminary follow-up studies in polyendocrine cases suggest that the presence of unusual organ antibodies, such as islet cell antibodies or adrenal antibodies in patients without overt Addison's disease or diabetes respectively are nevertheless often predictive of subsequent clinical disease. This is however in contrast to observations based on thyroid or gastric antibodies in population studies which suggest that only about 10% of serologically positive persons will ultimately develop clinical symptoms (Gordin and Lamberg 1975).

Neufeld and Blizzard (1980) have advanced a new classification of auto-immune endocrine diseases based upon the clinically expressed endocrine diseases in the patients and their relatives (Table 5.4). These suggested subdivions may provide impetus for determining possible genetic differences between the various categories proposed by these workers. The application of currently available and soon-to-be forthcoming techniques for studying immunogenetics and lymphocyte functions should shed considerable light on these remarkable clinical entities.

5.9 Other Possible Auto-immune Endocrinopathies

Immunofluorescent antibodies have been discovered against endocrine cells of the gastro-intestinal tract, producing secretin, and gastric inhibitory peptide (Doniach and Bottazzo 1981). Moreover, antibodies have been found by Bottazzo and Lendrum (1976) against human pancreatic glucagon and somatostatin cells of the islets of Langerhans. Likewise, antibodies to mast cells have now been described (Rizzetto and Doniach 1973). The precise significance of these findings has yet to be determined.

5.10 Summary

While there are several causes of adrenal insufficiency, the most common cause in Europe and North America now is idiopathic Addison's disease, which is now etablished as an auto-immune disorder. The evidence for this statement rests upon many lines of investigation, including the histology of the condition, the finding of auto-antibodies and cell-mediated immunity against the adrenal cortex in many patients with this condition, the association of other organ-specific auto-immune diseases, experimental observations, and studies of the HLA antigens and the genetics of the disorder. Histologically, the condition is characterized by mononuclear cell infiltrations, with lymphocytes, plasma cells, macrophages and occasionally germinal centres. Anti-adrenal antibodies can be demonstrated in about two-thirds of patients with auto-immune Addison's disease. In addition, other organ-specific auto-antibodies are found quite frequently. Evidence of cell-mediated immunity has also been demonstrated against adrenal antigen in this disorder, utilizing the leucocyte migration inhibition test, signifying sensitization of T-lymphocytes against adrenal antigen.

An increased incidence of HLA-B8 and HLA-Dw3 has been demonstrated in Caucasians with auto-immune Addison's disease. Family studies have indicated that this disorder tends to aggregate in families, and may occur in identical twins. There is evidence that this condition can be inherited in at least two (autosomal dominant and recessive) and possibly three (X-linked recessive) ways. Moreover, there is a markedly increased incidence of auto-immune diseases in first- and second-degree relatives of patients with auto-immune Addison's disease. These include premature ovarian failure due to auto-immune oophoritis, auto-immune thyroid disease, pernicious anaemia, diabetes mellitus, hypoparathyroidism, alopecia totalis or areata, vitiligo, myaesthenia gravis and others.

It is not clear whether auto-immune oophoritis ever occurs on its own. There has been a suggestion that auto-immune oophoritis occurs as result of cross-reacting cell mediated and humoral immunity, with the prime reaction against steroid-producing cells in the adrenal gland, but cross-reacting with other steroid-producing cells elsewhere, wherever they may be. This of course could not account for the association of one organ-specific auto-immune disorder with those organ-specific auto-immune diseases in which the antigens are clearly separate, such as pernicious anaemia, myaesthenia gravis and others.

It is curious that the incidence of the other organ-specific auto-immune diseases is much higher in patients with auto-immune adrenalitis than it is in relation to auto-immune thyroid disease; conversely, auto-immune thyroid disease is much more common in the general population. It would therefore appear that the disorder in immunoregulation responsible for Addison's disease is much more uncommon, but much more profound, and much more likely to be associated with other similar defects in immunoregulation. This particularly appears to be the case when Addison's disease is associated with hypoparathyroidism and mucocutaneous candidiasis.

There is evidence that there may be a generalized defect in suppressor T-lymphocytes in patients with polyglandular auto-immune failure. The author would speculate that it is at least equally likely that there are multiple inherited defects in suppressor T-lymphocytes, but not necessarily a generalized suppressor T cell deficiency state. The exception to this suggestion is likely to be those cases with mococutaneous candidiasis, since there is some preliminary evidence that this particular category may be genetically dissimilar to those who do not have this mucocutaneous complication. The means of cellular destruction may be via antibody-dependent "killer" cell activity. Investigators are now finding auto-antibodies to various endocrine secretory cells of the gastro-intestinal tract and to such hormone-producing cells as pancreatic glucagon and somatostatin cells. Whether antibodies related to these particular cells have pathophysiological consequences remains to be determined, and thus the pathophysiological significance of these antibodies is not yet known. However, it is clear that in many of the other disorders listed above, such as auto-immune thyroiditis, hypoparathyroidism, adrenalitis, diabetes mellitus and others, antibodies may appear years before there are any overt manifestations of the appropriate disorder. Such antibodies, therefore, may represent occult forms of the appropriate diseases. While it is known, for example, that only 10 % of asymptomatic persons with auto-antibodies to the thyroid actually develop overt auto-immune thyroid disease, nevertheless it is also known that the presence of thyroid auto-antibodies in asymptomatic people has a close relationship to the actual presence of lymphocytic infiltration within the thyroid gland. Thus the presence of antibodies even in the absence of overt disease may well have pathological significance, and may have some predictive and prognostic value.

5.11 References

Addison T (1868) On the constitutional and local effects of disease of the suprarenal capsules. In: Wilk S, Daldy Th (eds) A collection of the published writings of the late Thomas Addison, M.D., physican to Guy's hospital, London. New Sydenham Society, pp 209–239

Altenahr E, Jenke W (1974) Experimental parathyroiditis in the rat by passive immunization. Virchows Arch [Pathol Anat] 363:333–342

Anderson JR, Goudie RB, Gray KG, Timbury GC (1957) Auto antibodies in Addison's disease. Lancet 1:1123–1124

Anderson JR, Goudie RB, Gray KG, Stuart-Smith DA (1968) Immunological features of idiopathic Addison's disease: an antibody to cells producing steroid hormones. Clin Exp Immunol 3:107–117

Andrada JA, Skelton FR, Andrada EC, Milgrom F, Witebsky E (1968) Experimental autoimmune adrenalitis in rats. Lab Invest 19:460–465

Andrada JA, Murray FT, Andrada EC, Ezrin C (1979) Cushing's syndrome and autoimmunity. Arch Pathol Lab Med 103:244–246

Arulanantham K, Dwyer JM, Genel M (1979) Evidence for defective immunoregulation in the syndrome of familial candidiasis endocrinopathy. N Engl J Med 300:164–168

Bammater F, Koegel R, DeHaller J, Muller AF (1966) Maladie d'Addison familiale. Helv Paediatr Acta 21:109–152

Barnett EV, Dumonde EDC, Glynn LE (1963) Induction of autoimmunity to adrenal gland. Immunology 6:382–402

Beaven DW, Nelson DH, Renold AE, Thorn GW (1959) Diabetes mellitus and Addison's disease: a report on eight patients and a review of 55 cases in the literature. N Engl J Med 261:443–354

Blizzard RM, Chee D, Davis W (1966) The incidence of parathyroid and other antibodies in the sera of patients with idiopathic hypoparathyroidism. Clin Exp Immunol 1:119–128

Bosch EP, Reith PE, Granner DK (1977) Myasthenia gravis and Schmidt syndrome. Neurology (Minneap) 27:1179–1180

Bottazzo GD, Lendrum R (1976) Separate autoantibodies to human pancreatic glucagon and somatostatin cells. Lancet 2:873–876

Brostoff J, Bor S, Feiwel M (1969) Autoantibodies in patients with vitiligo. Lancet 2:177–178

Bundey S, Doniach D, Soothill JF (1972) Immunological studies in patients with juvenile onset myasthenia gravis and in their relatives. Clin Exp Immunol 11:321–332

Carpenter CCJ, Solomon N, Silverberg SG, Bledsoe T, Northcutt RC, Klinenberg JR, Bennett IL, McGehee-Harvey A (1964) Schmidt's syndrome (thyroid and adrenal insufficiency): a review of the literature and a report of fifteen new cases including ten instances of coexistent diabetes mellitus. Medicine (Baltimore) 43:153–180

Colover J, Glynn LE (1958) Experimental iso-immune adrenalitis. Immunology 1:172–178

Cooper BT, Holmes GKT, Cooke WT (1978) Coeliac disease and immunological disorders. Br Med J 1:537–539

DeCock DJ, DeGraeff J, Smeenk D, Querido A (1957) Chronische, Primäre Bijnierinsufficiëntie (Chronic primary adrenal insufficiency). Ned Tijdschr Geneeskd 101:2426–2437

Doniach D, Bottazzo GF (1981) Polyendocrine autoimmunity. In: Franklin EC (ed) Clinical immunology update. Elsevier/North Holland, New York, pp 96–109

Doniach D, Roitt IM (1964) An evaluation of gastric and thyroid auto-immunity in relation to haematologic disorders. Semin Haematol 1:313–343

Doniach D, Roitt IM, Taylor KB (1965 a) Autoimmunity in pernicious anemia and thyroiditis: a family study. Ann NY Acad Sci 124:605–625

Doniach D, Nilsson LR, Roitt IM (1965 b) Autoimmune thyroiditis in children and adolescents. II. Immunological correlations and parent study. Acta Paediatr Scand 54:260–274

Doniach D, Grant D, Newns GH (1972) Multi-endocrine autoimmune disorder in mother and son. Proc Soc Med 65:488–490

Edmonds M, Lamki L, Killinger DW, Volpé R (1973) Autoimmune thyroiditis, adrenalitis and ophoritis. Am J Med 54:782–787

Eisenbarth G, Wilson P, Ward F, Lebovitz HE (1978) HLA type and occurence of disease in familial polyglandular failure. N Engl J Med 298:92–94

Eisenbarth GS, Wilson PW, Ward F, Buckley C, Lebovitz H (1979) The polyglandular failure syndrome: disease inheritance, HLA type, and immune function. Ann Intern Med 91:528–533

Faber J, Cohn D, Kirkegaard C, Christy M, Siersbaek-Nielsen K, Friis T, Nerup J (1979) Subclinical hypothyroidism in Addison's disease. Acta Endocrinol (Copenh) 91:674:679

Farid NR, Larsen B, Payne R, Noel EP, Sampson L (1980) Immunogenetics of polyglandular autoimmune disease. 62nd Meeting Endocrine Society, Washington, D. C., June 18-20 1980, Abstract 82 (to be published)

Frey HMM, Vogt JH, Nerup J (1973) Familial polyendocrinopathy. Acta Endocrinol (Copenh) 72:401–416

Galbraith RM, Fudenberg HH (1977) Autoimmunity in chronic active hepatitis and diabetes mellitus. Clin Immunol Immunopathol 8:116–149

Gambaro C (1962) Iposurrealismo familare. Pediatr Int 12:335–339

Gamlen TR, Aynsley-Green A, Irvine WJ, McCallum CJ (1977) Immunological studies in the neonate of a mother with Addison's disease and diabetes mellitus. Clin Exp Immunol 28:192–195

Gharib H, Hodgson SF, Castineau CF, Scholz DA, Smith LA (1972) Reversible hypothyroidism in Addison's disease. Lancet 2:734–736

Gordin A, Lamberg BA (1975) Natural course of symptomless autoimmune thyroiditis. Lancet 2:1234–1238

Gorsuch AN, Dean BM, Bottazzo GF, Lister J, Gudworth AG (1980) Evidence that type I diabetes and thyrogastric autoimmunity have different genetic determinants. Br Med J 280:145–147

Gottesman IS, Shewchuk AB, Burrow GN (1980) Premature ovarian failure in twenty chromosomally competent women. Annu Meeting, Obst et Gyne col Canada, Jasper, Alberta, June 10–14,1980, Abstract 31 (to be published)

Heggarty H (1968) Addison's disease in identical twins. Br Med J 1:559

Hoenig EM, Hirano A, Levine S, Ghatak NR (1970) The early development and fine structure of allergic adrenalitis. Lab Invest 22:198–205

Irino T, Grollman A (1968) Induction of adrenal insufficiency in the rat by sensitization with homologous tissue. Metabolism 17:717–724

Irvine WJ (1977) Autoimmunity in endocrine disease. In: Besser GM (ed) Advanced medicine, vol 13. Pitman, Tunbridge Wells pp 115–140

Irvine WJ (1978) The immunology and genetics of autoimmune endocrine disease. In: Rose NR, Bigazzi PE, Warner NL (eds) Genetic control of autoimmune endocrine disease. Elsevier/North Holland, New York, pp 77–100

Irvine WJ, Barnes EW (1972) Adrenocortical insufficiency. Clin Endocrinol Metab 1:549–594

Irvine WJ, Barnes EW (1975 a) Addison's disease, ovarian failure and hypoparathyroidism Clin Endocrinol Metab 4:379–434

Irvine WJ, Barnes EW (1975 b) Addison's disease and associated conditions: with particular reference to premature ovarian failure, diabetes mellitus and hypoparathyroidism. In: Gell PGH, Coombs RRA, Lachmann, PS (eds) Clinical aspects of immunology, 3rd ed. Blackwels, Oxford, Chapter 46, pp 1301–1354

Irvine WJ, Scarth L (1969) Antibody to the oxyphil cells of the human parathyroid in idiopathic hypoparathyroidism. Clin Exp Immunol 4:505–510

Knowles HC (1960) The incidence and development of diabetes mellitus. In: Williams RH (ed) Diabetes. Hoeber, New York, pp 360–369

Kracht J, Fisher K, Moebius G (1962) Durch Autoaggression hervorgerufene Veränderungen der Nebenniere. Verh Dtsch Ges Pathol 46:152–157

Kunin AS, McKay BR, Burns SL, Halberstam MJ (1963) The syndrome of hypoparathyroidism and adrenocortical insufficiency, a possible sequel of hepatitis; case report and review of the literature. Am J Med 34:856–866

Levine S, Wenk EJ (1968) The production and passive transfer of allergic adrenalitis. Am J Pathol 52:41–53

Liddle GW (1974) The adrenals part I. In: Williams RH (ed) Textbook of endocrinology, 5th ed. Saunders, Toronto, pp 223–283

Ludwig H, Mayr WR, Pacher M, Schernthaner G, Koller K, Eibl M, Erd W (1975) HL-A antigens in idiopathic Addison's disease. Z Immunitaetsforsch 149:423–427

Lupulescu A, Pop A, Merculiev E, Neacsu C, Heitmanek C (1965) Experimental iso-immune hypoparathyroidism in rats. Nature 206:415–416

Lupulescu A, Potorac E, Pop A, Heitmanek C, Merculiev E, Chisiu N, Oprisan R, Neacsu C (1968) Experimental investigations on immunology of the parathyroid gland. Immunology 14:475–482.

McHardy-Young S, Lessof MH, Maisey MN (1972) Serum TSH and thyroid antibody studies in Addison's disease. Clin Endocrinol (Oxf) 1:45–46

McNatty KP, Short RV, Barnes EW, Irvine WJ (1975) The cytotoxic effect of serum from patients with Addison's disease and autoimmune ovarian failure on human granulosa cells in culture. Clin Exp Immunol 22:378–384

Milcou SM, Pop A, Lupulescu A, Taga M (1959) L'auto-immunisation experimentale de la surrenale chez le lapin. Ann Endocrinol (Paris) 20:799–804

Moulias R, Goust JM (1971) Contributation à l'étude d'un nouveau test d'hypersensibilité retardée in vitro chez l'homme: le test de migration des leucocytes. Thesis, University of Paris

Moulias R, Goust JM, DeVillechabrolle A, Buffet C, Muller Berat CN (1970) Le test de migration des leucocytes du sang périphérique (TML); un nouveau test d'hypersensibilité retardée "in vitro" chez l'homme. II. Utilisation dans les affections auto-immunes humaines. Resultats préliminaires et interprétation. Presse Med. 78:2315–2318

Moulias R, Goust JM, Muller-Berat CN (1971) Hypoparathyroidism and cell-mediated immunity. Lancet 1:1239-1242

Moulias R, Goust JM, Bernard S, Croisier B, Attali A, Berthaux P (1974) Humoral and cellular thyroid autoimmunity in diabetes mellitus. In: Bastenie PA, Gepts W (eds) Immunity and autoimmunity in diabetes mellitus. Excerpta Medica, Amsterdam, pp 140–148

Murthy GG, Peress NS, Khan SA (1976) A demonstration of antibodies to testicular basement membrane by immunofluorescence in a patient with multiple endocrine deficiency. J Clin Endocrinol Metab 42:637–641

Nerup J, (1974 a) On the clinical and immunological association of diabetes mellitus and Addison's disease. In: Bastenie PA, Gepts W (eds) Immunity and autoimmunity in diabetes mellitus. Excerpta Medica, Amsterdam, pp 149–152

Nerup J (1974 b) Addison's disease – serological studies. Acta Endocrinol (Copenh) 76:142–158

Nerup J, Bendixen G (1969 a) Anti-adrenal cellular hypersensitivity in Addison's disease. II. Correlation with clinical and serological findings. Clin Exp Immunol 5:341–353

Nerup J, Benedixen G (1969 b) Anti-adrenal cellular hypersensitivity an Addison's disease. III. Species specifity and subcellular localization of the antigen. Clin Exp Immunol 5:355–364

Nerup J, Andersen V, Bendixen G (1970) Anti-Adrenal cellular hypersensitivity in Addison's disease. IV. In vivo and in vitro investigations of the mitochondrial fraction. Clin Exp Immunol 6:733–739

Neufeld M, Blizzard RM (1980) Polyglandular autoimmune disease. In: Pinchera A (ed) Autoimmune aspects of endocrine disorders. Academic Press, New York, pp 357–366

Neufeld M, MacLaren N, Blizzard R (1980) Autoimmune polyglandular syndrome. Pediatr Ann 9:43–53

Nothiger F (1967) Familiärer Morbus Addison. Z Kinderheilkd 99:14–32

Ogle JW (1886) On disease of the brain as a result of diabetes mellitus. St. George's Hosp 1:157–188

Okita N, Kidd A, Row VV, Volpé R (1980 a) Sensitization of T lymphocytes in Graves' and Hashimoto's diseases. J Clin Endocrinol 51:316–320

Okita N, Kidd A, Row VV, Volpé R (1981) Suppressor T lymphocyte deficiency in Graves' disease and Hashimoto's thyroiditis. J Clin Endocrinol Metab 52: 528–533
Petri M, Nerup J (1971) Addison's adrenalitis. Studies on diffuse lymphocytic adrenalitis (idiopathic Addison's disease) and focal lymphocytic infiltration in a control material. Acta Pathol Microbiol Scand [A] 79:381–388
Pozzilli P, Sensi M, Gorsuch A, Bottazzo GF, Cudworth AG (1979) Evidence for raised K cell levels in type I diabetes. Lancet 2:173–175
Pozzilli P, Adreani D, Sensi M, Wolf E, Taylor M, Bottazzo GF, Cudworth AG (1980) K cells and antibody dependent cytotoxicity in autoimmune polyendocrine disease. 6th Internat Endocrinol Congr, Melbourne, Australia, February 10–16, 1980 Abstract 639, p 539 (to be published)
Rimoin DL, Schimke RN (1971) Genetic disorders of the endocrine glands. Mosby, St Louis
Ritchie WT (1908) The specificity and potency of adrenolytic and thymolytic sera. J Pathol Bacteriol 12:140–153
Rizzetto M, Doniach D (1973) Human antibodies to mast cells. Clin Exp Immunol 14:327–334
Ruehsen M de R, Blizzard M, Garcia Bunuel R, Jones GS (1972) Autoimmunity and ovarian failure. Am J Obstet Gynecol 112:693–703
Schmidt MB (1936) Eine biglandulare Erkrankung (Nebennieren und Schilddrüse) bei Morbus Addisonii. Verh. Dtsch Ges Pathol 21:212–216
Schwartz WL (1973) Hypothyroidism and Addison's disease totally corrected by adrenal replacement therapy. Calif Med 118:57–60
Simmonds JP, Lister J (1978) Auto-immune Addison's disease in identical twins. Postgrad Med J 54:552–554
Smith ME, Gough J, Galpin OP 1963) Addison's disease in identical twins. Br Med M 2:1316
Spinner MW, Blizzard RM, Childs B (1968) Clinical and genetic heterogeneity in idiopathic Addison's disease and hypoparathyroidism. J Clin Endocrinol Metab 28:795–804
Spinner MW, Blizzard RM, Giggs J, Abbey H, Childs B (1969) Familial distribution of organ specific antibodies in the blood of patients with Addison's disease and hypoparathyroidism and their relatives. Clin Exp Immunol 5:461–468
Steiner JW, Langer B, Schatz DL, Volpé R (1960) Experimental immunological adrenal injury: a response to injections of autologous and homologous adrenal antigens in adjuvant. J Exp Med 112:187–202
Stuart-Mason A, Meade TW, Lee JAH, Morris JN (1968) Epidemiological and clinical picture of Addison's disease. Lancet 2:744–747
Symington T (1969) Functional pathology of the human adrenal gland. Livingstone, Edinburgh London
Thomsen M, Platz P, Anderson OO, Christy M, Lyngsoe J, Nerup J, Rasmussen K, Ryder LP, Staub Nielsen L, Svejgaard A (1975) MLC typing in juvenile diabetes mellitus and idiopathic Addison's disease. Transpant Rev 22:125–147
Toccafondi R, Borghi A (1962) Morbo de Addison familiare (iposurrealismo chronico "parzialmente compensato" insoste in padrie e figlio dopo l'influenza asiatica). Acta Genet Med Gemellol (Roma) 11:407–417
Topliss DJ, White EL, Stockigt JR (1980) Significance of thyrotrophin excess in untreated primary adrenal insufficiency. J Clin Endocrinol Metab 50:52–56
Tunbridge WMG (1979) The epidemiology of hypothyroidism. Clin Endocrinol Metab 8:21–27
Turkington RW, Lebovitz HE (1967) Extra-adrenal endocrine deficiencies in Addison's disease. Am J Med 43:499–507
Ungar B, Mathews JD, Tait BD, Cowling DC (1977) HLA patterns in pernicious anaemia. Br Med J 1:798–800
Vladimarsson H, Higgs JM, Wells RS, Yamamura M, Hobbs JR, Holt PJL (1973) Immune abnormalities associated with chronic mucocutaneous candidiasis. Cell Immunol 6:348–361
Verghese MW, Ward FE, Eisenbarth GS (1980) Decreased suppressor cell activity in patients with polyglandular failure. Clin Res 28:270 A
Volpé R (1977) The role of autoimmunity in hypoendocrine and hyperendocrine function. Ann Intern Med 87:86–99
Wall JR, Fang SL, Walters BA, Strakosch CR, Ingbar SH, Bravermann LE (1978) Multi-system immunologically mediated disease: T lymphocyte deficiency and thyroid immunologic disease – a report of four cases. Aust N Z J Med 8:290–294
Walsh CH, Cooper BT, Wright AD, Malins JM, Cooke WT (1978) Diabetes mellitus and coeliac disease: a clinical study. Q J Med 47:89–100

Werdelin O (1972) The origin, nature and specificity of mononuclear cells in experimental autoimmune inflammations. Acta Pathol Microbiol Scand [A] [Suppl] 232:1–91

Werdelin O, Boehme DH (1969) Immunization and BSVS mice with heterologous and homologous adrenal gland. Immunology 16:205–215

Werdelin O, Wick G, McCluskey RT (1971) The fate of newly formed lymphocytes migrating from an antigen-stimulated lymphnode in rats with allergic adrenalities. Lab Invest 25:279–286

Whittingham S (1974) Pernicious anaemia, diabetes mellitus and Addison's disease In: Brent L, Holborow J (eds) Progress in immunology II, vol 5: Clinical aspects II. Elsevier/North Holland, Amsterdam, pp 301-303

Wick G (1975) Experimental animal models in autoimmune endocrine disease. Clin Endocrinol Metab 4:241–266

Wigzell H, Bing H, Fischknecht H, Peterson P, Sege K (1978) Possible role of auto-anti-idiotypic immunity in autoimmune disease. In: Rose NR, Bigazzi PE, Warner NL (eds) Genetic control of autoimmune disease. Elsevier/North Holland, New York, pp 327–342

Witebsky E, Klinke J (1933) Die sereologische Spezifität des Nebennierenmarks. Z Immunitaetsforsch Exp Ther 78:509–523

Witebsky E, Milgrom F (1962) Immunological studies on adrenal glands. II. Immunization with adrenals of the same species. Immunology 5:67–78

Wuepper KD, Wegienka LC, Fudenberg HH (1969) Immunologic aspects of adrenocortical insufficiency. Am J Med 46:206–216

6 Immunological Aspects of Male Infertility

In this series of monographs on endocrinology, Mancini (1976) published a superb monograph on the status in this field, and other excellent reviews have been published (Rumke and Hekman 1975; Troen and Nankin 1977). Thus it would seem redundant to attempt to write a prolonged review on this topic. Moreover there is little or no genetic relationship between the disorders which will be discussed in this chapter and those documented in previous chapters. Furthermore little is known about pathogenetic mechanisms pertaining to the conditions under discussion here. It is therefore the intention of the author to write a brief summary, since the field has not changed dramatically since these reviews were written.

Immune mechanisms have been implicated in as many as 30% of cases of idiopathic infertility. The initial observation in this regard was made by Meaker (1922), who found that sera from two sterile women could agglutinate and immobilize the spermatozoa of their respective husbands. Moreover, Wilson (1954) and Rumke (1954) independently examined serum samples of human males for their capacity to agglutinate and immobilize spermatozoa suggesting a possible role of sperm agglutinins in infertility. Rumke (1954) described two patients with extreme oligospermia, whose sera possessed sperm agglutinins in high titres. Subsequently, Rumke examined the sera of over 2000 male patients in an infertility unit, along with the sera of 416 patients of pregnant women (Rumke and Hellinga 1959). Only about 3 % of the infertile males showed agglutinins of a least 1:32, whereas none of the fertile males showed such agglutinins. In Wilson's study (1954) there were two men whose spermatozoa showed spontanous agglutination and early loss of motility, and the agglutinating factor was considered to be due to the presence of antibodies to spermatozoa.

Fjallbrant (1968) found that high titres of antispermatozoa antibodies correlated well with infertility, although Li (1974) detected sperm agglutinins in the sera of pregnant women. Infertile males may have agglutinins in their semen, resulting in clumping of their spermatozoa. A less common but more specific antibody is the complement-fixing sperm-immobilizing antibody, which has not been found in patients with documented fertility (Rumke and Hekman 1975). The mechanism by which sperm antibodies produce infertility is not clearly understood. They do not generally cause azospermia or alter testicular histology. Sperm agglutinins and sperm-immobilizing antibodies may act by reducing the ability of sperm to penetrate cervical mucus (Kahn and Flier 1980). Mancini (1976) postulates that immunological factors may affect male fertility by impairment of the germinal epithelium and of seminal spermatozoa. In the latter case, antibodies must reach the seminal plasma via the accessory glands. This may lead to hypo-or azospermatogenesis when the testis is affected or immobilization and agglutination of spermatozoa if the interaction takes place in some other segment of the genital tract. Presumably local antibody production and the stimulation of the proximal lymph nodes may initiate a new release of antigens due to the interaction of germinal cells with antibodies, thus inducing a self-perpetuating circuit of self-destruction of germinal cells and seminal spermatozoa. Mancini points out that during this process more than one type of humoral antibody and cellular immunity may develop, thus making it more difficult to be certain of the precise mechanisms operative in infertility.

For further details with respect to the experimental and clinical aspects of male infertility, the reader is referred to the excellent monograph by Mancini (1976) and to the reviews by Rumke and Hekman (1975), by Troen and Nankin (1977), and by Rumke (1980). It should be emphasized, however, that in general antibodies against spermatozoa do not seem to relate to the other organ-specific auto-immune diseases, nor have there been as yet epidemiologic, genetic, or HLA studies in large groups of infertile male patients possessing such antibodies. Such studies are awaited with interest.

6.1 References

Fjallbrant B (1968) Sperm antibodies and sterility in men. Acta Obstet Gynecol Scand [Suppl 4] 47:5–38

Kahn CR, Flier JS (1980) Immunologic aspects of endocrine disease. In: Parker CW (ed) Clinical immunology, vol II. Saunders, Philadelphia, pp 815–866

Li TS (1974) Sperm immunology, infertility and fertility control. Obstet Gynecol 44:607–623

Mancini RE (1976) Immunologic aspects of testicular function. Springer, Berlin Heidelberg New York (Monographs on endocrinology, vol 9)

Meaker SR (1922) Some aspects of the problem of sterility. Boston Med Surg J 187:535–539

Rumke P (1954) The presence of sperm antibodies in the serum of two patients with oligospermia. Vox Sang 4:135–140

Rumke P (1980) Auto- and isoimmune reactions to the antigens of the gonads and genital tract. In: Fougereau M, Dausset J (eds) Immunology 80. Progress in immunology IV. Academic Press, London pp 1065–1092

Rumke P, Hekman A (1975) Auto- and isoimmunity to sperm in infertility. Clin Endocrinol Metab 4:473–496

Rumke P, Hellinga G (1959) Autoantibodies against spermatozoa in sterile men. Am Clin Pathol 32:357–363

Troen P, Nankin HR (1977) The testis in normal and infertile men. Raven, New York

Wilson L (1975) Sperm agglutinins in human semen and blood. Proc Soc Exp Biol Med 85:652–655

7 Epilogue

7.1 Introduction

From the foregoing chapters it is clear that there are many important unanswered questions and needs for future development. Many of these undoubtedly will come from laboratories dealing with basic immunology, and not necessarily from laboratories with an intrinsic interest in endocrine diseases. The types of questions to be answered fall into the following categories:

7.1.1 Genetics and Epidemiology

While there have been population studies done in relation to organ-specific auto-immune diseases, these have been comparatively few and comparatively localized. Much larger epidemiological studies are required with suitable controls so as to elucidate clear statistics vis-a-vis the proportion of people in the general population who have a given disease in occult as well as overt form, the proportion of the population at risk for the disease, the genetic relationship of one auto-immune disease to another, the genetic factors which determine the length of time before the disease becomes expressed, and the genetic factors which determine the severity of the disease. The studies are most relevant to diabetes mellitus and to auto-immune thyroid disease, since these constitute the largest number of patients with auto-immune endocrine disease.

7.1.2 Histocompatibility Antigens

With the availability of current techniques, it is possible to establish risks for many of the auto-immune disorders. It is feasible that this could be carried out in population studies early in life, so as to identify thôse members of the population at special risk. However, it is equally clear that the presently identified HLA genes are not specific "disease susceptibility" genes, although they may be very closely related by linkage disequilibrium. Hence it will be important to ultimately establish new techniques which may allow us to determine the precise gene or genes responsible for each of the disorders dealt with in his monograph. Finally, it will be even more important to determine the mechanism by which the gene expresses itself in terms of the disorder of immunoregulation.

In relation to histocompatibility genes, emphasis on family studies would be required, with comparisons of multiplex families versus single patient families, inquiries into the numbers of genes involved and mode of inheritance, all with the broad goal of defining the populations at risk with high probability.

7.1.3 Definition of the Role of the Antigen

Definition of the role of the antigen will be important. There is increasing evidence that there is no need for antigenic alteration prior to the initiation of at least some of these conditions, and that the disorder of immunoregulation is sufficient. However, this point remains to be proven, and it is clear that much more precise definition of the nature of the antigen or antigens involved in each disorder will be necessary. Is there a role for viruses in altering the target cell antigen? Is there a role for other modifiers of the antigen? While the author tends to the view that there does not appear to be any neccesity for antigenic alteration in many of these disease, many investigators are not yet satisfied about this point, and indeed in some of the entities discussed, e. g. diabetes mellitus, antigenic alteration may play an initiating role in some cases. Undoubtedly as techniques for purification of antigen improve, more will be learned about the interaction of the immune system with the appropriate antigen.

7.1.4 T-Lymphocyte Studies

Further studies of the role of T-lymphocytes are required. While there appears to be evidence that there may be specific defects in suppressor T-lymphocytes involved in each of the organ-specific auto-immune diseases, this remains to be proven beyond doubt. If indeed this point is established, then it will be important to determine the mechanism by which this occurs, i. e. what is the molecular defect in a suppressor T-lymphocyte population, or in suppressor T-lymphocytes generally? What is the role of chemical modifiers of suppressor T-lymphocyte function, e. g. prostaglandins, histamine, cortisol concentrations? Are there other important chemical mediators which affect suppressor T-lymphocyte function? The role of receptors for mediators such as histamine or lymphocyte populations also requires further clarification.

The role of helper T-lymphocytes also needs further clarification. Once again, there appears to be evidence that specific helper T-lymphocytes have to be sensitized to the specific antigen, as we have seen in Chap 2. However, there is also some evidence that non-specific helper T-lymphocytes can activate specific B-lymphocytes, at least under the stimulation of non-specific mitogens. Does this finding have any biological importance? How many helper T-lymphocytes are required to "turn on" the specific B-lymphocytes? What is the mechanism of co-operation between helper T-lymphocytes and B-lymphocytes?

What is the role of T-lymphocytes in producing cell damage? Can they do this alone, by the production of lymphokines? Does it always require the co-operation of B-lymphocytes with the production of antibodies? Does lymphocyte-dependent antibody-mediated cytotoxicity depend on T-lymphocytes?

Moreover, studies are necessary into the structure, specificity and mode of action of the lymphokines produced by T-lymphocytes and their precise role in the control of the immune processes relative to the auto-immune disease.

7.1.5 Studies of Antibodies

Further studies are required into the nature of the interaction of anti-receptor antibodies which can cause the antibodies to be agonists or antagonists, or even in some instances to produce secondary changes in the receptors. The mechanism of antibody-induced cellular destruction requires further clarification. Can antibodies ever produce cellular destruction alone? Must they do so as immune complexes? Must they do so in co-operation with lymphocytes or "killer" cells? What is the role of anti-idiotypic antibodies in immunoregulation with specific reference to organ-specific auto-immune diseases?

7.1.6 Non-Specific Cellular and Chemical Elements

What is the precise role for macrophages in these auto-immune disorders? Also the roles of complement, prostaglandins, corticosteroids, histamine, other hormones, and other chemical mediators, all need further study.

7.1.7 Sex Incidence

Since the organ-specific auto-immune diseases occur predominantly in women, is there a role for oestrogens in lymphocytic regulation, as has been suggested? Alternatively, is there a role for the X chromosome?

7.1.8 Tolerance

Is it possible to re-establish tolerance? Is it possible to generate specific suppressor T-lymphocytes which could be introduced into the body? Is it possible to produce suppressor factors in vitro which could prove to be therapeutically useful? Is it possible to induce anti-idiotypic antibodies which might potentially interrupt the cycle of the immune process and permit specific immunotherapy?

7.1.9 Future Therapeutic Possibilities

It is possible that in the short run further work on the use of immunosuppressive drugs and those which enhance the immune process will have limited value as possible therapy. In the long run, however, what is required is a full understanding of the genetic background of these conditions and the mechanism of gene expression in relation to the actual disorder of immunoregulation. Once this is completely comprehended, it might be possible to attempt means of altering the immunoregulatory disorder so as to re-establish tolerance. While this is indeed a long-term objective, it is within the realm of possibility. There may be means by which specific suppressor T-lymphocytes could be generated and reintroduced into the body. Suppressor factors could be produced which may prove to be therapeutically useful. The induction of anti-idiotypic antibodies might potentially interrupt the cycle of auto-antibody generation, and permit specific immunotherapy, as opposed to presently available non-specific immunosuppression for the treatment of auto-immune disorders. In addition, there is at least the potential of disease prevention, based upon a full understanding of the genetics and the risk in any given family of having a child with auto-immune disease. Thus, while techniques are not now available for such benefits, the general outline of what could be possible is actually becoming visible.

7.1.10 Radio-immunoassay

The employment of increasingly purified substances as antigens will ultimately lead to the harvesting of more specific antibodies. This will allow the measurements of these antigens in biological fluids and the characterization of their metabolism. The advances in prostaglandin metabolism, for example, have come through such techniques. The recently discovered hybridoma techniques to produce monoclonal antibodies can produce antibodies in high yield and with exquisite specificity. The applications of such antibodies in radioimmunoassay and immunologic dissection of complex biological systems hold great promise for increasing the rate and effectiveness of identifying new chemical signals and their metabolism.

Subject Index

Other Volumes: in This Series:

Volume 19: P. Mauvais-Jarvis, F. Kuttenn, I. Mowszowicz
Hirsutism
1981. 32 figures, 10 tables. XI, 110 pages
ISBN 3-540-10509-3

Volume 18: I.J. Chopra
Triiodothyronines in Health and Disease
With a contribution by V. Cody
1981. 76 figures, 18 tables. IX, 145 pages
ISBN 3-540-10400-3

Volume 17: J. Chayen
The Cytochemical Bioassay of Polypeptide Hormones
1980. 72 figures, 7 tables. XIV, 208 pages
ISBN 3-540-10040-7

Volume 16: J.E.A. McIntosh, R.P. McIntosh
Mathematical Modelling and Computers in Endocrinology
1980. 73 figures, 56 tables. XII, 337 pages
ISBN 3-540-09693-0

Volume 15: A.T. Cowie, I.A. Forsyth, I.C. Hart
Hormonal Control of Lactation
1980. 64 figures, 7 tables. XIV, 275 pages
ISBN 3-540-09680-9

Volume 14: J.H. Clark, E.J. Peck, Jr.
Female Sex Steroids
Receptors and Function
1979. 116 figures, 18 tables. XII, 245 pages
ISBN 3-540-09375-3

Volume 13: H.F. De Luca
Vitamin D - Metabolism and Function
1979. 14 figures. VIII, 80 pages
ISBN 3-540-09182-3

Volume 12
Glucocorticoid Hormone Action
Editors: J.D. Baxter, G.G. Rousseau
1979. 176 figures, 58 tables. XIX, 638 pages
ISBN 3-540-08973-X

Volume 11: S. Ohne
Major Sex-Determining Genes
1979. 34 figures, 6 tables. XIII, 140 pages
ISBN 3-540-08965-9

Volume 10: W.I.P. Mainwaring
The Mechanism of Action of Androgens
1977. 12 figures, 17 tables. XI, 178 pages
ISBN 3-540-07941-6

Springer-Verlag
Berlin
Heidelberg
New York

Volume 9: R.E. Mancini

Immunologic Aspects of Testicular Functions

1976. 36 figures, 8 tables. IX, 114 pages
ISBN 3-540-07496-1

Volume 8: E. Gurpide

Tracer Methods in Hormone Research

1975. 35 figures. XI, 188 pages
ISBN 3-540-07039-7

Volume 7: E.W. Horton

Prostaglandins

1972. 97 figures. XI, 197 pages
ISBN 3-540-05571-1

Volume 6: K. Federlin

Immunopathology of Insulin

Clinical and Experimental Studies
1971. 53 figures. XIII, 185 pages
ISBN 3-540-05408-1

Volume 5: J. Müller

Regulation of Aldosterone Biosynthesis

1971. 19 figures. VII, 137 pages
ISBN 3-540-05213-5

Volume 4: U. Westphal

Steroid-Protein Interactions

1971. 144 figures. XIII, 567 pages
ISBN 3-540-05313-3

Volume 3: F.G. Sulman

Hypothalamic Control of Lactation

In collaboration with numerous experts.
1970. 58 figures. XII, 235 pages
ISBN 3-540-04973-8

Volume 2: K.B. Eik-Nes, E.C. Horning

Gas Phase Chromatography of Steroids

1968. 85 figures. XV, 382 pages
ISBN 3-540-04277-6

Volume 1: S. Ohno

Sex Chromosomes and Sex-linked Genes

1967. 33 figures. X, 192 pages
ISBN 3-540-03934-1

Springer-Verlag
Berlin
Heidelberg
New York

MIX
Papier aus verantwortungsvollen Quellen
Paper from responsible sources
FSC® C105338

If you have any concerns about our products,
you can contact us on
ProductSafety@springernature.com

In case Publisher is established outside the EU,
the EU authorized representative is:
Springer Nature Customer Service Center GmbH
Europaplatz 3, 69115 Heidelberg, Germany

Printed by Libri Plureos GmbH
in Hamburg, Germany